Strategies to Alleviate Human Zinc Deficiency

Ratnesh Das
Dr. Harisingh Gour Central University, India

Megha Das
Dr. Harisingh Gour Central University, India

IGI Global
Scientific Publishing
Publishing Tomorrow's Research Today

Vice President of Editorial Melissa Wagner
Director of Acquisitions Mikaela Felty
Director of Book Development Jocelynn Hessler
Production Manager Mike Brehm
Cover Design Jose Rosado

Published in the United States of America by
IGI Global Scientific Publishing
701 East Chocolate Avenue
Hershey, PA, 17033, USA
Tel: 717-533-8845
Fax: 717-533-7115
Website: https://www.igi-global.com E-mail: cust@igi-global.com

Library of Congress Cataloging-in-Publication Data

Names: Das, Ratnesh, editor. | Das, Megha, 1978- editor.
Title: Strategies to alleviate human zinc deficiency / edited by Ratnesh Das, Megha Das.
Description: Hershey, PA : Medical Information Science Reference, [2025] | Includes bibliographical references and index. | Summary: "This book summarizes the role of zinc in human health, its bioavailability, causes and consequences of deficiency, and strategies to alleviate the deficiency. Zinc deficiency is one of the major problems in developing world. Humans mainly depend on the daily intake of zinc through diet as no storage system for zinc exists in body"-- Provided by publisher.
Identifiers: LCCN 2024039270 (print) | LCCN 2024039271 (ebook) | ISBN 9798369353554 (h/c) | ISBN 9798369353561 (s/c) | ISBN 9798369353578 (eISBN)
Subjects: LCSH: Zinc deficiency diseases. | Zinc deficiency diseases--Treatment.
Classification: LCC RC627.Z5 S77 2024 (print) | LCC RC627.Z5 (ebook) | DDC 616.3/96--dc23/eng/20241108
LC record available at https://lccn.loc.gov/2024039270
LC ebook record available at https://lccn.loc.gov/2024039271

British Cataloguing in Publication Data
A Cataloguing in Publication record for this book is available from the British Library.

Table of Contents

Detailed Table of Contents

Zinc is an essential micronutrient and plays an important role in various physiological functions including immunity, wound healing, DNA synthesis, and cell signaling. This chapter gives a detailed outline of the biochemical functions of Zinc, a cofactor for many enzymes plus transcription factors taking part in primary metabolic pathways. The chapter also goes into details about dietary sources of Zinc and other factors contributing to its bioavailability. The consequences of Zinc deficiency have been outlined, including its effect on immune function, growth and development, cognitive function, and reproductive health. We have delved into methods of controlling Zinc deficiency: be it food fortification, biofortification, dietary supplements or dietary diversity. So, this chapter basically talks about how incredibly important Zinc is for human health and how desperately crucial it is to act on Zinc deficiency through well-targeted interventions, as well as smart policymaking. All these efforts are geared towards ensuring that we pave way for healthy generations across the globe.

Zinc was adjudged as an essential micronutrient for human health in the mid-20th century. It is required for gene transcription, enzyme activity, nucleic acid, protein and lipid metabolism. Its role at microcellular level makes it an integral part of the milieu interieur. So, its deficiency involves every system of the body, but evident burnt is on integument, skeletal, gastro-intestinal, central nervous, immune and reproductive systems. The zinc deficiency in growth period may even lead to growth deprivation. Zinc deficiency may be inherited or acquired. It may be attributed to zinc deficient diet, decreased intake, malabsorption, accentuated physiological metabolic requirements or increased loss. The zinc deficiency may be observed on

This chapter highlights the significance of zinc deficiency as a pressing public health issue in developing countries. It explores the root causes, including inadequate dietary intake, frequent infectious diseases, and overall malnutrition. Furthermore, the review examines various strategies to combat zinc deficiency and manage its consequences. These strategies include promoting dietary diversification, fortifying staple foods with zinc, developing biofortified crops with higher inherent zinc content, implementing targeted zinc supplementation programs, and launching educational initiatives. The review emphasizes the need for a multi-faceted approach that tackles both dietary and non-dietary factors. This comprehensive strategy holds promise for achieving sustainable improvements in zinc nutrition and public health outcomes in developing countries.

Zinc, vital for growth, immunity, wound healing, and DNA synthesis, faces global deficiency issues, especially in regions with limited dietary diversity. About 17.3% of the world is at risk, with vulnerable groups including pregnant women and the elderly. Deficiency leads to growth impairment, weakened immunity, and increased infection susceptibility, affecting both physical and cognitive health. Supplementation, in forms like zinc gluconate and zinc citrate, is crucial, with dosages tailored to age groups. It aids growth, reduces respiratory infections' severity, and may alleviate common cold symptoms if taken early. In acute diarrhea, zinc can shorten illness duration, while in conditions like age-related macular degeneration (AMD) and Wilson's disease, it plays a vital role in management. However, excessive intake may cause adverse effects like gastrointestinal discomfort and copper deficiency. Zinc supplementation is essential for public health strategies to prevent deficiency and ensure overall well-being, particularly in high-risk populations.

Zinc deficiency is a global health issue, especially in developing countries where diets often lack diversity and essential nutrients. Alleviating zinc deficiency requires a multifaceted approach involving dietary diversification, biofortification, and zinc supplementation. Dietary diversification, with a varied diet rich in zinc-containing foods like meat, seafood, dairy, legumes, nuts, seeds, and whole grains, is essential for meeting zinc requirements and mitigating health effects. Biofortification, which enhances the zinc content of staple crops through breeding or biotechnology, offers a sustainable solution to improve zinc intake and address deficiency-related health issues. Zinc supplementation provides targeted interventions for vulnerable populations, supporting growth, immune function, and overall well-being, and helps manage diseases like acute respiratory infections and Wilson's disease. By integrating dietary diversification, biofortification, and supplementation, we can effectively manage zinc deficiency and improve global health outcomes.

Preface

INTRODUCTION

Zinc, though classified as a trace element, exerts an outsized influence on human health. This essential micronutrient serves as a critical cofactor in over 300 enzymatic reactions, underpinning vital physiological processes ranging from immune competence to neurocognitive development. Despite its fundamental importance, zinc deficiency remains one of the most prevalent yet underrecognized micronutrient deficiencies worldwide, particularly affecting vulnerable populations in resource-limited settings where dietary diversity is constrained and access to fortified foods remains inadequate.

This volume, Strategies to Alleviate Human Zinc Deficiency, represents a comprehensive effort to bridge the gap between our scientific understanding of zinc metabolism and practical interventions to address its deficiency. We present a systematic examination of evidence-based approaches including food fortification, biofortification of staple crops, targeted supplementation protocols, and dietary modification strategies - all contextualized within sustainable public health frameworks. The book's multidisciplinary perspective integrates cutting-edge research from molecular nutrition, clinical medicine, and global health policy.

Our aspirations for this work extend beyond academic discourse. We aim to equip healthcare providers with actionable clinical insights, empower policymakers with data-driven intervention models, and provide researchers with a consolidated knowledge base to advance the field. Most importantly, we seek to translate complex scientific concepts into practical solutions that can improve health outcomes in communities most burdened by zinc deficiency.

The intended readership encompasses clinicians managing zinc-related disorders, public health professionals designing nutrition interventions, agricultural scientists developing biofortified crops, and policymakers shaping micronutrient strategies.

We also welcome engaged readers from allied health fields and concerned global citizens seeking deeper understanding of this critical health issue.

We dedicate this work to our parents late Mr. Rajeshwar and Mrs. Sunbeam Das, along with Ritika and Ritvik Das. We are profoundly grateful to the international team of contributors whose expertise across multiple disciplines has enriched this volume. Their collective wisdom has helped create what we hope will serve as both a definitive reference and a catalyst for meaningful action against this silent epidemic of zinc deficiency.

ORGANIZATION OF THE CONTENT

The book's structure follows a logical progression from fundamental science to practical applications, with each chapter building upon the last to create a comprehensive understanding of zinc deficiency and its solutions.

The opening chapter establishes the essential biochemical foundations, detailing zinc's unique role as a catalytic and structural component of numerous metalloenzymes and transcription factors. It explores the nutrient's critical functions in immune response, DNA synthesis, and cellular signalling, while emphasizing the body's lack of specialized zinc storage systems - a biological reality that necessitates regular dietary intake.

Subsequent chapters delve deeper into the pathophysiology of deficiency states. The molecular mechanisms by which zinc insufficiency leads to oxidative stress, impaired wound healing, and immune dysfunction are examined in detail, with particular attention to the nutrient's role in maintaining genomic stability and modulating inflammatory responses. The clinical manifestations chapter provides a systematic review of deficiency signs across organ systems, from the characteristic dermatological presentations to more subtle neurological and reproductive consequences.

The epidemiological sections present rigorous analyses of zinc deficiency's global burden, challenging traditional paradigms that viewed this as solely a developing world problem. Recent data reveal concerning prevalence rates even in affluent nations, tied to dietary shifts toward processed foods and increasing rates of conditions like inflammatory bowel disease that impair zinc absorption.

The intervention chapters offer practical guidance on implementing supplementation programs, with careful consideration of dosage regimens, delivery platforms, and monitoring protocols tailored to different age groups and physiological states. The food-based strategies section compares the relative merits and challenges of fortification versus biofortification approaches, while the final synthesis chapter presents an integrated framework for combining these interventions within national nutrition policies.

CONCLUSION

In bringing this volume to completion, we are struck by both the complexity of zinc's biological roles and the remarkable potential of targeted interventions to alleviate deficiency states. The collective work presented here underscores that zinc insufficiency is not merely a nutritional concern, but a multifaceted public health challenge requiring coordinated action across scientific, agricultural, and policy domains.

The evidence is clear: addressing zinc deficiency can yield disproportionate benefits for global health, from reducing childhood mortality to slowing the progression of chronic diseases. What remains is the translation of this knowledge into sustained action. We hope this book will serve as both a roadmap and an inspiration for all stakeholders committed to achieving optimal zinc status worldwide - not as an end in itself, but as a fundamental step toward health equity and human development.

Ratnesh Das
Harisingh Gour Central University, India

Megha Das
Harisingh Gour Central University, India

Acknowledgement

The completion of this book has been a profound journey made possible through the collective support and contributions of many remarkable individuals. At the outset, we wish to express our deepest gratitude to our beloved parents, the late Mr. Rajeshwar Das and Mrs. Sunbeam Das, whose enduring values, unconditional love, and emphasis on education laid the foundation for all our endeavors. This work stands as a humble tribute to their memory and the legacy they left behind.

Our heartfelt thanks go to Ritika and Ritvik, whose steadfast support, boundless patience, and constant encouragement sustained us through every phase of this demanding yet rewarding process. Their understanding during the long hours of research and writing provided the emotional anchor we needed to see this project through to completion.

We are profoundly honored to acknowledge Prof. Neelima Gupta, Hon'ble Vice Chancellor of Dr. Harisingh Gour Vishwavidyalaya, Sagar (M.P.), for her visionary leadership and unwavering commitment to academic excellence. Her guidance and encouragement proved invaluable at every stage of this work, and for this we remain deeply grateful.

We extend our sincere appreciation to all our chapter contributors whose expertise and dedication have enriched the content of this book. The dedication of researchers and healthcare professionals working in the field of nutrition has been a constant source of inspiration, and we are indebted to their pioneering work which forms the backbone of this publication. The editorial team deserves special recognition for their meticulous attention to detail and professional expertise in refining the manuscript.

Finally, we express our gratitude to our readers whose interest in this critical subject matter motivates us to continue our work in addressing global nutritional challenges. To all who have supported this endeavor in any capacity - through knowledge sharing, encouragement, or simply by believing in its importance - we remain eternally thankful. This book is as much yours as it is ours.

Chapter 1
Understanding Zinc and Its Importance in Human Health

Safdar Hussain
University of the Punjab, India

Nosheen Mushtaq
Lahore University of Biological and Applied Sciences, Pakistan

ABSTRACT

Zinc is an essential micronutrient and plays an important role in various physiological functions including immunity, wound healing, DNA synthesis, and cell signaling. This chapter gives a detailed outline of the biochemical functions of Zinc, a cofactor for many enzymes plus transcription factors taking part in primary metabolic pathways. The chapter also goes into details about dietary sources of Zinc and other factors contributing to its bioavailability. The consequences of Zinc deficiency have been outlined, including its effect on immune function, growth and development, cognitive function, and reproductive health. We have delved into methods of controlling Zinc deficiency: be it food fortification, biofortification, dietary supplements or dietary diversity. So, this chapter basically talks about how incredibly important Zinc is for human health and how desperately crucial it is to act on Zinc deficiency through well-targeted interventions, as well as smart policymaking. All these efforts are geared towards ensuring that we pave way for healthy generations across the globe.

DOI: 10.4018/979-8-3693-5355-4.ch001

INTRODUCTION

Zinc is an important micronutrient, playing a multifaceted role in the enzymatic activity of gene expression and cellular signaling pathways, hence being an essential factor for a variety of biological functions. As a cofactor, it is indispensable for the catalytic activity of more than 300 enzymes, including enzymes responsible for digestion, metabolism, and DNA synthesis (Vallee & Falchuk, 1993). It stabilizes the structure of proteins and cell membranes, hence protecting them from oxidative damage (Vallee & Auld, 1990). In gene expression, for example, Zn acts with transcription factors, among which are Zn finger proteins, that regulate the transcription of specific genes by binding to DNA. This interaction is crucial in processes such as cell proliferation, differentiation, and apoptosis (Laity et al., 2001). Moreover, it is included in cellular signaling pathways, where it acts as a second messenger. It controls multiple signaling molecules and pathways related to immune responses, cell growth, and apoptosis (Yamasaki et al., 2007). The ability of Zn to modulate these pathways underlines its significance in maintaining cellular homeostasis and general health. A deficiency in this metal can disturb these processes and result in health problems ranging from immune dysfunction to developmental problems (M. Hambidge et al., 2000).

The total amount of zinc in the body is approximately 2.5 g and 1.5 g in men and women respectively (Ryu MS, 2020), most of which is stored in bones and skeletal muscles ("Dietary Reference Intakes for Vitamin A, Vitamin K, Arsenic, Boron, Chromium, Copper, Iodine, Iron, Manganese, Molybdenum, Nickel, Silicon, Vanadium, and Zinc," 2001). The average daily intake of zinc through natural dietary sources for an adult is approximately 10-15 mg/day (National Institutes of Health, 2022). This intake can vary based on dietary habits, age, sex, and geographical location. Zinc deficiency is typically diagnosed when plasma or serum zinc levels are below 70 µg/dL (11 µmol/L) (Allen et al., 2006a). Dietary Zn comes from a wide variety of food sources, which include meat, shellfish, dairy products, legumes, seeds, nuts, and whole grains. Red meat and poultry are good sources of bioavailable Zn, while phytates in plant foods inhibit Zn bioavailability (King et al., 2000; Sandström, 1997). Once ingested, Zn is mainly absorbed from the small intestine, particularly in the jejunum and ileum. There are two major mechanisms for the absorption of dietary Zn: the carrier-mediated transport system and passive diffusion. Carrier-mediated transport, which is important at low dietary Zn intake, involves some specific proteins that mediate Zn uptake into enterocytes; one of these proteins is ZIP4 (Lichten & Cousins, 2009). Within these cells, Zn can be stored, utilized, or transported into the bloodstream via another protein, ZnT1. A number of factors affect Zn absorption, such as dietary inhibitors like phytates and enhancers including some amino acids and organic acids (Lönnerdal, 2000). The status of Zn in the body also influences the efficiency of absorption; higher needs or lower Zn levels are associated with an increase in the efficiency of uptake. All of these processes are tightly regulated to ensure that Zn homeostasis is maintained for its many physiological functions (Cousins, 1985).

Zn deficiency can be caused by the interaction of dietary intake, absorptive impairment, increased losses, and physiological requirements. It has a wide range of clinical manifestations, such as immune dysfunction, delayed wound healing, growth retardation in children, loss of hair, and neurological deficits (Prasad, 2009). The subtlety of Zn deficiency makes its diagnosis often difficult, due to overlapping signs and symptoms of other nutritional and medical conditions. Solutions to alleviate Zn deficiency will have to be multi-pronged and context-specific. In the first instance, diet diversification including Zn-rich foods such as meat, shellfish, dairy, and fortified cereals, is a basic strategy for preventing deficiency. In areas where dietary intake is insufficient, zinc supplementation may be effective, particularly for at-risk populations including pregnant women, young children, and the elderly (Bhutta et al., 2013). Correcting underlying causes such as malabsorption syndromes or chronic diseases also remains a key strategy. Some public health interventions that combine education, food fortification, and supplementation appear effective in decreasing zinc deficiency (Hotz & Brown, n.d.). In addition, improving agricultural practices to bio-fortify crops with zinc could also yield sustainable solutions. As such, these may be effective in combating Zn deficiency and the health impacts of such deficiency.

BIOCHEMICAL/PHYSIOLOGICAL FUNCTIONS OF ZINC

The majority of Zn's biochemical functions are broad, varied, and essential to many physiological processes hence it is an integral component of human health. It is indispensable as a cofactor for over 300 enzymes catalyzing vital biochemical reactions (Prasad, 2013). Carbonic anhydrase that maintains the acid-base balance and alcohol dehydrogenase responsible for detoxification of alcohols through oxidation are some of the key Zn-dependent enzymes in cellular metabolism (Vallee & Auld, 1990). By participating in DNA synthesis, it plays a crucial role together with other enzymes like DNA polymerases which facilitates DNA replication and repair thus maintaining genomic stability and correct cell division (MacDonald, 2000). As a cofactor for enzymes such as thymulin in the immune system, it influences T-cell function and cytokine production (Prasad, 2008). Also being helpful to cells against oxidative damage as it supports antioxidant enzymes like superoxide dismutase (Oteiza & Mackenzie, 2005). These biochemical functions highlight Zn's indispensability in maintaining cellular health, facilitating proper immune responses, and ensuring efficient metabolic and genetic processes. A deficiency in Zn can disrupt these enzymatic functions, leading to widespread health issues and compromised biological functions (K. M. Hambidge, 2010).

Figure 1. Physiological functions of Zn

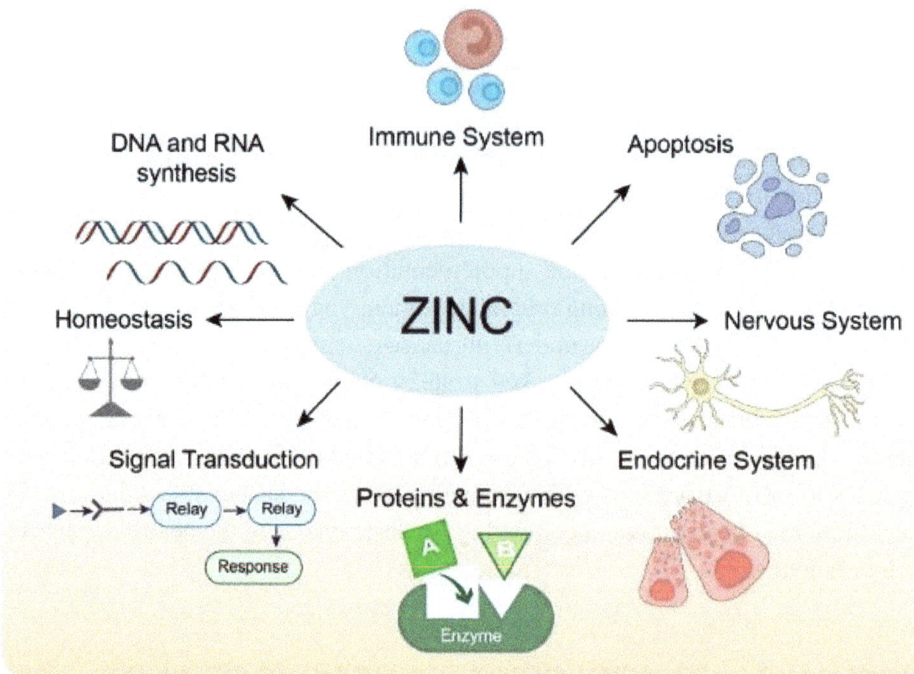

(Li et al., 2023)

Zn is fundamental in maintaining the structural integrity and stability of proteins, as well as in regulating gene expression and cell signaling pathways, thus playing a multifaceted role in cellular physiology. Structurally, Zn stabilizes proteins by forming Zn fingers, which are small protein motifs that create strong interactions with DNA, RNA, and other proteins, thereby maintaining their proper configuration and functionality (Berg & Shi, 1996). Such stabilization is essential for several transcription factors, enzymes and structural proteins so that their shape will be maintained while still biologically active. In gene expression Zn fingers allow transcription factors to bind to specific DNA sequences thereby controlling the transcription of genes necessary in cell growth, differentiation and apoptosis (Klug, 1999). This regulation ensures precise control over genetic programming and cellular function. In cellular signaling pathways Zn acts as a secondary messenger modulating various signaling molecules and their pathways including immune response, cell proliferation and apoptosis (Hara et al., 2017). Consequently, by influencing these pathways Zn helps maintain cellular homeostasis as well as coordinating appropriate cellular responses to internal or external stimuli. Disruptions in Zn availability can therefore impair protein function, gene regulation, and signal transduction, leading to a cascade of cellular dysfunctions and disease states (Outten & O'Halloran, 2001).

ZINC DEFICIENCY: CAUSES AND CONSEQUENCES

Inadequate dietary intake is the primary cause of Zn deficiency, with certain populations at higher risk, including pregnant women, infants, and elderly individuals (Krebs, 1998). Poor soil quality, food processing methods, and dietary restrictions can further exacerbate deficiency (Hotz & Brown, n.d.).

Zn deficiency can have profound consequences on human health, manifesting in a range of physiological and clinical symptoms. One of the most significant physiological impacts is immune dysfunction where zinc deficiency undermines the body's ability to mount an adequate immune response. This predisposes an individual to infections including bacterial, viral, and fungal agents. Clinically, it leads to more sicknesses and a longer recovery period (Shankar & Prasad, 1998). Moreover, Zn deficiencies have been shown to lead to impaired growth as well as delayed development specifically in children. This is because Zn plays a crucial role in cell division and protein synthesis processes that are vital for growth and tissue development (Brown et al., 2002). Cognitive function also suffers from poor nutrition such that deficiencies of Zn affect learning disabilities in individuals which leads to impairment of memory leading to inefficient brain functions thus underscoring the importance of Zn in neural development and neurotransmission.

The impact of Zn deficiency on reproductive health is significant, affecting both males and females. In males, Zn is crucial for spermatogenesis and testosterone synthesis, with deficiencies potentially leading to reduced fertility and hypogonadism. In females, Zn is vital for ovulation and overall reproductive health, and deficiencies can result in complications such as irregular menstrual cycles and impaired fetal development. Pregnant women with Zn deficiency are at a higher risk of complications, including preterm birth and low birth weight (King, 2000). These reproductive issues underscore Zn's essential role in ensuring healthy reproductive and developmental outcomes.

Figure 2. Physiological and clinical symptoms of Zn deficiency

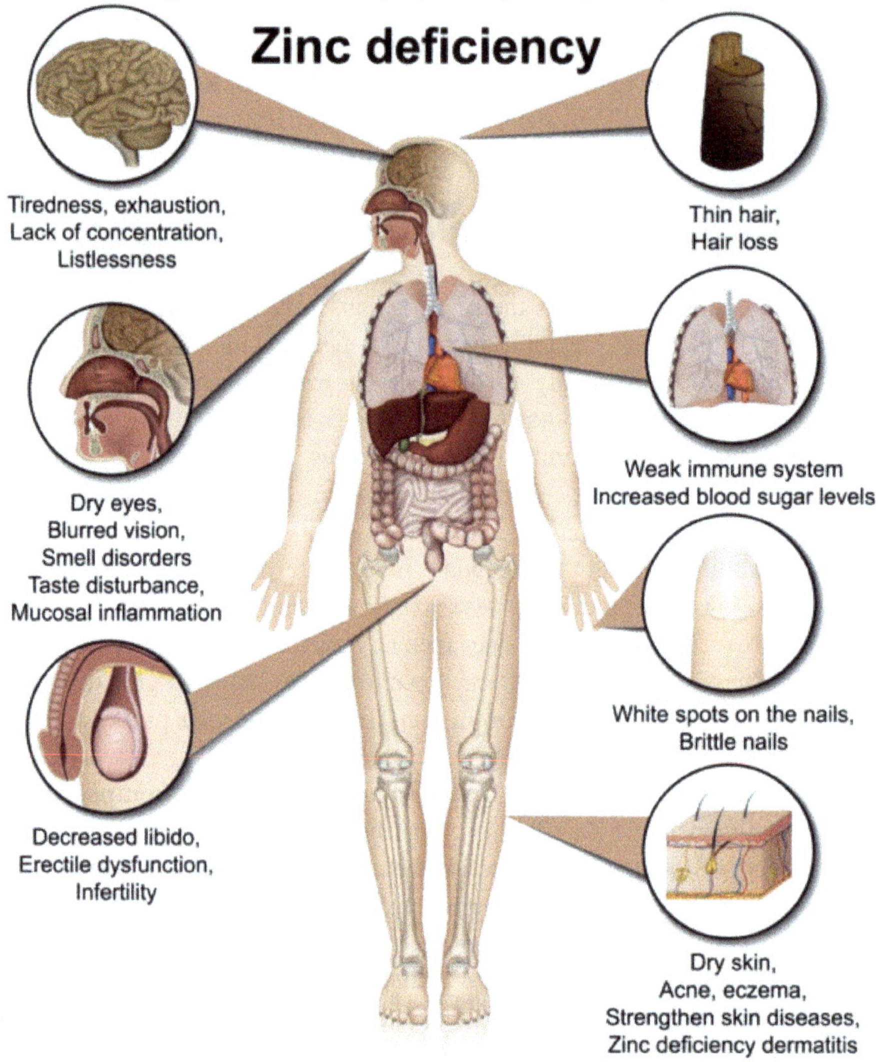

(Https://Nutrition4ibd.Com/Articles/First-Signs-of-Low-Zinc-a-Zinc-Deficiency/, n.d.)

Zn deficiency is linked to several specific disease states. In children, diarrhea both triggers and results from a lack of Zn thereby worsening the deficiency while weakening the immune system (Bhutta et al., 1999). Zinc deficient individuals have more frequent and severe respiratory infections including pneumonia due to compromised mucosal barriers and immune function. Besides, impaired wound healing occurs frequently because Zn plays a critical role in collagen synthesis, cell replication, immune response needed for tissue repair (Lansdown, 1996). These connections illustrate how extensive, and devastating are consequences of zinc deficiency, emphasizing the need for adequate Zn intake through diet or supplementation to prevent and mitigate these health issues.

DIETARY SOURCES AND ABSORPTION MECHANISMS OF ZINC

Zn is an indispensable element and is obtained from a variety of dietary sources, both from animal and plant origin. Animal-based sources include red meat, poultry, seafood (particularly oysters), dairy products, and eggs, which are Zn rich and offer high bioavailability (Solomons, 2001).

Legumes, nuts, seeds, whole grains and fortified cereals are considered plant-based options. Nevertheless, the bioavailability of Zn from plant foods is typically lower than animal foods, due to factors such as the presence of phytic acid that impedes Zn absorption (Sandström, 1997).

Zinc's bioavailability is impacted by several food ingredients. Phytates can bind zinc and prevent the gastrointestinal tract from absorbing it; they are present in whole grains, seeds, legumes, and some vegetables (R. S. Gibson, 2006). In a similar vein, consuming a lot of fiber might also hinder the absorption of zinc.

Zn's bioavailability may be further decreased by competing with other dietary elements, such as high calcium and iron levels, for absorption.

Figure 3. Dietary sources of Zn

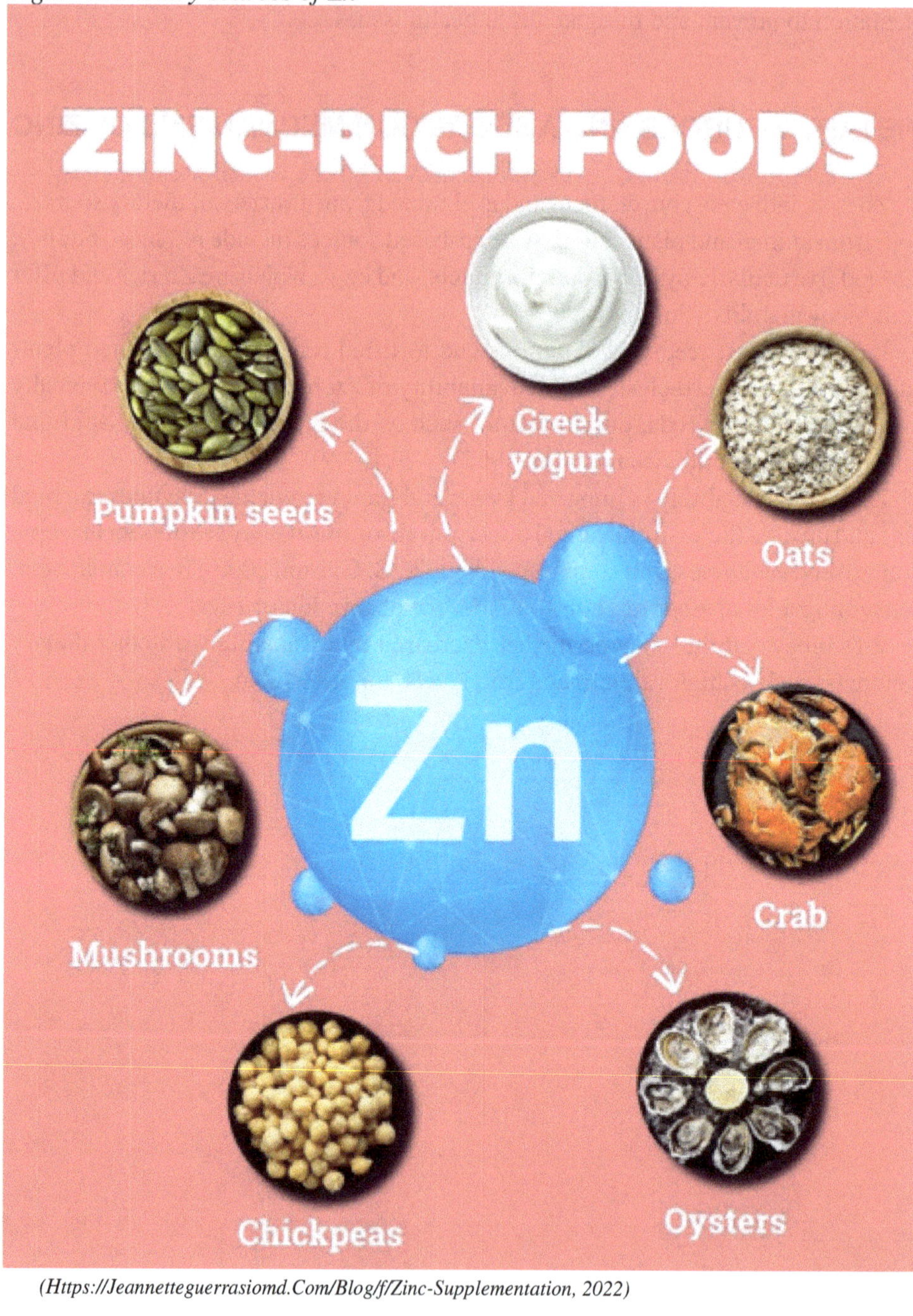

(Https://Jeanneteguerrasiomd.Com/Blog/f/Zinc-Supplementation, 2022)

On the other hand, some food items, notably animal proteins and organic acids like citric acid, can improve the absorption of zinc by combining with zinc to form soluble complexes (Lönnerdal, 2000; Solomons, 2001).

Zn absorption takes place mainly in the small intestine, especially in the jejunum and the ileum, mediated by certain Zn transporters and regulatory proteins. ZIP4 is a transporter protein that facilitates the entry of Zn into the intestinal cells (enterocytes) (Wang et al., 2002). On entering the cell, Zn may be stored in vesicles, used in cellular functions, or released into the bloodstream with the help of another protein called ZnT1 (Palmiter & Huang, 2004).

The regulation of the transporters is very important in maintaining Zn homeostasis, such that the body may adjust the absorption rates due to dietary intake and physiological needs. At low Zn levels, the expression of ZIP4 is upregulated to enhance absorption, while high Zn levels can downregulate ZIP4 in order to avoid excess accumulation (Cousins, 2010).

Figure 4. Absorption mechanisms of Zn

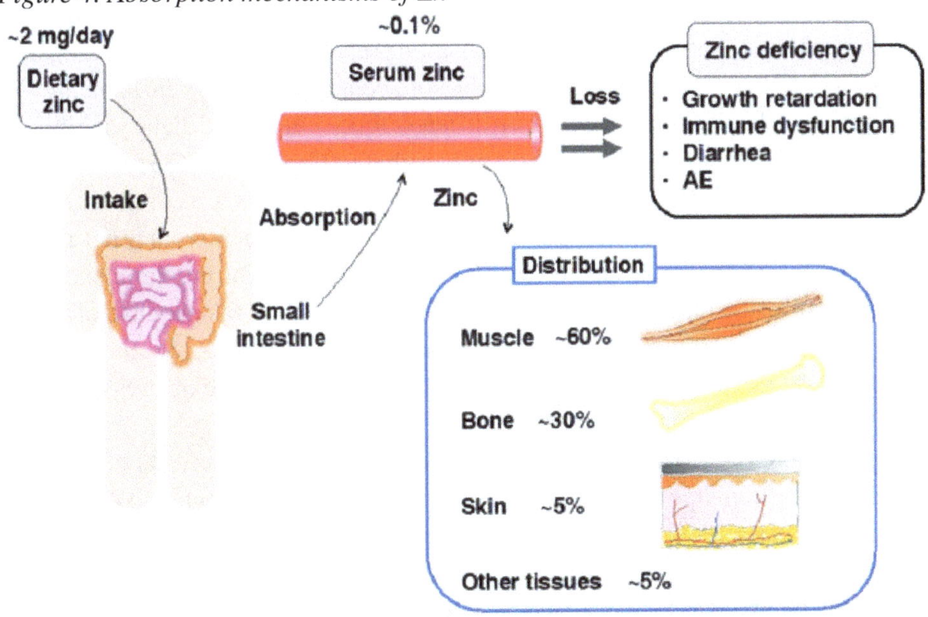

(Takagishi et al., 2017)

Traditional food processing methods enhance Zn absorption from plant foods. Soaking, for example, reduces the content of phytate in grains, seeds, and legumes. Sprouting also decreases the content of phytate and increases the amount of some amino acids and organic acids that enhance the bioavailability of Zn (Hotz & Gibson, 2007). Fermentation involves the biodegradation of phytates by the action of microorganisms, thereby liberating minerals. The application of these food-processing techniques can significantly improve Zn absorption from plant sources, thereby protecting against Zn deficiency, particularly in populations that depend mainly on plant food sources for their nutrient intake (R. Gibson et al., 1998).

ASSESSING ZINC STATUS

Accurate assessment of Zn status is essential for identifying individuals at risk of deficiency and monitoring intervention outcomes. Various methods, including dietary assessment, biochemical markers, and functional tests, are utilized to evaluate Zn status. Each method for assessing Zn status comes with its own set of challenges and limitations, emphasizing the importance of employing multiple approaches for a comprehensive evaluation (King, 2011).

Dietary Assessment: This method involves estimating Zn intake through food records, recalls, or dietary surveys. However, accurately assessing Zn intake can be challenging due to factors like incomplete food composition databases, inaccuracies in portion size estimation, and variations in food preparation methods. Additionally, relying solely on dietary assessment may not account for factors influencing Zn absorption, such as bioavailability from different food sources and dietary inhibitors like phytates (International Zinc Nutrition Consultative Group (IZiNCG) et al., 2004).

Biochemical Markers: Blood plasma or serum Zn levels are commonly used biochemical markers for assessing Zn status. However, these markers may not always accurately reflect Zn status due to homeostatic regulation. During deficiency, the body may prioritize maintaining normal serum Zn levels at the expense of tissue Zn levels, leading to false-negative results. Additionally, serum Zn levels can fluctuate in response to various factors, such as recent dietary intake or stress, making interpretation challenging (King, 2011).

Functional Tests: Functional tests assess the physiological effects of Zn deficiency, such as impaired immune function or abnormal taste perception. While these tests provide valuable insights into the functional consequences of Zn deficiency, they may lack specificity and sensitivity. For example, immune function tests may be influenced by factors other than Zn status, such as overall health or concurrent infections. Taste perception tests may also be subjective and variable among individuals (K. M. Hambidge, 2010).

Employing multiple assessment methods can help mitigate the limitations of each approach and provide a more comprehensive understanding of Zn status. Combining dietary assessment with biochemical markers and functional tests allows for triangulation of data, enhancing the accuracy and reliability of the assessment. Additionally, considering individual factors such as age, sex, physiological status, and dietary habits is essential for interpreting results accurately. Overall, a multidimensional approach to assessing Zn status is crucial for identifying individuals at risk of deficiency and monitoring intervention outcomes effectively (King, 2011).

INTERVENTIONS AND STRATEGIES TO ALLEVIATE ZINC DEFICIENCY

Addressing Zn deficiency on a population level requires a multifaceted approach that integrates various strategies to enhance Zn intake and address nutritional gaps.

Food Fortification is a cost-effective and scalable intervention that involves adding Zn to commonly consumed foods such as flour, rice, or salt. Fortification programs can target vulnerable groups such as pregnant women, children, and individuals in regions where dietary Zn intake is low. By fortifying widely consumed foods, fortification programs can reach a large portion of the population and help alleviate Zn deficiency (Allen et al., 2006b).

Biofortification is another promising strategy for addressing Zn deficiency, particularly in regions where access to diverse and nutrient-rich foods is limited. Biofortification involves breeding crops to increase their Zn content through traditional plant breeding techniques or genetic modification. Zn-biofortified crops, such as Zn-enhanced rice, wheat, or maize, offer a sustainable and cost-effective solution to improve Zn intake, especially for rural communities dependent on staple crops for their diets. Integrating biofortified crops into agricultural systems can help increase dietary Zn intake and reduce the prevalence of Zn deficiency over the long term (Bouis, n.d.).

Supplementation programs play a crucial role in addressing Zn deficiency, particularly in populations where dietary diversification and fortification may be challenging to implement. Zn supplements, in the form of tablets, syrups, or powders, can provide individuals at risk of deficiency with the recommended daily intake of Zn. Supplementation programs are often targeted towards specific groups, such as pregnant women, infants, and young children, who have increased Zn requirements for growth and development. Additionally, supplementation programs can be integrated into existing health and nutrition programs, such as antenatal care or child health services, to reach vulnerable populations effectively (Bhutta et al., 2013).

Dietary Diversification is a fundamental strategy for promoting Zn intake and addressing deficiency on a population level. Encouraging individuals to consume a diverse diet that includes Zn-rich foods such as meat, fish, dairy products, legumes, nuts, seeds, and whole grains can help improve Zn intake and overall nutritional status. Nutrition education and awareness campaigns are essential components of dietary diversification strategies, as they empower individuals and communities to make informed food choices and adopt healthier eating habits. By promoting dietary diversity, health authorities can help reduce the risk of Zn deficiency and improve overall health outcomes on a population level (M. Hambidge et al., 2000).

Figure 5. Strategies to alleviate Zn deficiency

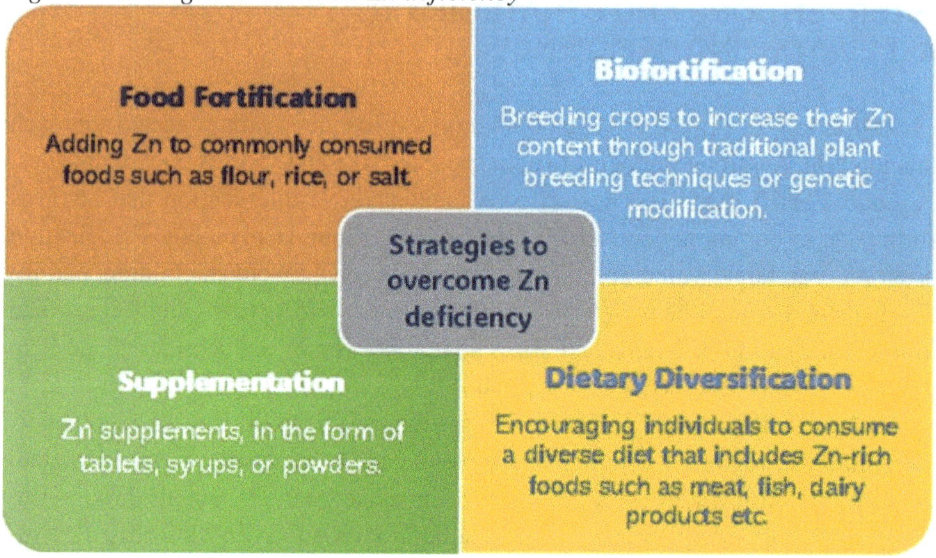

For maximum impact and assurance of sustainability, these strategies should be integrated into comprehensive health and nutrition programs. Their implementation, monitoring, and evaluation require effective collaborative efforts of government agencies, NGOs, healthcare providers, agricultural sectors, and community stakeholders. The successes of interventions are assured through community engagement, capacity building, and empowerment, which foster ownership and participation at the community level. Investing in research, monitoring, and surveillance systems is important for tracking progress, identifying gaps, and informing evidence-based policies and programs (R. S. Gibson & Ferguson, 1998).

CONCLUSION

Zn deficiency remains a significant global health concern, with far-reaching implications for individuals and communities worldwide. By recognizing the importance of Zn and implementing targeted interventions, we can work towards reducing the burden of Zn deficiency and improving health outcomes for populations globally.

This chapter highlights the multifaceted nature of Zn's role in the body, from its involvement in enzymatic activity and gene expression to its impact on immune function, growth and development, cognitive function, and reproductive health. Through a nuanced understanding of Zn's physiological functions, healthcare professionals can better identify individuals at risk of deficiency and tailor interventions to address their specific needs. Moreover, by exploring various strategies such as food fortification, biofortification, supplementation, and dietary diversification, we can adopt a comprehensive approach to promoting adequate Zn intake and mitigating deficiency on a population level.

The importance of collaboration and concerted efforts cannot be overstated in addressing the global burden of Zn deficiency. Healthcare professionals, researchers, policymakers, and the general public, all have vital roles to play in raising awareness, advocating for effective interventions, and implementing sustainable solutions. By fostering partnerships and leveraging resources effectively, we can create environments that support healthy lifestyles and ensure access to Zn-rich foods and interventions for those in need.

In essence, "Understanding Zn: Its Importance in Human Health" underscores the significance of Zn in promoting optimal health outcomes and underscores the urgency of addressing Zn deficiency on a global scale. Through education, advocacy, and targeted interventions, we can strive towards a healthier future for all, where adequate Zn intake is prioritized, and individuals can thrive and reach their full potential.

REFERENCES

Allen, L. (2006a). World Health Organization., & Food and Agriculture Organization of the United Nations. *Guidelines on food fortification with micronutrients*. World Health Organization.

Allen, L. (2006b). World Health Organization., & Food and Agriculture Organization of the United Nations. *Guidelines on food fortification with micronutrients*. World Health Organization.

Berg, J. M., & Shi, Y. (1996). The Galvanization of Biology: A Growing Appreciation for the Roles of Zinc. *Science*, *271*(5252), 1081–1085. DOI: 10.1126/science.271.5252.1081 PMID: 8599083

Bhutta, Z. A., Black, R. E., Brown, K. H., Gardner, J. M., Gore, S., Hidayat, A., Khatun, F., Martorell, R., Ninh, N. X., Penny, M. E., Rosado, J. L., Roy, S. K., Ruel, M., Sazawal, S., & Shankar, A. (1999). Prevention of diarrhea and pneumonia by zinc supplementation in children in developing countries: Pooled analysis of randomized controlled trials. *The Journal of Pediatrics*, *135*(6), 689–697. DOI: 10.1016/S0022-3476(99)70086-7 PMID: 10586170

Bhutta, Z. A., Salam, R. A., & Das, J. K. (2013). Meeting the challenges of micronutrient malnutrition in the developing world. In *British Medical Bulletin* (Vol. 106, Issue 1, pp. 7–17). DOI: 10.1093/bmb/ldt015

Bouis, H. E. (n.d.). *S32*. www.harvestplus.org

Brown, K. H., Peerson, J. M., Rivera, J., & Allen, L. H. (2002). Effect of supplemental zinc on the growth and serum zinc concentrations of prepubertal children: A meta-analysis of randomized controlled trials. *The American Journal of Clinical Nutrition*, *75*(6), 1062–1071. DOI: 10.1093/ajcn/75.6.1062 PMID: 12036814

Brown, K. H., Rivera, J. A., Bhutta, Z., Gibson, R. S., King, J. C., Lönnerdal, B., Ruel, M. T., Sandtröm, B., Wasantwisut, E., & Hotz, C. (2004). International Zinc Nutrition Consultative Group (IZiNCG) technical document #1. Assessment of the risk of zinc deficiency in populations and options for its control. *Food and Nutrition Bulletin*, *25*(1, Suppl 2), S99–S203.

Cousins, R. J. (1985). *Absorption, Transport, and Hepatic Metabolism of Copper and Zinc: Special Reference to Metallothionein and Ceruloplasmin*. www.physiology.org/journal/physrev

Cousins, R. J. (2010). Gastrointestinal Factors Influencing Zinc Absorption and Homeostasis. *International Journal for Vitamin and Nutrition Research, 80*(45), 243–248. DOI: 10.1024/0300-9831/a000030 PMID: 21462106

Gibson, R., Ferguson, E., & Lehrfeld, J. (1998). Complementary foods for infant feeding in developing countries: Their nutrient adequacy and improvement. *European Journal of Clinical Nutrition, 52*(10), 764–770. DOI: 10.1038/sj.ejcn.1600645 PMID: 9805226

Gibson, R. S. (2006). Zinc: The missing link in combating micronutrient malnutrition in developing countries. *The Proceedings of the Nutrition Society, 65*(1), 51–60. DOI: 10.1079/PNS2005474 PMID: 16441944

Gibson, R. S., & Ferguson, E. L. (1998). Nutrition intervention strategies to combat zinc deficiency in developing countries. *Nutrition Research Reviews, 11*(1), 115–131. DOI: 10.1079/NRR19980008 PMID: 19087462

Hambidge, K. M. (2010). Micronutrient bioavailability: Dietary Reference Intakes and a future perspective. *The American Journal of Clinical Nutrition, 91*(5), 1430S–1432S. DOI: 10.3945/ajcn.2010.28674B PMID: 20200261

Hambidge, M., Cousins, R. J., & Costello, R. B. (2000). Introduction. *The Journal of Nutrition, 130*(5), 1341S–1343S. DOI: 10.1093/jn/130.5.1341S PMID: 10801940

Hara, T., Takeda, T. A., Takagishi, T., Fukue, K., Kambe, T., & Fukada, T. (2017). Physiological roles of zinc transporters: Molecular and genetic importance in zinc homeostasis. *The Journal of Physiological Sciences; JPS, 67*(2), 283–301.

Hotz, C., & Brown, K. H. (2004). Assessment of the risk of zinc deficiency in populations and options for its control.

Hotz, C., & Gibson, R. S. (2007). Traditional Food-Processing and Preparation Practices to Enhance the Bioavailability of Micronutrients in Plant-Based Diets1. *The Journal of Nutrition, 137*(4), 1097–1100. DOI: 10.1093/jn/137.4.1097 PMID: 17374686

Institute of Medicine. (2001). *Dietary Reference Intakes for Vitamin A, Vitamin K, Arsenic, Boron, Chromium, Copper, Iodine, Iron, Manganese, Molybdenum, Nickel, Silicon, Vanadium, and Zinc*. The National Academies Press., DOI: 10.17226/10026

King, J. C. (2000). Physiology of pregnancy and nutrient metabolism. *The American Journal of Clinical Nutrition, 71*(5), 1218S–1225S. DOI: 10.1093/ajcn/71.5.1218s PMID: 10799394

King, J. C. (2011). Zinc: An essential but elusive nutrient. *The American Journal of Clinical Nutrition, 94*(2), 679S–684S. DOI: 10.3945/ajcn.110.005744 PMID: 21715515

King, J. C., Shames, D. M., & Woodhouse, L. R. (2000). Zinc Homeostasis in Humans. *The Journal of Nutrition, 130*(5), 1360S–1366S. DOI: 10.1093/jn/130.5.1360S PMID: 10801944

Klug, A. (1999). Zinc finger peptides for the regulation of gene expression. *Journal of Molecular Biology, 293*(2), 215–218. DOI: 10.1006/jmbi.1999.3007 PMID: 10529348

Krebs, N. F. (1998). Zinc supplementation during lactation. *The American Journal of Clinical Nutrition, 68*(2, SUPPL.), 509S–512S. Advance online publication. DOI: 10.1093/ajcn/68.2.509S PMID: 9701169

Laity, J. H., Lee, B. M., & Wright, P. E. (2001). Zinc finger proteins: New insights into structural and functional diversity. *Current Opinion in Structural Biology, 11*(1), 39–46. DOI: 10.1016/S0959-440X(00)00167-6 PMID: 11179890

Lansdown, A. B. G. (1996). Zinc in the healing wound. *Lancet, 347*(9003), 706–707. DOI: 10.1016/S0140-6736(96)90072-0 PMID: 8601997

Li, Z., Liu, Y., Wei, R., Yong, V. W., & Xue, M. (2023). The Important Role of Zinc in Neurological Diseases. In *Biomolecules* (Vol. 13, Issue 1). MDPI. DOI: 10.3390/biom13010028

Lichten, L. A., & Cousins, R. J. (2009). Mammalian Zinc Transporters: Nutritional and Physiologic Regulation. *Annual Review of Nutrition, 29*(1), 153–176. DOI: 10.1146/annurev-nutr-033009-083312 PMID: 19400752

Lönnerdal, B. (2000). Dietary factors influencing zinc absorption. *The Journal of Nutrition, 130*(5, SUPPL.), 1378S–1383S. Advance online publication. DOI: 10.1093/jn/130.5.1378S PMID: 10801947

MacDonald, R. S. (2000). The Role of Zinc in Growth and Cell Proliferation. *The Journal of Nutrition, 130*(5), 1500S–1508S. DOI: 10.1093/jn/130.5.1500S PMID: 10801966

National Institutes of Health. (2022, January 3). *Zinc: Fact Sheet for Health Professionals*. Office of Dietary Supplements. https://ods.od.nih.gov/factsheets/Zinc-HealthProfessional

Oteiza, P. I., & Mackenzie, G. G. (2005). Zinc, oxidant-triggered cell signaling, and human health. *Molecular Aspects of Medicine*, *26*(4–5), 245–255. DOI: 10.1016/j.mam.2005.07.012 PMID: 16115673

Outten, C. E., & O'Halloran, T. V. (2001). Femtomolar Sensitivity of Metalloregulatory Proteins Controlling Zinc Homeostasis. *Science*, *292*(5526), 2488–2492. DOI: 10.1126/science.1060331 PMID: 11397910

Palmiter, R. D., & Huang, L. (2004). Efflux and compartmentalization of zinc by members of the SLC30 family of solute carriers. *Pflügers Archiv*, *447*(5), 744–751. DOI: 10.1007/s00424-003-1070-7 PMID: 12748859

Prasad, A. S. (2008). Zinc in Human Health: Effect of Zinc on Immune Cells. *Molecular Medicine (Cambridge, Mass.)*, *14*(5–6), 353–357. DOI: 10.2119/2008-00033.Prasad PMID: 18385818

Prasad, A. S. (2009). Zinc: Role in immunity, oxidative stress and chronic inflammation. *Current Opinion in Clinical Nutrition and Metabolic Care*, *12*(6), 646–652. DOI: 10.1097/MCO.0b013e3283312956 PMID: 19710611

Prasad, A. S. (2013). Discovery of Human Zinc Deficiency: Its Impact on Human Health and Disease. *Advances in Nutrition*, *4*(2), 176–190. DOI: 10.3945/an.112.003210 PMID: 23493534

Ryu, M. S. A. T. (2020). *Present Knowledge in Nutrition* (Bernadette P. Marriott, Diane F. Birt, Virginia A. Stalling, & Allison A. Yates, Eds.; 11th ed). Wiley-Blackwell.

Sandström, B. (1997). Bioavailability of zinc. *European Journal of Clinical Nutrition*, *51*(Suppl 1), S17–S19. PMID: 9023474

Shankar, A. H., & Prasad, A. S. (1998). Zinc and immune function: The biological basis of altered resistance to infection. *The American Journal of Clinical Nutrition*, *68*(2), 447S–463S. DOI: 10.1093/ajcn/68.2.447S PMID: 9701160

Solomons, N. W. (2001). Dietary Sources of Zinc and Factors Affecting its Bioavailability. *Food and Nutrition Bulletin*, *22*(2), 138–154. DOI: 10.1177/156482650102200204

Takagishi, T., Hara, T., & Fukada, T. (2017). Recent Advances in the Role of SLC39A/ZIP Zinc Transporters In Vivo. *International Journal of Molecular Sciences*, *18*(12), 2708. DOI: 10.3390/ijms18122708 PMID: 29236063

Vallee, B. L., & Auld, D. S. (1990). Zinc coordination, function, and structure of zinc enzymes and other proteins. *Biochemistry*, *29*(24), 5647–5659. DOI: 10.1021/bi00476a001 PMID: 2200508

Vallee, B. L., & Falchuk, K. H. (1993). The Biochemical Basis of Zinc Physiology. In *REVIEWS* (Vol. 73, Issue 1). DOI: 10.1152/physrev.1993.73.1.79

Wang, K., Zhou, B., Kuo, Y.-M., Zemansky, J., & Gitschier, J. (2002). A Novel Member of a Zinc Transporter Family Is Defective in Acrodermatitis Enteropathica. In *Am* (Vol. 71). J. Hum. Genet. DOI: 10.1086/341125

Yamasaki, S., Sakata-Sogawa, K., Hasegawa, A., Suzuki, T., Kabu, K., Sato, E., Kurosaki, T., Yamashita, S., Tokunaga, M., Nishida, K., & Hirano, T. (2007). Zinc is a novel intracellular second messenger. *The Journal of Cell Biology*, *177*(4), 637–645. DOI: 10.1083/jcb.200702081 PMID: 17502426

Chapter 2
Cutaneous Markers and Systemic Manifestations of Zinc Deficiency

Rajesh Datt Mehta
Rajasthan University of Health Sciences, India

Shashwat Datt Mehta
https://orcid.org/0000-0002-6852-8683
Rajasthan University of Health Sciences, India

ABSTRACT

Zinc was adjudged as an essential micronutrient for human health in the mid-20th century. It is required for gene transcription, enzyme activity, nucleic acid, protein and lipid metabolism. Its role at microcellular level makes it an integral part of the milieu interieur. So, its deficiency involves every system of the body, but evident burnt is on integument, skeletal, gastro-intestinal, central nervous, immune and reproductive systems. The zinc deficiency in growth period may even lead to growth deprivation. Zinc deficiency may be inherited or acquired. It may be attributed to zinc deficient diet, decreased intake, malabsorption, accentuated physiological metabolic requirements or increased loss. The zinc deficiency may be observed on the integument as cutaneous markers and there are systemic manifestations too. Diagnosis of symptoms and signs should help the clinicians to manage the deficient status and its consequences.

DOI: 10.4018/979-8-3693-5355-4.ch002

INTRODUCTION

Human body comprises 3-4% of its weight as trace elements and minerals. These are essential micronutrients required as cofactors for micro-cellular enzymes as well as prosthetic groups for metalloproteins.

Zinc, though begins with the last alphabet but does have a key role in homeostasis through about 200 metalloenzymes; mandatory in synthesis and degradation of nucleic acids and fatty acids (Prasad, 2013). It is necessary for human beings since intrauterine life for growth maintenance and for the optimum functioning of skin and its appendages, immune, central nervous, gastrointestinal, musculoskeletal and reproductive systems; later in life. (Roohani & Hurrell, 2013)

Zinc is distributed in human body in muscles, bones, skin, liver and other tissues in different proportions. (Figure 1)

Figure 1. Zinc distribution in human body (Concept – Mani Datt Mehta)

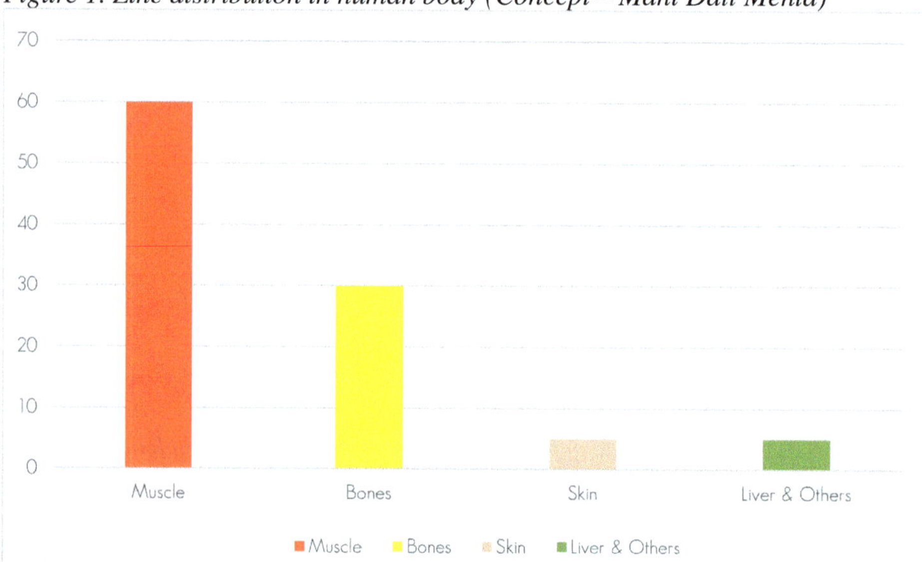

Sources

Zinc is found in breast milk, dairy products, non-vegetarian eatables, sea food, legumes, whole grains and green leafy vegetables. (Morel & Schaefer, 2018, p. 804)

Absorption

Zinc in the form of liquid suspensions is better absorbed as compared to solid diets. Absorption of zinc is directly proportional to the zinc content in the diet, i.e. more the zinc in the diet, better would be the absorption until reaching a maximum limit. Zinc deficient individuals tend to absorb this micronutrient more efficiently when compared to zinc sufficed individuals.

The free zinc ions from diet bind to certain ligands before being transported to the enterocytes in small gut with the help of transcellular transporter, ZIP4 and thereafter reach the portal circulation. (Table 1) Then, they are released from liver into the systemic circulation where majority of the zinc ions get bound to serum albumin; available to fulfil the tissue demands whenever needed. (Krebs, 2000)

Table 1. Zinc transporters in various cells and their functions

Zinc transporter	Site	Function
ZIP 2 & ZIP 4	Keratinocytes (KC)	Proliferation & differentiation of KCs
ZIP 10	Epidermal progenitors	Epidermogenesis
ZnT5	Mast cells	Inflammatory cytokine release
ZIP 8	T cells	Release of γ-interferon
ZIP 7 & ZIP 13	Fibroblasts	Dermal formation & TGFβ signalling
ZIP 13 & ZIP 14	Adipocytes	Inhibits beige fat lobule differentiation and curbs excessive inflammation

Epidemiology

Globally about 1/5th of the population suffers from inadequate zinc in their diet. Paediatric age group is at higher risk (5 out of 5 lac children) developing zinc associated deficiency with no sex or ethnic predilection. (Wessells & Brown, 2012)

Pathogenesis of Zinc Deficiency

Zinc deficiency may be inherited or acquired. (Yan & Oboite, 2024, p.61.25-27) Acquired zinc deficiency is more prevalent as compared to its inherited version. The inherited version is because of mutation in transporter gene whereas the acquired variant is regulated by

(i) deceased dietary ingestion
(ii) decreased intestinal absorption
(iii) increased excretion
(iv) special conditions

A. The Decreased Ingestion is Multifactorial:
- Anorexia nervosa
- Alcoholics
- Pure vegan dietary recipes
- Poor supplement in parenteral nutrition

B. Absorption Status is Checked by:
- 'Phytates', in grains and legumes decrease the zinc absorption; this interference is absent in non- vegetarian diet.
- Gastrointestinal diseases (chronic recurrent diarrhoea, celiac disease, inflammatory bowel syndrome, short bowel syndrome, gastric bypass surgical interventions)

C. Increased Elimination:
- Pregnancy
- Alcoholics
- Infections
- Renal disorders
- Burns

D. Special Conditions:
- Premature infants (high metabolic demands of zinc, decreased zinc absorption by immature gut epithelium, increased cutaneous, gastrointestinal and renal excretion)
- Top fed bovine milk infants (higher molecular weight protein in bovine source decreases zinc absorption as compared to breastfed infants)
- Breast fed infants (mothers with mutant zinc transporter genes in mammary glands, leading to decreased secretion of zinc in breast milk)
- Certain drugs (diuretics, sodium valproate, penicillamine) may contribute to zinc deficiency

Zinc Deficiency and Integumentary Organelles

In human body skin is the third zinc rich organ. The various cutaneous organelles play pivotal role in zinc deficient conditions.

Langerhans Cells

These are the epidermal 'antigen presenting cells'. Langerhans cells homeostasis is dependent upon appropriate levels of zinc. There are two hypotheses for deranged Langerhans function in zinc deficiency. The first one is impaired expression of transforming growth factor -beta 1 (TGF-β1), in the epidermis of hypozincemia individuals as compared to the healthy ones. It is because zinc finger transcription factors are essential for TGF-β1 signalling. Secondly, zinc deficiency triggers Langerhans cells' apoptosis. Epidermal Langerhans cells were absent in the cutaneous lesions of autosomal recessive condition, acrodermatitis enteropathica. (Ogawa & Kinoshita, 2018)

Melanocytes

Rudolf and Rudolf, 2017 found that increased intracellular zinc has a role in the amplification of mitochondrial and lysosomal activity in human melanocytes. The melanocytes' proliferation and autophagy are also augmented with zinc as facilitator micronutrient. So, zinc may have definite role in pathogenesis of vitiligo and melanoma.

Mast Cells

In addition to being a proliferation activist for different cell lines in skin, zinc does have a very crucial function of transducing extracellular stimulus into intracellular signalling. The cytosolic zinc in mast cells mediates the production of inflammatory cytokines by overexpression of ZnT5 mRNA, leading to activation of the NFkB pathway. (Kabu & Yamasaki, 2006)

Dendritic Cells

Dendritic cell maturation is regulated by zinc and zinc transporters. Reduced free intracellular zinc upregulates the expression of major histocompatibility complex of class II (MHC-II).

T-Cells

Zinc deficiency leads to thymic atrophy inducing decreased double positive thymocytes and ultimately the mature single T cells (Golden & Jackson, 1977). The zinc transporter ZIP 8's (SLC39A8) over expression in lysosomes of T cells, promotes IFN - gamma secretion. It proves that zinc is essential for the proper T cell generation and IFN production. (Aydemir & Liuzzi, 2009)

Endothelial Cells

Malavolta and Costarelli, 2017 observed that chelation of zinc causes demise of endothelial cells furthermore, chronic exposure to zinc speeds up senescence of these cells. It reiterates the role of adequate zinc in viability of endothelial cells and angiogenesis. (Oikawa & Ichihara, 2015)

Fibroblasts

Zinc promotes formation of fibroblasts through crucial functions of ZIP7 and ZIP13 in connective tissue homeostasis. ZIP7 in fibroblasts is essential for proper activity of dermis. (Fukuda & Civic, 2008)

Adipocytes

Zinc transporter ZIP13 is involved in regulation of adipocyte's physiology. ZIP13 facilitates beige adipocytes' differentiation, thereby preventing obesity. ZIP 14 and zinc finger prints in adipocytes get upregulated after adipocyte hypertrophy and hyperplasia by the action of inflammatory cytokines. This ultimately suppresses the excessive inflammatory response. (Troche & Aydemir, 2016)

Cutaneous Markers of Zinc Deficiency

Acrodermatitis Enteropathica (AE)

Loss of function mutation of zinc transporter, ZIP14 is responsible for causation of the inherited variant of acrodermatitis enteropathica (Schmitt & Kury, 2009).

The three symptoms making the classical triad of acrodermatitis enteropathica are:

1. Alopecia
2. Eczematous lesions
3. Diarrhoea

Pathogenesis of AE in Zinc Deficiency

Irritant exposure in zinc deficient individuals leads to decreased expression of TGF-β1 in epidermis which causes absence of Langerhans cells. Subsequently, due to absence of CD39 expressing LCs, there is excessive ATP production which remain unhydrolyzed; resulting in inflammatory response in form of acrodermatitis enteropathica. (Figure 2)

Figure 2. Schematic diagram of AE pathophysiology (Concept – Mani Datt Mehta)

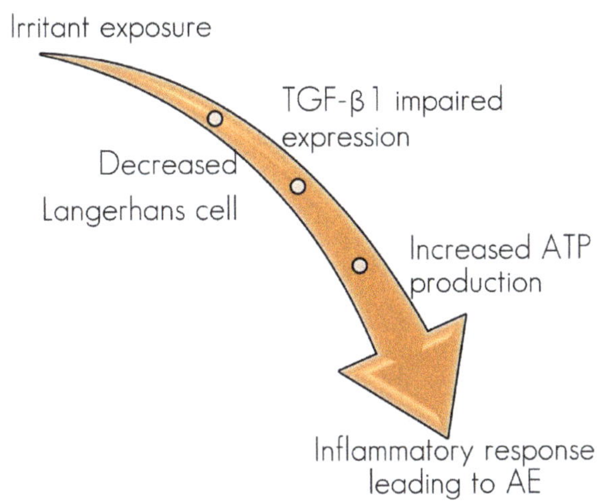

Clinical Manifestations of Inherited Acrodermatitis Enteropathica

- **Acral Eruptions**. These are eczematous lesions present symmetrically as plaques to begin with. Later on, these may become vesiculobullous, pustular or even turn eroded with crusted margins. Skin lesions around mouth i.e. perioral cutaneous eruptions are, U -shaped (grossly resembling a 'horse shoe ') as these spare the upper lip (Figure 3). The periorificial and acral eczematous lesions may have altered morphology in the immunocompromised children because of superadded infections by Staphylococcus aureus and Candida albicans.
- **Alopecia.** The patches of hair loss, 'alopecia' are observed on the scalp. The hair is otherwise dry and brittle in character.
- **Other Non-specific Cutaneous Findings.** The occasional associated dermatological findings with classical acrodermatitis enteropathica are angular

cheilitis, paronychia, hypopigmented patches and deranged wound healing. Transient zinc deficiency seen in breast fed infants with low maternal zinc in milk may have papulosquamous plaques on face and trunk. Old children and adolescents show psoriasiform plaques on extensor surface of limbs.

- **Systemic Associations with Acrodermatitis Enteropathica.** Though observed rarely, these are growth retardation, hypogonadism in males, dysgeusia, comprised dark adaptation and nephrotic syndrome.

Clinical Features of Acquired Acrodermatitis Enteropathica

Risk Factors for acquired zinc deficiency are: (Osmani & Smidt, 2021)

a. Pregnancy
b. Phytate rich diet (mineral's binding character)
c. Vegan & ketogenic diet
d. Alcoholics
e. Immunocompromised status (HIV etc)
f. Chronic kidney disease
g. Drugs (Penicillamine etc.)

The patients' clinical presentation is more or less the same as that of inherited variant. Lesions are either moist or dry erythematous patches around perioral, peri-genital and perineal regions, which may turn vesiculobullous, pustular or desquamative. The external surfaces of limbs usually have psoriasiform plaques. Oral mucosae may show frank glossitis and angular cheilitis with raw oral cavity. The nails can have the evident transverse ridges, 'Beau's lines', paronychia and onychodystrophy. The associated ophthalmic findings include blepharitis, conjunctivitis and photophobia. (Morel & Schaefer, 2018) Scalp usually shows diffuse alopecia, the remnant hair being dry, lustreless, brittle and few may have kinking. Moreover, patients with chronic condition may show disturbed sleeping habits and irritable behaviour. (Mohanan & Gupta, 2012)

Classical triad of 3 Ds is seen in 20% of the patients suffering from hypozincemia.

-Diarrhoea
-Depression (apathy)
-Dermatitis (erosive type)

In addition, paediatric patients may show delayed milestones resulting into growth retardation and hypogonadism.

Figure 3. Clinical pictures of acrodermatitis enteropathica (Credit – Dr R D Mehta)

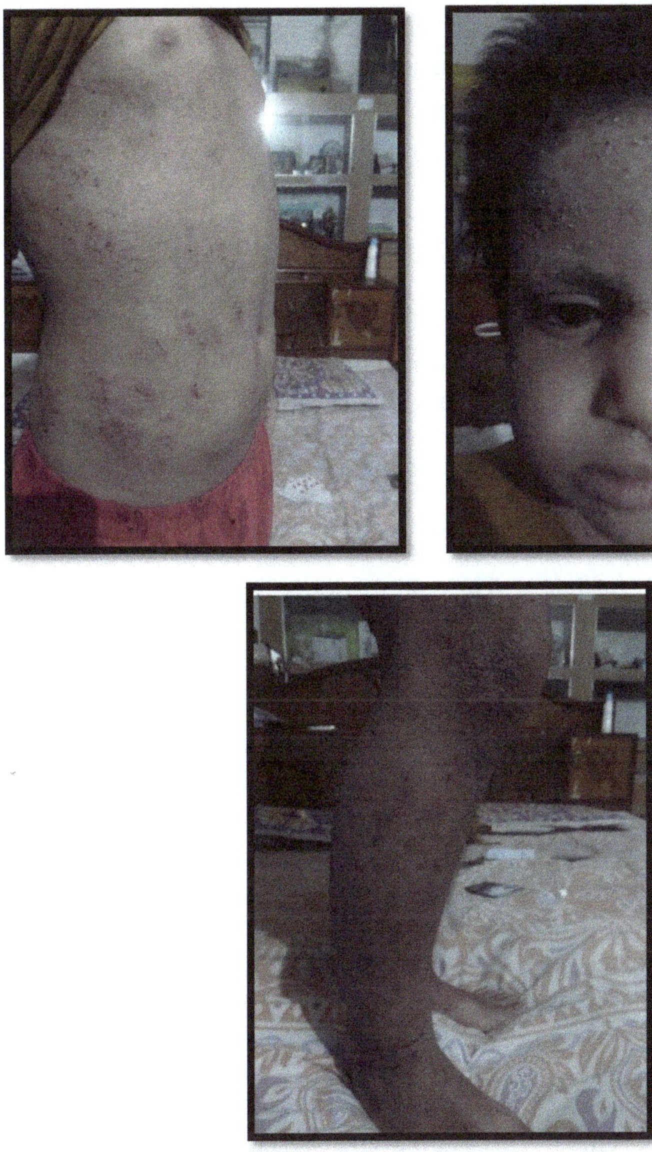

Clinical Mimickers of Acrodermatitis Enteropathica

The clinical presentation in various cutaneous diseases may look like acrodermatitis enteropathica. The differential diagnosis includes

- Psoriasis
- Seborrhoeic dermatitis
- Biotin deficiency
- Protein malnutrition, kwashiorkor type
- Allergic contact dermatitis
- Irritant contact dermatitis
- Acrodermatitis dysmetabolica, associated with maple urine disease, methylmalonic aciduria, propionic aciduria, glutaric aciduria and citrullinemia.

Sequalae of Acrodermatitis Enteropathica

Severe zinc deficiency if remains untreated may culminate into fatal outcome because of opportunistic infections. Thus, prevention, early detection and prompt management is pivotal to combat the serious consequences.

Investigation Protocol

Biochemical analysis. Serum zinc levels below 70 micro grams /dl in fasting state and 65 micro grams in non-fasting conditions are the deficiency markers.

Maternal serum and breast milk zinc levels besides infant 's serum assay for zinc reaffirms the clinical diagnosis of transient zinc deficiency due to low zinc in breast milk.

Ideal time for assessment is morning hours. The collection kit i.e. needle, cannula, tubes or stoppers should not contain zinc. The hemolyzed samples are to be discarded.

Certain conditions like mental stress, trauma, inflammatory comorbidities, hypoalbuminemia and altered serum alkaline phosphatase, do have definitive impact on assessed serum zinc levels.

Histopathology. The skin biopsy from the cutaneous lesions of acrodermatitis enteropathica stained with hematoxylin - eosin, under light microscopy (40 X) are not disease specific. But might act as a corroborative finding to support the clinical diagnosis of zinc deficiency. Microscopic peep-in reveals psoriasiform hyperplasia comprising of confluent parakeratosis, spongiosis, focal dyskeratotic changes and epidermal pallor in upper region.

Ehlers -Danlos Syndrome

The Ehlers - Danlos Syndrome, spondylocheiro dysplastic variant is because of homozygous loss of function mutation in the ZIP13 transporter gene. ZIP 13 is localised to fibroblasts in connective tissue. This mutation is acquired in autosomal recessive pattern. Its clinical features include hyper-elastic thin skin and hypermobile small joints. (Giunta & Elcioglu, 2008)

Transient Neonatal Zinc Deficiency

Eczematous lesions amongst neonates are present, over perioral, perianal and peri-genital regions, as that of, acrodermatitis enteropathica. Similarly, diffuse alopecia and diarrhoea also coexist. The reason behind transient neonatal zinc deficiency is found to be mutation of ZnT2. This ZnT2 regulates zinc concentration in breast milk, hence its mutation leads to decreased zinc content in breast milk. (Itsumura & Inamo, 2013)

Pellagra

Vitamin B3 (niacin, nicotinic acid and nicotinamide) and tryptophan deficiency lead to pellagra. The clinical manifestations of pellagra are denoted as, '4 Ds' i.e. dermatitis, diarrhoea, dementia and death (in untreated worst cases). Cutaneous lesions are on the photo exposed parts as erythematous, scarlet dermatitic rash. These plaques may turn hyperpigmented, scaly and crusted with shellac surface. The diagnostic characteristic feature of pellagra is 'Casal necklace', i.e. hyperpigmented well demarcated band around neck. Palmo-plantar painful fissuring, cheilitis, glossitis, perianal, perioral and vaginal erosions may be associated with pellagra. Vannucchi and Favaro (1995) could establish the role of zinc deficiency in development of pellagra. It may be attributed to decreased Langerhans cells because of zinc deficiency.

Alopecia

The non scarring diffuse alopecia is hallmark of zinc deficiency. It is associated with acrodermatitis enteropathica and seen otherwise also with deficient zinc serum levels. The alopecia is telogen effluvium type in which there is premature transition of hair follicles from anagen to telogen phase of the hair cycle. Patients of alopecia exhibit decreased serum and hair zinc levels. The hair shaft in trichoscopy reveals irregular pattern because of poor cystine incorporation during keratinization. Another proof of associated zinc deficiency in alopecia is clinical recovery perceived with supplementation of Zn. (Finner & Kil, 2013)

Alopecia Areata

Bhat and Manzoor (2009) could asses the lower zinc levels in patients of alopecia areata, an autoimmune cutaneous disorder. The monitoring of serum zinc levels may be an important prognostic tool in cases of alopecia areata. Zinc supplementation has been found to be invaluable adjuvant to conventional therapy for alopecia areata. (Fatteh & Atef, 2016)

Epidermodysplasia Verruciformis (EV)

The autosomal recessive cutaneous disorder usually of paediatric age group immunosuppressed individuals e.g. transplant recipients, lymphoma and HIV patients. It clinically presents as polymorphic widespread pinkish or hypopigmented guttate macules mimicking verruca plana. Sometimes, thin plaques of it, look like pityriasis versicolor. Lazarczyk and Pons (2008) established that truncating mutations in TMC6 (EVER1) and TMC8 (EVER2) and their complex with ZnT1 causes aberrant replication of EV related oncogenic β HPV 5,8. It may end up in non-melanoma skin cancers like squamous cell carcinoma. Hence dysregulation of ZnT1 might provoke oncogenicity in otherwise a benign skin disease. (Orth, 2008)

Wound Healing

Schwartz and Marsh (2005) could establish way back, the critical mechanism of wound healing and role of various zinc related molecules. Zinc promotes wound healing and strengthens cutaneous immunity. Chronic zinc deficiency has been found to be associated with delayed and poor wound healing. It might be attributed to frequent superadded cutaneous infections due to the compromised cutaneous immunity. So, zinc happens to be an integral part of wound management either when applied locally or consumed orally.

G- protein coupled receptor 39,'GPR39' acts as zinc sensing receptor. It promotes epithelial repair through stem cells located in different skin appendages. (Gonzales & Fuchs, 2017)

UV Damage

Zinc does have potent antioxidant property so its deficiency may lead to UV induced skin damage. The deficiency of zinc has been found to be associated with various photo-induced dermatopathies such as Pleomorphic light eruptions, phytophotodermatitis, melasma, etc. (Roston & DeBuys, 2002)

Miscellaneous Skin Disorders

Ogawa and Kinoshita (2018) enlisted quite a number of dermatological diseases which were proven to have a definitive role of zinc deficiency as key etiological factor. Zinc is known to be an important immunomodulator and inflammatory regulator. Therefore, its deficiency leads to the inflammatory and autoimmune conditions like atopic dermatitis, lichen planus, Behcet's disease, pemphigus vulgaris, bullous pemphigoid, epidermolysis bullosa and pigmentary disorders.

Management of Zinc Deficiency

The clinical diagnosis of zinc deficiency with cutaneous symptoms and signs, confirmed with investigative support is to be corrected by treatment.

Combating zinc deficiency

The community medicine approach to deal with zinc deficiency should include the following steps; (Figure 4)

- Dietary modification
- Dietary diversification
- Supplementation
- Fortification
- Bio fortification.

Figure 4. Preventive strategies for zinc deficiency management (Concept- Mani Datt Mehta)

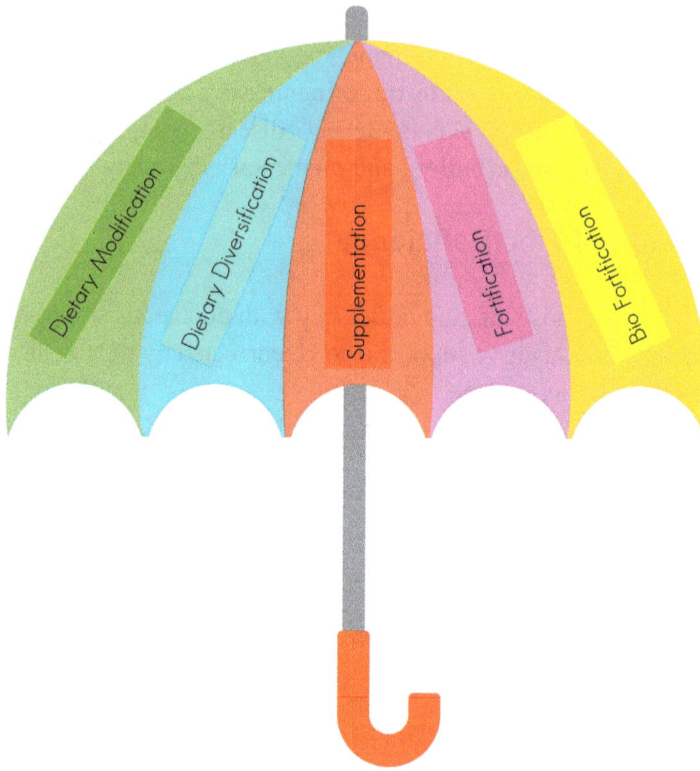

The required dose schedule is followed as per WHO norms (Table 2)

Table 2. Recommended daily dietary intake of elemental zinc

Age	Recommended intake
< 4 years	2-3 mg/day
4-8 years	4-5 mg/ day
9-14 years	7-8 mg/ day
14+ years (female)	8-9 mg/day
14 + years (male)	10-11 mg/ day
Pregnant & Lactating	11-12 mg/day

Adverse drug reactions may be observed if the dose exceeds 50 mg / day, in form of nausea, gastritis, vomiting, abdominal discomfort and diarrhoea. The dosage beyond 150 mg/ day, would cause decreased absorption of iron and copper, the other essential micronutrients. It may also impair the immune system, lipid metabolism and genito-urinary functions.

Zinc formulations preferred for management are as given in Figure 5.

* 50 mg elemental zinc equates 220 mg zinc sulphate
* 50 mg elemental zinc is also equivalent to 50 mg of zinc gluconate

Figure 5. Recommended zinc formulations (Concept – Mani Datt Mehta)

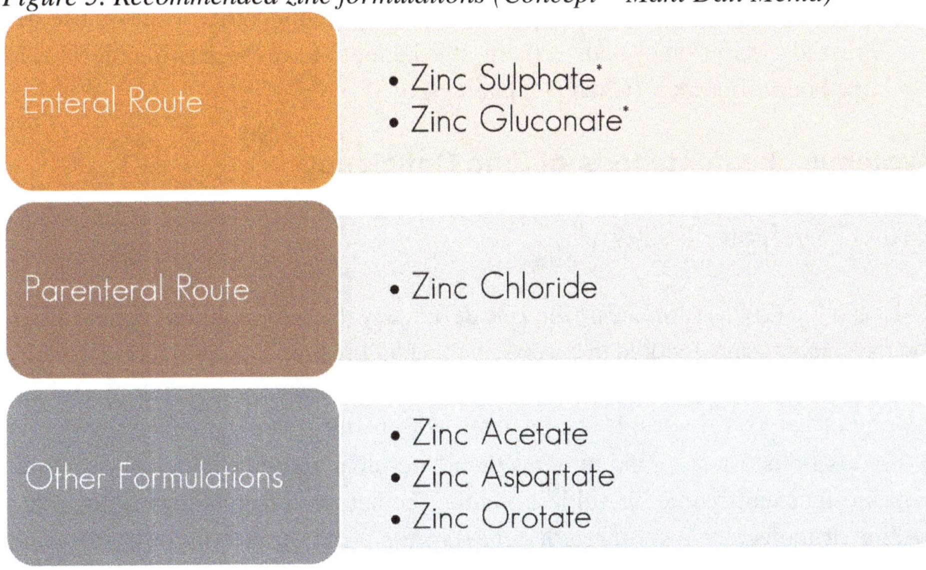
Enteral Route
• Zinc Sulphate*
• Zinc Gluconate*
Parenteral Route
• Zinc Chloride
Other Formulations
• Zinc Acetate
• Zinc Aspartate
• Zinc Orotate

Dose and Duration

Acrodermatitis enteropathica:
Zinc supplement 3mg/ kg/ day of elemental zinc - Life long
Transient zinc deficiency:
3mg /kg/ day of elemental zinc supplement - During breastfeeding only.
Acquired zinc deficiency:
0.5- 1.0 mg /kg/ day elemental zinc - Paediatric age group
15- 30 mg/day elemental zinc - Adult population
* Higher doses are required for malabsorption induced zinc deficiency.

Drug Interactions With Zinc Supplement

(i)Antibiotics of quinolone and tetracycline group if consumed with zinc, interfere with each-other's absorption. Zinc and antibiotic's absorption stand decreased, leading to unfruitful zinc supplementation. The issue can be dealt by spacing the ingestion of the antibiotics either 2 hours prior or 6 hours later. (Donaldson & Decker, 2014)

(ii) Diuretics (chlorthalidone and hydrochlorothiazide) if taken with zinc supplement, increase the urinary excretion of zinc, thereby may lead to serum zinc deficiency. (Suliburska & Skrypnik, 2018)

(iii)Penicillamine and zinc supplement, if ingested together would cause decreased absorption of both of them. It is better to have these two molecules at one hour difference. (Chen & Chuang, 2015)

Systemic Manifestations of Zinc Deficiency

Neuro Psychiatry System

Li and Liu (2023) summed up the zinc deficiency related conditions of neurology and psychiatry. Zinc is stored in cortex, telencephalon, hippocampus and amygdala. Zinc metabolism has definitive basic regulatory mechanism in physiology and pathology of nervous tissues. It is associated with neurogenesis, immune regulation and redox homeostasis. Zinc initiates the anatomical and physiological evolution of brain since embryonic life till last breath. The neuronal metabolism is governed by zinc at molecular level through gene expression via transcription factors and activated enzymes. The neuronal synaptic activity and plasticity is maintained by appropriate amount of zinc at cellular level.

Cerebrovascular Accident (CVA). The ischemic stroke is the second most common killer medical condition after cardiac ailments. Zinc does have potent anti-atherogenic properties because of antioxidant and endothelial stabilizing characters. It was substantiated with zinc supplementation that it induces endothelial repair, promotes endothelial integrity and hence attenuates the progression of CVA along with speeding up the recovery. Therefore, zinc holds a strong preventive role in ischemic stroke. (Munshi & Babu, 2010)

Intracerebral Haemorrhage. Zinc has got important role in the intrinsic pathway of coagulation as it binds with factor XII. Its deficiency leads to prolonged bleeding time. It culminates into impaired coagulation mechanism and faulty fibrin formation.

Therefore, zinc deficiency increases the risk of intracerebral haemorrhage and poor prognosis. (Vu & Fredenburg, 2013)

Alzheimer's Disease. Xie and Wu (2020) reiterated that Alzheimer's disease, a neurodegenerative condition is associated with a change in the expression level of zinc transporters (ZnT and Zrt-/Irt-like protein transporters). This zinc dyshomeostasis has got key role in development of Alzheimer's disease. Xu and Xiao (2019) found that extracellular elevation of zinc levels lead to the deposition of amyloid (Aβ protein) and neurofibrillary tangles, thus initiating the pathogenesis of Alzheimer's disease at molecular level.

Traumatic Brain Injury. Appropriate zinc levels are required to manage the traumatic brain injury as zinc deficiency inhibits the neuronal proliferation and promotes cellular death by activating p53. (Seth & Corniola, 2015). Cope and Morris (2012) proved that zinc supplementation in diet may boost resistance against traumatic brain injury and improve behavioural outcomes like memory and spatial learning.

Epilepsy. Manford (2017) describes epilepsy as chronic and recurrent convulsions because of abnormal, excessive and synchronised neuronal excitation. The elemental zinc happens to be neurotoxic as well as neuroprotective depending upon the serum levels, so may have pro-seizure and anti-convulsant effects (Gower & Levenson, 2012). The clinical data by Seven and Basaran, 2012, suggested that hypozincemia increases the oxidative stress and then frequency of seizures due to inadequate scavenging by glutathione peroxidase and superoxide dismutase; which are zinc dependent free-radical scavengers.

Depression. Takeda (2011) discussed the probable pathogenesis of depression suggesting that zinc deficiency regulates the hypothalamo-pituitary-adrenocortical axis, leading to altered hippocampal functions. The clinical studies substantiated that serum zinc levels and severity of depression are inversely related, even the efficacy of anti-depressants is governed by body's zinc status. (Swardfager & Herrmann, 2013) Zinc deficiency may decrease cognitive function, learning aptitude, memory and emotional stability.

Cardiovascular System

Hara and Yoshigai (2023) have thrown light on essentiality of zinc in maintaining the milieu interior of cardiovascular system. The basic research and various clinical studies have reaffirmed the role of homeostasis of zinc at molecular level through signalling mechanism in cardiac physiology and pathologies. Serum zinc level has deemed value as important biomarker for various cardiovascular disorders. The zinc transporters of slc30a and slc39a have been found to have regulatory and modulatory role in monitoring the cardiovascular functions. These are: ZnT1, ZnT5, Znt7, ZIP7, ZIP2, ZIP8 and ZIP13.

Cardiovascular Diseases Related to Diabetes. In particular the risk of diabetes mellitus type 2 (DM type 2) related cardiovascular diseases (CVD) was found to be significantly decreased in patients with normozincemia. Pompano and Boy (2021) established that long duration and small dose supplementation of zinc showed better outcomes as compared to short duration and large doses in preventing the cardiovascular events related to DM type 2. ZnT8 and metallothioneins are found to have regulatory role in the pathogenesis of DM2 associated CVDs. Choi and Liu (2018) categorically described the essentiality of zinc in various cardiovascular diseases attached with diabetes.

Hypertension and Atherosclerosis. Homeostatic role of zinc has been defined in etiology of arterial hypertension. In arterial hypertension, there is redistribution of zinc in the intracellular. Extracellular compartments and tissues. Korichneva (2006) mentioned the role of zinc in cell oxidant and antioxidant event, maintaining balance between the two. The decrease in zinc levels increases the production of reactive oxygen species (ROS), leading to decreased nitric oxide (NO) by the endothelial cells. The low NO levels provoke atherosclerosis, in turn augmenting the blood pressure.

Myocardial Infarction. Zinc is believed to have cardioprotective role in myocardial ischemia/infarct via preservation of protein kinase C (PKC) isoforms and reperfusion injury salvage kinase (RISK) pathways. The raised zinc quartiles are associated with decreased prevalence rate of MI. (Karagulova & Yue, 2007) Nonetheless, serum zinc has both diagnostic and prognostic relevance in case of myocardial infarction; showing inverse trends with the cardiac biomarkers like CK-MB and cardiac troponin T. (Huang & Teng, 2018)

Atrial Fibrillation. It is commonly encountered in patients who have undergone cardiac surgeries like CABG (coronary artery bypass grafting) and the postoperative low zinc levels are associated with higher chances of developing atrial fibrillation. (Yan & Zou, 2012)

Congestive Heart Failure (CHF). Efeovbokhan and Bhattacharya (2014) could find relation between zinc deficiency and congestive heart failure in children and patients with dilated cardiomyopathy. The disturbed zinc levels lead to oxidative stress and weakened anti-oxidative defense mechanisms which could have attenuated the progression of CHF. (Kamalov & Holewinski, 2009)

Respiratory System

Luan and Ding (2023) comprehended role of zinc status and respiratory diseases in human beings. Various mechanisms involved in the pathogenesis of respiratory conditions are dependant on properties of zinc as antioxidant, anti-inflammatory, immunomodulator, antiviral etc. It also exerts inhibitory effect on malignant cells and regulates the lipid metabolism.

Covid Pneumonia. The covid-19 pandemic of recent past had tragic pathology of SARS-CoV-2 induced pneumonia as the major cause of mortality. Panchariya and Khan, 2021 suggested the role of zinc in inhibiting viral replication by forming a stable Zn^{2+}-Mpro complex. Hypozincemia favours the release of pro-inflammatory cytokines in serum, i.e. TNF-α, IL-6,7,8 and CRP; promoting severe lung damage. (Conti & Ronconi, 2020). Moreover, it was associated with increased chances of complications, longer stays at the hospital and greater risk of mortality. On the same lines, an eligible vaccine candidate for covid infections is Zn-chitosan; though trials are going on.

Chronic Obstructive Pulmonary Disease (COPD). Anti-inflammatory and anti-oxidant impact of micronutrient zinc help to improve the clinical status of COPD patients by delaying its progression. Cadmium containing cigarette smoke induces oxidative stress, lung inflammation and emphysema in COPD; which can be countered by zinc due to its competitive binding with ZIP8 which is known to reduce the toxic effects of cadmium on lung epithelial cells (Tanwar & Zhang, 2019). Yao and Ren (2021) focused on the role of zinc in activating the mitochondrial autophagy pathways; thus protecting the bronchial epithelial cells in patients with COPD caused by environmental pollutants.

Bronchial Asthma. Zinc has an action of inhibiting the proliferation and differentiation of CD4+ cells into Th1 and Th2 cells; which play an important role in the pathogenesis of allergic asthma. Zinc supplementation inhibits the NF-kB regulated inflammatory cascade, thus reducing hyperresponsiveness of the airways and decreasing the serum IgE levels. (Morgan & Ledford, 2011). Thirdly, ZIP1 and ZIP2, zinc transporters on the alveolar macrophages promote the clearance of inflammatory mediators of bronchial asthma, thereby curbing the inflammatory reactions.

Non-Small Cell Lung Cancer (NSCLC). Zinc supplementation has got key role in inhibiting the progression and invasion of NSCLC. Zinc along with Cupric oxide nanoparticles suppress the tumour growth via the ROS dependent NF-kB pathway. (Xu & Yuan, 2019). Zinc can be used as an adjuvant with various chemotherapeutic agents to enhance their efficacy as anti-tumour drugs.

Gastrointestinal System

Zinc enhances the epithelial barrier of gastrointestinal mucosa, making it therapeutically a significant molecule in GI diseases. (Sonja & Katherine, 2014)

Primary causes of zinc deficiency

- Zinc deficient diet
- Diet rich in phytates
- Malabsorption syndromes
- Excessive use of Proton pump inhibitors

Consequences of epithelial barrier dysfunction

- Diarrhoea
- Food allergies
- Inflammatory Bowel Disease
- Celiac Sprue
- GI cancers

Renal System

Tokuyama and Kanda (2021) established that adequate serum zinc levels are required to protect the renal anatomy and physiology. Zinc supplementation to compensate for the hemodialysis induced hypozincemia can attenuate the glomerular and tubulointerstitial damage, thus it helps in arresting the progression of ESRD (end stage renal disease).

Fukushima and Horike (2009) proposed that improvement in serum zinc levels remediates the response to erythropoietin therapy in CKD patients. It also decreases microalbuminuria associated with Type 2 Diabetes Mellitus. Therefore, enhancing the serum zinc levels prevents the deterioration of renal disorders. (Parham & Amini, 2008)

Endocrine System

Baltaci and Mogulkoc (2019) summarized the role of zinc in augmentation of growth hormone synthesis, maintenance of thyroid hormone levels and regulation of insulin secretion by pancreas. Hence, zinc deficiency may play a role in growth retardation, thyroid dysfunction and impaired glucose metabolism.

Reproductive System

In Males. Adequate levels of zinc has shown to improve the sperm function by enhancing the sperm motility and capacitation to fertilize the oocyte; which is supported by the evidence of higher levels of zinc in fertile groups as compared to the infertile men. Zinc deficiency is linked with decreased testicular volume and failure of spermatogenesis. Nevertheless, the supplementation of zinc has been proven to improve the results of in-vitro assisted reproductive techniques. (Allouche-Fitoussi & Breitbart, 2020)

In Females. Nasiadek and Stragierowicz (2020) suggested that zinc supplementation improves the features of PCOS (polycystic ovarian syndrome) especially in patients with associated insulin resistance and dyslipidemia. It is also proved to be beneficial in alleviating the intensity of pain in primary dysmenorrhoea.

ACKNOWLEDGEMENT

Miss. Mani Datt Mehta (MBBS, final year student, SKGMC, Sikar, Rajasthan University of Health Sciences, Jaipur, India)

REFERENCES

Abdel Fattah, N. S., Atef, M. M., & Al-Qaradaghi, S. M. (2016). Evaluation of serum zinc level in patients with newly diagnosed and resistant alopecia areata. *International Journal of Dermatology*, *55*(1), 24–29. DOI: 10.1111/ijd.12769 PMID: 26147750

Allouche-Fitoussi, D., & Breitbart, H. (2020). The role of zinc in male fertility. *International Journal of Molecular Sciences*, *21*(20), 7796. DOI: 10.3390/ijms21207796 PMID: 33096823

Aydemir, T. B., Liuzzi, J. P., McClellan, S., & Cousins, R. J. (2009). Zinc transporter ZIP8 (SLC39A8) and zinc influence IFN-γ expression in activated human T cells. *Journal of Leukocyte Biology*, *86*(2), 337–348. DOI: 10.1189/jlb.1208759 PMID: 19401385

Baltaci, A. K., Mogulkoc, R., & Baltaci, S. B. (2019). Review: The role of zinc in the endocrine system. *Pakistan Journal of Pharmaceutical Sciences*, *32*(1), 231–239. PMID: 30772815

Bhat, Y. J., Manzoor, S., Khan, A. R., & Qayoom, S. (2009). Trace element levels in alopecia areata. *Indian Journal of Dermatology, Venereology and Leprology*, *75*(1), 29–31. DOI: 10.4103/0378-6323.45216 PMID: 19172027

Chen, J. C., Chuang, C. H., Wang, J. D., & Wang, C. W. (2015). Combination therapy using chelating agent and zinc for Wilson's disease. *Journal of Medical and Biological Engineering*, *35*(6), 697–708. DOI: 10.1007/s40846-015-0087-7 PMID: 26692828

Choi, S., Liu, X., & Pan, Z. (2018). Zinc deficiency and cellular oxidative stress: Prognostic implications in cardiovascular diseases. *Acta Pharmacologica Sinica*, *39*(7), 1120–1132. DOI: 10.1038/aps.2018.25 PMID: 29926844

Conti, P. R. O. N. C. O. N. I., Ronconi, G., Caraffa, A. L., Gallenga, C. E., Ross, R., Frydas, I., & Kritas, S. K. (2020). Induction of pro-inflammatory cytokines (IL-1 and IL-6) and lung inflammation by Coronavirus-19 (COVI-19 or SARS-CoV-2): Anti-inflammatory strategies. *Journal of Biological Regulators and Homeostatic Agents*, *34*(2), 327–331.

Cope, E. C., Morris, D. R., Scrimgeour, A. G., & Levenson, C. W. (2012). Use of zinc as a treatment for traumatic brain injury in the rat: Effects on cognitive and behavioral outcomes. *Neurorehabilitation and Neural Repair*, *26*(7), 907–913. DOI: 10.1177/1545968311435337 PMID: 22331212

Donaldson, M., & Touger-Decker, R. (2014). Vitamin and mineral supplements: Friend or foe when combined with medications? *The Journal of the American Dental Association*, *145*(11), 1153–1158. DOI: 10.14219/jada.2014.78 PMID: 25359648

Efeovbokhan, N., Bhattacharya, S. K., Ahokas, R. A., Sun, Y., Guntaka, R. V., Gerling, I. C., & Weber, K. T. (2014). Zinc and the prooxidant heart failure phenotype. *Journal of Cardiovascular Pharmacology*, *64*(4), 393–400. DOI: 10.1097/FJC.0000000000000125 PMID: 25291496

Finner, A. M. (2013). Nutrition and hair: Deficiencies and supplements. *Dermatol. Clin.*, *31*(1), 167-172. doi:10:1016/j.det.2012.08.015

Fukuda, T., Civic, N., Furuichi, T., Shimoda, S., Mishima, K., Higashiyama, H., Idaira, Y., Asada, Y., Kitamura, H., Yamasaki, S., Hojyo, S., Nakayama, M., Ohara, O., Koseki, H., Santos, H. G. D., Bonafe, L., Ha-Vinh, R., Zankl, A., Unger, S., & Hirano, T. (2008). The zinc transporter SLC39A13/ZIP13 is required for connective tissue development; it's involvement in BMP/TGF-beta, signalling pathways. *PLoS One*, *3*(11), e3642. DOI: 10.1371/journal.pone.0003642 PMID: 18985159

Fukushima, T., Horike, H., Fujiki, S., Kitada, S., Sasaki, T., & Kashihara, N. (2009). Zinc deficiency anemia and effects of zinc therapy in maintenance hemodialysis patients. *Therapeutic Apheresis and Dialysis*, *13*(3), 213–219. DOI: 10.1111/j.1744-9987.2009.00656.x PMID: 19527468

Giunta, C., Elcioglu, N. H., Albrecht, B., Eich, G., Chambaz, C., Janecke, A. R., Yeowell, H., Weis, M., Eyre, D. R., Kraenzlin, M., & Steinmann, B. (2008). Spondylocheiro dysplastic form of the Ehlers -Danlos syndrome -An autosomal -recessive entity caused by mutation in the zinc transporter gene SLC39A13. *American Journal of Human Genetics*, *82*(6), 1290–1305. DOI: 10.1016/j.ajhg.2008.05.001 PMID: 18513683

Golden, M. H., Jackson, A. A., & Golden, B. E. (1977). Effect of zinc on thymus of recently malnourished children. *Lancet*, *2*(8047), 1057–1059. DOI: 10.1016/S0140-6736(77)91888-8 PMID: 72960

Gonzales, K. A. U., & Fuchs, E. (2017). Skin and it's regenerative powers: An alliance between stem cells and their niche. *Developmental Cell*, *43*(4), 387–401. DOI: 10.1016/j.devcel.2017.10.001 PMID: 29161590

Gower-Winter, S. D., & Levenson, C. W. (2012). Zinc in the central nervous system: From molecules to behavior. *BioFactors (Oxford, England)*, *38*(3), 186–193. DOI: 10.1002/biof.1012 PMID: 22473811

Hara, T., Yoshigai, E., Ohashi, T., & Fukada, T. (2023). Zinc in cardiovascular functions and diseases: Epidemiology and molecular mechanisms for therapeutic development. *International Journal of Molecular Sciences*, *24*(8), 7152. DOI: 10.3390/ijms24087152 PMID: 37108314

Huang, L., Teng, T., Zhao, J., Bian, B., Yao, W., Yu, X., Wang, Z., Xu, Z., & Sun, Y. (2018). The relationship between serum zinc levels, cardiac markers and the risk of acute myocardial infarction by zinc quartiles. *Heart Lung and Circulation*, *27*(1), 66–72. DOI: 10.1016/j.hlc.2017.01.022 PMID: 28408092

Itsumura, N., Inamo, Y., Okazaki, F., Teranishi, F., Narita, H., Kambe, T., & Kodama, H. (2013). Compound heterozygous mutations in SLC30A2/ZnT2 results in low milk zinc concentration. A novel mechanism for zinc deficiency in a breast fed infant. *PLoS One*, *8*(5), e64045. DOI: 10.1371/journal.pone.0064045 PMID: 23741301

Kabu, K., Yamasaki, S., Kamimura, D., Ito, Y., Hasegawa, A., Sato, E., Kitamura, H., Nishida, K., & Hirano, T. (2006). Zinc is required for Fc epsilon RI-mediated mast cell activation. *The Journal of Immunology : Official Journal of the American Association of Immunologists*, *177*(2), 1296–1305. DOI: 10.4049/jimmunol.177.2.1296 PMID: 16818790

Kamalov, G., Holewinski, J. P., Bhattacharya, S. K., Ahokas, R. A., Sun, Y., Gerling, I. C., & Weber, K. T. (2009). Nutrient dyshomeostasis in congestive heart failure. *The American Journal of the Medical Sciences*, *338*(1), 28–33. DOI: 10.1097/MAJ.0b013e3181aaee63 PMID: 19593100

Karagulova, G., Yue, Y., Moreyra, A., Boutjdir, M., & Korichneva, I. (2007). Protective role of intracellular zinc in myocardial ischemia/reperfusion is associated with preservation of protein kinase C isoforms. *The Journal of Pharmacology and Experimental Therapeutics*, *321*(2), 517–525. DOI: 10.1124/jpet.107.119644 PMID: 17322024

Kil, M. S., Kim, C. W., & Kim, S. S. (2013). Analysis of serum zinc and copper concentration in hair loss. *Annals of Dermatology*, *25*(4), 405–409. DOI: 10.5021/ad.2013.25.4.405 PMID: 24371385

Korichneva, I. (2006). Zinc dynamics in the myocardial redox signaling network. *Antioxidants & Redox Signaling*, *8*(9-10), 1707–1721. DOI: 10.1089/ars.2006.8.1707 PMID: 16987023

Krebs, N. F. (2000). Overview of zinc absorption and excretion in the human gastrointestinal tract. *The Journal of Nutrition, 130*(5), 1374S–1377S. DOI: 10.1093/jn/130.5.1374S PMID: 10801946

Lazarczyk, M., Pons, C., Mendoza, J. A., Cassonnet, P., Jacob, Y., & Favre, M. (2008). Regulation of cellular zinc balance as a potential mechanism of EVER- mediated protection against pathogenesis by cutaneous oncogenic human papillomaviruses. *The Journal of Experimental Medicine, 205*(1), 35–42. DOI: 10.1084/jem.20071311 PMID: 18158319

Li, Z., Liu, Y., Wei, R., Yong, V. W., & Xue, M. (2023). The important role of zinc in neurological diseases. *Biomolecules, 13*(1), 28. DOI: 10.3390/biom13010028 PMID: 36671413

Luan, R., Ding, D., Xue, Q., Li, H., Wang, Y., & Yang, J. (2023). Protective role of zinc in the pathogenesis of respiratory diseases. *European Journal of Clinical Nutrition, 77*(4), 427–435. DOI: 10.1038/s41430-022-01191-6 PMID: 35982216

Malavolta, M., Costarelli, L., Giacconi, R., Basso, A., Piacenza, F., Pierpaoli, E., Provinciali, M., Ogo, O. A., & Ford, D. (2017). Changes in Zn homeostasis during long term culture of primary endothelial cells and effects of Zn on endothelial cell senescence. *Experimental Gerontology, 99*, 35–45. DOI: 10.1016/j.exger.2017.09.006 PMID: 28918363

Manford, M. (2017). Recent advances in epilepsy. *Journal of Neurology, 264*(8), 1811–1824. DOI: 10.1007/s00415-017-8394-2 PMID: 28120042

Mohanan, S., Gupta, D., Chandrashekhar, L., Thappa, D. M., & Rajesh, N. G. (2012). Acquired zinc deficiency in an adult female. *Indian Journal of Dermatology, 57*(6), 492–494. DOI: 10.4103/0019-5154.103073 PMID: 23248371

Morel, L. N., Schaefer, S. M., & Hivnor, C. M. (2018). Nutritional diseases. In Bolognia, J. L., Schaffer, J. V., & Cerroni, L. (Eds.), *Dermatology* (4th ed., p. 804). Elsevier.

Morgan, C. I., Ledford, J. R., Zhou, P., & Page, K. (2011). Zinc supplementation alters airway inflammation and airway hyperresponsiveness to a common allergen. *Journal of Inflammation (London, England), 8*(1), 36. DOI: 10.1186/1476-9255-8-36 PMID: 22151973

Munshi, A., Babu, S., Kaul, S., Shafi, G., Rajeshwar, K., Alladi, S., & Jyothy, A. (2010). Depletion of serum zinc in ischemic stroke patients. *Methods and Findings in Experimental and Clinical Pharmacology, 32*(6), 433–436. DOI: 10.1358/mf.2010.32.6.1487084 PMID: 20852753

Nasiadek, M., Stragierowicz, J., Klimczak, M., & Kilanowicz, A. (2020). The role of zinc in selected female reproductive system disorders. *Nutrients, 12*(8), 2464. DOI: 10.3390/nu12082464 PMID: 32824334

Ogawa, Y., Kinoshita, M., Shimada, S., & Kawamura, T. (2018). Zinc and skin disorders. *Nutrients, 10*(2), 199. DOI: 10.3390/nu10020199 PMID: 29439479

Orth, G. (2008). Host defenses against human papillomaviruses: Lessons from epidermodysplasia verruciformis. *Current Topics in Microbiology and Immunology, 321*, 59–83. DOI: 10.1007/978-3-540-75203-5_3 PMID: 18727487

Osmani, S., Smidt, A. C., Phan, C. M., & Johnson, D. W. (2021). Acquired acrodermatitis enteropathica from a ketogenic diet. *JAAD Case Reports, 9*, 75–77. DOI: 10.1016/j.jdcr.2021.01.016 PMID: 33665283

Panchariya, L., Khan, W. A., Kuila, S., Sonkar, K., Sahoo, S., Ghoshal, A., Kumar, A., Verma, D. K., Hasan, A., Khan, M. A., Jain, N., Mohapatra, A. K., Das, S., Thakur, J. K., Maiti, S., Nanda, R. K., Halder, R., Sunil, S., & Arockiasamy, A. (2021). $Zinc^{2+}$ ion inhibits SARS-CoV-2 main protease and viral replication in vitro. *Chemical Communications (Cambridge), 57*(78), 10083–10086. DOI: 10.1039/D1CC03563K PMID: 34514483

Parham, M., Amini, M., Aminorroaya, A., & Heidarian, E. (2008). Effect of zinc supplementation on microalbuminuria in patients with type 2 diabetes: A double blind, randomized, placebo-controlled, cross-over trial. *The Review of Diabetic Studies; RDS, 5*(2), 102–109. DOI: 10.1900/RDS.2008.5.102 PMID: 18795212

Pompano, L. M., & Boy, E. (2021). Effects of dose and duration of zinc interventions on risk factors for Type 2 Diabetes and cardiovascular disease: A systematic review and meta-analysis. *Advances in Nutrition, 12*(1), 141–160. DOI: 10.1093/advances/nmaa087 PMID: 32722790

Prasad, A. S. (2013). Discovery of human zinc deficiency: Its impact on human health and disease. *Advances in Nutrition, 4*(2), 176–190. DOI: 10.3945/an.112.003210 PMID: 23493534

Roohani, N., Hurrell, R., Kelishadi, R., & Schulin, R. (2013). Zinc and its importance in human health: An integrative review. *Journal of Research in Medical Sciences : the Official Journal of Isfahan University of Medical Sciences, 18*(2), 144–157. PMID: 23914218

Roston, E. F., DeBuys, H. V., Madey, D. L., & Pinnell, S. R. (2002). Evidence supporting zinc as an important antioxidant for skin. *International Journal of Dermatology, 41*(9), 606–611. DOI: 10.1046/j.1365-4362.2002.01567.x PMID: 12358835

Rudolf, E., & Rudolf, K. (2017). Increases in Intracellular zinc enhance proliferative signalling as well as mitochondrial and lysosomal activity in human melanocytes. *Cellular Physiology and Biochemistry*, *43*(1), 1–16. DOI: 10.1159/000480306 PMID: 28848213

Schmitt, S., Kury, S., Giraud, M., Dreno, B., Kharfi, M., & Bezieau, S. (2009). An update on mutations of the SLC39A4 gene in acrodermatitis enteropathica. *Human Mutation*, *30*(6), 926–933. DOI: 10.1002/humu.20988 PMID: 19370757

Schwartz, J. R., Marsh, R. G., & Draelos, Z. D. (2005). Zinc and skin health: Overview of physiology and pharmacology. *Dermatologic Surgery*, *31*(7 Pt 2), 837–847. DOI: 10.1111/j.1524-4725.2005.31729 PMID: 16029676

Seth, R., Corniola, R. S., Gower-Winter, S. D., Morgan, T. J.Jr, Bishop, B., & Levenson, C. W. (2015). Zinc deficiency induces apoptosis via mitochondrial p53- and caspase-dependent pathways in human neuronal precursor cells. *Journal of Trace Elements in Medicine and Biology*, *30*, 59–65. DOI: 10.1016/j.jtemb.2014.10.010 PMID: 25467851

Seven, M., Basaran, S. Y., Cengiz, M., Unal, S., & Yuksel, A. (2013). Deficiency of selenium and zinc as a causative factor for idiopathic intractable epilepsy. *Epilepsy Research*, *104*(1-2), 35–39. DOI: 10.1016/j.eplepsyres.2012.09.013 PMID: 23103062

Skrovanek, S., DiGuilio, K., Bailey, R., Huntington, W., Urbas, R., Mayilvaganan, B., Mercogliano, G., & Mullin, J. M. (2014). Zinc and gastrointestinal disease. *World Journal of Gastrointestinal Pathophysiology*, *5*(4), 496–513. DOI: 10.4291/wjgp.v5.i4.496 PMID: 25400994

Suliburska, J., Skrypnik, K., Szulinska, M., Kupsz, J., Markuszewaki, L., & Bogdanski, P. (2018). Diuretics, Ca antagonists and angiotensin converting enzyme inhibitors affect zinc status in hypertensive patients on monotherpy: A randomized trial. *Nutrients*, *10*(9), 1284. DOI: 10.3390/nu10091284 PMID: 30208601

Swardfager, W., Herrmann, N., Mazereeuw, G., Goldberger, K., Harimoto, T., & Lanctôt, K. L. (2013). Zinc in depression: A meta-analysis. *Biological Psychiatry*, *74*(12), 872–878. DOI: 10.1016/j.biopsych.2013.05.008 PMID: 23806573

Tada-Oikawa, S., Ichihara, G., Suzuki, Y., Izuoka, K., Wu, W., Yamada, Y., Mishima, T., & Ichihara, S. (2015). Zn (II) released from zinc oxide nano/micro particles suppresses vasculogenesis in human endothelial colony forming cells. *Toxicology Reports*, *2*, 692–701. DOI: 10.1016/j.toxrep.2015.04.003 PMID: 28962405

Takeda, A. (2011). Zinc signaling in the hippocampus and its relation to pathogenesis of depression. *Molecular Neurobiology*, *44*(2), 166–174. DOI: 10.1007/s12035-010-8158-9 PMID: 21161611

Tanwar, V. S., Zhang, X., Jagannathan, L., Jose, C. C., & Cuddapah, S. (2019). Cadmium exposure upregulates SNAIL through miR-30 repression in human lung epithelial cells. *Toxicology and Applied Pharmacology*, *373*, 1–9. DOI: 10.1016/j.taap.2019.04.011 PMID: 30998937

Tokuyama, A., Kanda, E., Itano, S., Kondo, M., Wada, Y., Kadoya, H., Kidokoro, K., Nagasu, H., Sasaki, T., & Kashihara, N. (2021). Effect of zinc deficiency on chronic kidney disease progression and effect modification by hypoalbuminemia. *PLoS One*, *16*(5), e0251554. DOI: 10.1371/journal.pone.0251554 PMID: 33974681

Troche, C., Aydemir, T. B., & Cousins, R. J. (2016). Zinc transporter Slc39a14 regulates inflammatory signalling associated with hypertrophic adiposity. *American Journal of Physiology. Endocrinology and Metabolism*, *310*(4), E258–E268. DOI: 10.1152/ajpendo.00421.2015 PMID: 26646099

Vannucchi, H., Favaro, R. M., Cunha, D. F., & Marchini, J. S. (1995). Assessment of zinc nutritional status of pellagra patients. *Alcohol and Alcoholism (Oxford, Oxfordshire)*, *30*(3), 297–302. PMID: 7545983

Vu, T. T., Fredenburg, J. C., & Weitz, J. I. (2013). Zinc: An important cofactor in haemostasis and thrombosis. *Thrombosis and Haemostasis*, *109*(3), 421–430. DOI: 10.1160/TH12-07-0465 PMID: 23306381

Wessells, K. R., & Brown, K. H. (2012). Estimating the global prevalence of zinc deficiency: Results based on zinc availability in national food supplies and the prevalence of stunting. *PLoS One*, *7*(11), e50568. DOI: 10.1371/journal.pone.0050568 PMID: 23209782

Xie, Z., Wu, H., & Zhao, J. (2020). Multifunctional roles of zinc in Alzheimer's disease. *Neurotoxicology*, *80*, 112–123. DOI: 10.1016/j.neuro.2020.07.003 PMID: 32717200

Xu, H., Yuan, R., Liu, X., Li, X., Qiao, G., Li, C., Gedanken, A., & Lin, X. (2019). Zn-doped CuO nanocomposites inhibit tumor growth by NF-κB pathway cross-linked autophagy and apoptosis. *Nanomedicine (London)*, *14*(2), 131–149. DOI: 10.2217/nnm-2018-0366 PMID: 30394176

Xu, Y., Xiao, G., Liu, L., & Lang, M. (2019). Zinc transporters in Alzheimer's disease. *Molecular Brain*, *12*(1), 106. DOI: 10.1186/s13041-019-0528-2 PMID: 31818314

Yan, A. C., & Oboite, N. M. (2024). Nutritional disorders affecting the skin. In C. Griffiths, J. Barker, T. Bleiker, W. Hussain & R. Simpson (Eds.), ROOK'S Textbook of Dermatology (10th ed., pp. 61.25-27) John Wiley & Sons Ltd DOI: 10.1002/9781119709268.rook061

Yan, Y. Q., & Zou, L. J. (2012). Relation between zinc, copper, and magnesium concentrations following cardiopulmonary bypass and postoperative atrial fibrillation in patients undergoing coronary artery bypass grafting. *Biological Trace Element Research, 148*(2), 148–153. DOI: 10.1007/s12011-012-9356-2 PMID: 22351155

Yao, R. Q., Ren, C., Xia, Z. F., & Yao, Y. M. (2021). Organelle-specific autophagy in inflammatory diseases: A potential therapeutic target underlying the quality control of multiple organelles. *Autophagy, 17*(2), 385–401. DOI: 10.1080/15548627.2020.1725377 PMID: 32048886

Chapter 3

The Public Health Significance of Human Zinc Deficiency in the Developing World

Suresh Gadapati
https://orcid.org/0009-0005-8227-7728
University of Hyderabad, India

ABSTRACT

Zinc deficiency has long been associated with developing countries, but it is now emerging as a significant public health concern in developed countries. This chapter delves into the underappreciated problem of zinc deficiency, looking at its prevalence, contributing factors, and long-term health consequences in this population. It emphasizes zinc's importance in immune function, growth, and development and its potential role in the emergence of chronic diseases. The chapter examines the dietary habits, medical conditions, and socioeconomic disparities contributing to zinc deficiency in developed countries. It emphasizes the public health implications, such as the significant healthcare burden of zinc deficiency-related conditions. Finally, the chapter proposes a multifaceted strategy to combat this "hidden hunger" and ensure optimal zinc status for all populations.

1. INTRODUCTION

Zinc is a vital micronutrient that has a significant impact on multiple physiological processes in the human body. It has a crucial function in immune responses, repairing DNA, advancing the cell cycle, and mending wounds(Maywald & Rink,

DOI: 10.4018/979-8-3693-5355-4.ch003

2022; Nalyotov et al., 2022). Zinc deficiency, affecting around 17% of the global population, can lead to compromised immune function, making individuals more susceptible to infections, and it varies from region to region(2019; Palacios et al., 2020). Studies have shown that a deficiency in zinc is associated with a range of health issues, including inhibited growth, diminished sexual function, a compromised immune system, and poor cognitive functions.(Chasapis et al., 2020). When consumed in adequate quantities, zinc's anti-inflammatory and antioxidant properties make it a potent preventive and therapeutic agent against infectious illnesses. Approximately 9% of the global population suffers from zinc insufficiency(Myers et al., 2015), and the Global Burden of Disease (GBD) study 2019 (GBD 2020) has identified nearly 2800 deaths associated with this deficiency(Murray et al., 2020). The GBD 2018 and GBD 2020 studies produced divergent estimations about the occurrence of micronutrient deficiencies(Fanzo et al., 2018; Skalny et al., 2021; Stanaway et al., 2018). Hess (2021) has attributed the difference in these findings to the use of different statistical approaches in the two research studies (Hess et al., 2022). The Lancet Nutrition series predicts that in some low- and middle-income countries, up to 50% of children may experience inadequate zinc levels. (Victora et al., 2021).It is crucial to maintain a sufficient consumption of zinc for excellent physical well-being and overall health. This emphasizes the importance of acknowledging and addressing zinc deficiency in order to enhance human health and mitigate the risk of illness.

2. AN EXPLORATION OF ZINC DEFICIENCY: AN UNRECOGNIZED MENACE IN DEVELOPING NATIONS

Zinc, an essential yet frequently disregarded micronutrient, plays a fundamental role in maintaining human health. It acts as a conductor in our body’s functions, exerting influence over a broad spectrum of processes, including immune function and cell division. However, in developing countries, a considerable segment of the population is confronted with a hidden danger: zinc deficiency.

2.1. The Essential Micronutrient

Zinc's Function in the Human Body Zinc exerts a significant and widespread impact on various physiological processes within the human body. Here is a brief overview of some of its primary functionalities:

Zinc functions as a defender in the immune system, assisting in the generation of white blood cells and antibodies that combat infections (Jin et al., 2024). It plays a crucial role in promoting growth and development at all stages of life, from enhancing bone strength to facilitating healthy cell division. This element serves as a co-factor for multiple enzymes, exerting an influence on various processes such as metabolism and wound healing (Chen et al., 2024; Lin et al., 2017). An insufficiency in this vital component disturbs this intricate equilibrium, resulting in a series of health complications (Sangeetha et al., 2022).

2.2. Factors Contributing to Zinc Deficiency: An Intricate Network

The causes of zinc deficiency in developing countries are complex and have multiple facets:

2.3. Dietary Disparity

Although Staple foods like cereals, contain calories, they often lack bioavailable zinc, which is the form that the body can easily absorbed (Lönnerdal, 2000). Dependence on these foods leads to a deficiency in zinc, which has a particularly negative impact on vulnerable groups such as children and pregnant women.

2.3.1.The Role of Phytates in Impeding Absorption

Plant-based diets, commonly consumed in numerous developing nations, frequently include phytates, which have the ability to attach to zinc and impede its assimilation (Bel-Serrat et al., 2014; Sandstead & Freeland-Graves, 2014).

2.3.2. Additional Contributing Factors

Chronic diarrhea, infectious diseases, and poverty can worsen zinc deficiency by increasing the amount of zinc lost or restricting access to a variety of foods that are rich in zinc (Carla Adriana Santos et al., 2017; Imdad et al., 2023).

2.4. Assessing Zinc Deficiency: Revealing the Subtle Menace

Identifying zinc deficiency can pose difficulties. Blood tests may not always provide a reliable indicator, as he body's depleted zinc stores can maintain stable zinc levels in the blood. Nevertheless, certain indications and manifestations, such as protracted wound healing, recurring infections, and impaired growth, can offer valuable insights (King et al., 2016; McDonald et al., 2020).

To address the issue of zinc deficiency in the developing world, it is important to comprehend the underlying causes and the difficulties associated with assessing it. This understanding will enable us to develop and implement effective strategies to combat this widespread public health problem.

3. ZINC DEFICIENCY'S IMPACT ON PUBLIC HEALTH: HINDERING DEVELOPMENT

Zinc deficiency is not simply a deficiency of a single nutrient; it is a covert crisis with extensive repercussions, especially in developing countries. This section examines the profound consequences of zinc deficiency on public health, emphasizing its wide-ranging repercussions on individuals, communities, and entire healthcare systems.

3.1. Impaired Immunity: A Compromise in the Body's Defensive Mechanisms

An alarming consequence of inadequate zinc levels is its detrimental impact on the immune system. Zinc plays a vital role in the synthesis and operation of leukocytes, which are the body's defenders against infections(Colvin et al., 2015; El-Sayed Saad et al., 2018).

Enhanced Vulnerability to Infections: Insufficient zinc levels compromise the immune response, rendering individuals more prone to a broader spectrum of infections, ranging from ordinary colds to diarrhea. Childhood mortality is heightened in developing nations where infectious diseases are already a major concern, due to the additional risk posed by zinc deficiency(Chekol Abebe et al., 2021; Haase & Rink, 2014).

3.2. Stunted Growth and Development: The Impairment of Growth and Development

Insufficient zinc levels significantly impede a child's development. It plays a critical role in cellular division and the synthesis of proteins, both of which are necessary for optimal growth. Children suffering from zinc deficiency frequently encounter physical growth retardation, resulting in stunted growth, diminished stature, and decreased muscle mass (Das et al., 2016; Escobedo-Monge et al., 2021; Islam et al., 2022; Stevens et al., 2022).

Zinc plays a crucial role in the development of the brain, particularly in relation to cognitive function. Inadequacy can result in challenges in acquiring knowledge, issues with remembering information, and hindered mental abilities (Gondal et al., 2021; Hussain et al., 2022; Liu et al., 2019; Mohammadi et al., 2021).

These repercussions not only impact individual well-being but also have a cascading influence on a nation's future labor force and overall progress.

3.3. Maternal and Child Health: A Complex and Potentially Problematic Issue

Pregnant women and their infants are especially susceptible to the adverse effects of zinc deficiency. Pregnancy Complications: Insufficient levels of zinc can heighten the likelihood of experiencing complications during pregnancy, including preeclampsia and preterm birth (Agedew et al., 2022; Berhe et al., 2019; Karimi et al., 2012; Wang et al., 2015).

Zinc plays a vital role in the development of the fetus, particularly in preventing low birth weight and birth defects. Inadequacy can result in infants with low birth weight, making them more vulnerable to health complications throughout their lives. These repercussions establish a harmful pattern, where the well-being of mothers affects the well-being of their offspring, thus perpetuating the burden of zinc deficiency from one generation to the next (Grieger & Clifton, 2014; Sanusi et al., 2021).

3.4. Societal Implications: A Collective Responsibility

Zinc deficiency has wide-ranging effects that extend beyond individual health, negatively affecting entire communities and healthcare systems (Chekol Abebe et al., 2021).In developing countries Overburdened healthcare systems face additional strain from increased illness rates caused by weakened immunity.

3.4.1. Decreased Productivity

Impaired cognitive function and inhibited growth result in a workforce that is less efficient, thus impeding economic progress (Okwuonu et al., 2021). By remedying zinc deficiency, we can enhance both individual well-being and pave the way for a more prosperous future for entire communities in the developing world.

4. STRATEGIES FOR DEALING WITH ZINC DEFICIENCY: PROVIDING INSIGHT INTO A PATH FORWARD

In order to address zinc deficiency in developing nations, it is crucial to implement a comprehensive approach that prioritizes enhancing dietary intake and tackling underlying causes. This section explores effective strategies to illuminate a path towards a future free from this invisible threat.

4.1. Diversifying the Range of Consumed Foods: Reevaluating Staple Food Items

4.1.1. Promoting Zinc-Rich Options

Promoting the cultivation and consumption of zinc-rich foods, such as legumes (beans, lentils), nuts, and animal products (meat, eggs), can significantly increase the zinc content in one's diet(Alcorta et al., 2021; Cakmak et al., 2017; Rehman et al., 2018).

4.1.2. Bioavailability Enhancers

Spreading information to communities about food preparation techniques that enhance the absorption of zinc, such as soaking legumes and consuming dairy products with plant-based meals, can further improve dietary strategies(Chardigny & Walrand, 2016; García-Maldonado et al., 2019; Subhasri et al., 2022).

4.2. Strengthening and Enhancing: Targeted Approaches

4.2.1. Fortifying Staple Foods

Enriching staple foods like flour with zinc can significantly increase consumption among entire populations. This approach is highly cost-effective and has the capacity to exert a substantial impact over a wide geographical region(Blanco-Rojo & Vaquero, 2019; Shah et al., 2016; Shubham et al., 2020).

Specific supplementation programs can be put in place to target the particular requirements of high-risk populations, including pregnant women, young children, and individuals with chronic illnesses, in order to guarantee adequate zinc levels(Alshaikh et al., 2022; Oh et al., 2020; Wegmüller et al., 2014).

4.3. Biofortification: A Vision for the Future

Developing crops with increased bioavailable zinc levels through selective breeding programs offers a practical and long-lasting solution for enhancing zinc content. This approach ensures a consistent zinc supply without relying on external fortification(Bashir et al., 2023; Praharaj et al., 2021).

4.4. Addressing Fundamental Causes: Disrupting the Recurring Pattern

In order to successfully combat zinc deficiency, it is imperative to address the root causes that contribute to its occurrence. Improving sanitation and hygiene practices can effectively reduce the occurrence of diarrhea and other communicable diseases, leading to a decrease in zinc depletion(Lindenmayer et al., 2014).

4.4.1. Combating Poverty

Insufficient financial resources often limit the ability to obtain a diverse range of zinc-rich foods. Investing in poverty alleviation initiatives can result in a domino effect, ultimately leading to improved dietary decision-making(Ahsan et al., 2021; Pinzón-Rondón et al., 2019).

4.5. Collaboration and education: An integrated strategy

Successful execution requires the collaboration of governments, healthcare professionals, agricultural experts, and communities. Ensuring long-term success largely depends on educational programs that foster awareness about zinc deficiency, its repercussions, and the benefits of maintaining a well-balanced diet. By implementing zinc supplementation strategies(Winichagoon, 2008; World Health Organization, 2006), we can establish a future where the adverse effects of zinc deficiency on the health and development of millions in the developing world are eradicated. The success of this fight depends on the necessity of having a unified position, however, the potential advantages - a stronger future for future generations - validate the significance of achieving victory in this conflict.

5. CONCLUSION

Zinc deficiency, a seemingly uncomplicated nutritional issue, emerges as a noteworthy public health problem in developing nations. The repercussions of this situation are apparent through a compromised immune system, hindered growth, and increased rates of maternal and child mortality, indicating a distinct and concerning scenario. Nevertheless, amidst these challenging circumstances, there exists an opportunity for progress. By implementing effective strategies such as expanding the variety of foods in our diet, adding essential nutrients to food, providing supplements, enhancing the nutritional content of crops through biofortification, and addressing the underlying causes, we can create a more optimistic path for the future.

We investment in zinc deficiency remedies not only to addressing a single nutrient deficiency; but also, to unlock a healthier future for millions of individuals. Augmented immune systems lead to a decrease in childhood mortality. Increased growth and development lead to a workforce that is more productive and proficient. A plentiful population enables economic advancement and a more robust healthcare system.

In order to address zinc deficiency, it is crucial to form a unified coalition that includes governments, healthcare professionals, agricultural experts, and communities. It is crucial to implement educational programs that enhance individuals' understanding and enable them to make informed choices regarding their dietary habits. By working together, we can eliminate zinc deficiency and ensure that it no longer poses a public health concern. Let us create a path towards a future where zinc symbolizes optimal health and well-being for all individuals.

ACKNOWLEDGEMENT

Suresh Gadapati and Shamanna B R are thankful to the University of Hyderabad, Telangana, for providing resources to complete this chapter.

REFERENCES

Agedew, E., Tsegaye, B., Bante, A., Zerihun, E., Aklilu, A., Girma, M., Kerebih, H., Wale, M. Z., & Yirsaw, M. T. (2022). Zinc deficiency and associated factors among pregnant women's attending antenatal clinics in public health facilities of Konso Zone, Southern Ethiopia. *PLoS One*, *17*(7), e0270971. DOI: 10.1371/journal.pone.0270971 PMID: 35797387

Ahsan, A. K., Tebha, S. S., Sangi, R., Kamran, A., Zaidi, Z. A., Haque, T., & Ali Hamza, M. S. (2021). Zinc Micronutrient Deficiency and Its Prevalence in Malnourished Pediatric Children as Compared to Well-Nourished Children: A Nutritional Emergency. *Global Pediatric Health, 8*, 2333794X2110503. DOI: 10.1177/2333794X211050316

Alcorta, A., Porta, A., Tárrega, A., Alvarez, M. D., & Vaquero, M. P. (2021). Foods for Plant-Based Diets: Challenges and Innovations. *Foods*, *10*(2), 293. DOI: 10.3390/foods10020293 PMID: 33535684

Alshaikh, B., Abo Zeed, M., Yusuf, K., Guin, M., & Fenton, T. (2022). Effect of enteral zinc supplementation on growth and neurodevelopment of preterm infants: A systematic review and meta-analysis. *Journal of Perinatology*, *42*(4), 430–439. DOI: 10.1038/s41372-021-01094-7 PMID: 34006967

Bashir, A., Khan, Q. U., Alem, A., Hendi, A. A., Zaman, U., Khan, S. U., Rehman, K., Khan, A. A., Ullah, I., Anwar, Y., & Abdelrahman, E. A. (2023). Zinc and potassium fertilizer synergizes plant nutrient availability and affects growth, yield, and quality of wheat genotypes. *Plants*, *12*(12), 2241. DOI: 10.3390/plants12122241 PMID: 37375867

Bel-Serrat, S., Stammers, A.-L., Warthon-Medina, M., Moran, V. H., Iglesia-Altaba, I., Hermoso, M., Moreno, L. A., & Lowe, N. M. (2014). Factors that affect zinc bioavailability and losses in adult and elderly populations. *Nutrition Reviews*, *72*(5), 334–352. DOI: 10.1111/nure.12105 PMID: 24739133

Berhe, K., Gebrearegay, F., & Gebremariam, H. (2019). Prevalence and associated factors of zinc deficiency among pregnant women and children in Ethiopia: A systematic review and meta-analysis. *BMC Public Health, 19*(1), 1–11. DOI: 10.1186/s12889-019-7979-3 PMID: 31829213

Blanco-Rojo, R., & Vaquero, M. P. (2019). Iron bioavailability from food fortification to precision nutrition. A review. *Innovative Food Science & Emerging Technologies, 51*, 126–138. DOI: 10.1016/j.ifset.2018.04.015

Cakmak, I., McLaughlin, M. J., & White, P. (2017). Zinc for better crop production and human health. *Plant and Soil, 411*(1–2), 1–4. DOI: 10.1007/s11104-016-3166-9

Chardigny, J.-M., & Walrand, S. (2016). Plant protein for food: Opportunities and bottlenecks. *OCL Oilseeds and Fats Crops and Lipids, 23*(4), 6-p.

Chasapis, C. T., Ntoupa, P.-S. A., Spiliopoulou, C. A., & Stefanidou, M. E. (2020). Recent aspects of the effects of zinc on human health. *Archives of Toxicology, 94*(5), 1443–1460. DOI: 10.1007/s00204-020-02702-9 PMID: 32394086

Chekol Abebe, E., Asmamaw Dejenie, T., Mengie Ayele, T., Dagnew Baye, N., Agegnehu Teshome, A., & Tilahun Muche, Z. (2021). The role of regulatory B cells in health and diseases: A systemic review. *Journal of Inflammation Research, 14*, 75–84. DOI: 10.2147/JIR.S286426 PMID: 33469337

Chen, B., Yu, P., Chan, W. N., Xie, F., Zhang, Y., Liang, L., Leung, K. T., Lo, K. W., Yu, J., Tse, G. M. K., Kang, W., & To, K. F. (2024). Cellular zinc metabolism and zinc signaling: From biological functions to diseases and therapeutic targets. *Signal Transduction and Targeted Therapy, 9*(1), 6. DOI: 10.1038/s41392-023-01679-y PMID: 38169461

Colvin, R. A., Lai, B., Holmes, W. R., & Lee, D. (2015). Understanding metal homeostasis in primary cultured neurons. Studies using single neuron subcellular and quantitative metallomics. *Metallomics, 7*(7), 1111–1123. DOI: 10.1039/c5mt00084j PMID: 25894020

Das, J. K., Achakzai, A. B. K., & Bhutta, Z. A. (2016). Stop stunting: Pakistan perspective on how this could be realized. *Maternal and Child Nutrition, 12*(S1, Suppl 1), 253–256. DOI: 10.1111/mcn.12285 PMID: 27187923

El-Sayed Saad, A. M., El-Gebally, E.-S. I., El-Mashad, G. M., & El-Hefnawy, S. M. (2018). Effect of zinc supplementation on serum zinc and leptin levels in children on regular hemodialysis. *Menoufia Medical Journal, 31*(2), 664–670.

Escobedo-Monge, M. F., Torres-Hinojal, M. C., Barrado, E., Escobedo-Monge, M. A., & Marugán-Miguelsanz, J. M. (2021). Zinc nutritional status in a series of children with chronic diseases: A cross-sectional study. *Nutrients, 13*(4), 1121. DOI: 10.3390/nu13041121 PMID: 33805416

Fanzo, J., Hawkes, C., Udomkesmalee, E., Afshin, A., Allemandi, L., Assery, O., Baker, P., Battersby, J., Bhutta, Z., & Chen, K. (2018). *2018 Global Nutrition Report: Shining a light to spur action on nutrition.* 88149.

García-Maldonado, E., Gallego-Narbón, A., & Vaquero, M. (2019). ¿ Son las dietas vegetarianas nutricionalmente adecuadas? Una revisión de la evidencia científica. *Nutrición Hospitalaria, 36*(4), 950–961. PMID: 31232583

Gondal, A. H., Zafar, A., Zainab, D., Toor, M., Sohail, S., Ameen, S., Ijaz, A. Ch. B., Hussain, I., & Haider, S. (2021). A detailed review study of zinc involvement in animal, plant and human nutrition. *Indian Journal of Pure & Applied Biosciences, 9*(2), 262–271. DOI: 10.18782/2582-2845.8652

Grieger, J. A., & Clifton, V. L. (2014). A review of the impact of dietary intakes in human pregnancy on infant birthweight. *Nutrients, 7*(1), 153–178. DOI: 10.3390/nu7010153 PMID: 25551251

Haase, H., & Rink, L. (2014). Multiple impacts of zinc on immune function. *Metallomics, 6*(7), 1175. DOI: 10.1039/c3mt00353a PMID: 24531756

Hess, S. Y., McLain, A. C., Lescinsky, H., Brown, K. H., Afshin, A., Atkin, R., & Osendarp, S. J. (2022). Basis for changes in the disease burden estimates related to vitamin A and zinc deficiencies in the 2017 and 2019 Global Burden of Disease Studies. *Public Health Nutrition, 25*(8), 2225–2231. DOI: 10.1017/S1368980021004821 PMID: 34889182

Hussain, A., Jiang, W., Wang, X., Shahid, S., Saba, N., Ahmad, M., Dar, A., Masood, S. U., Imran, M., & Mustafa, A. (2022). Mechanistic Impact of Zinc Deficiency in Human Development. *Frontiers in Nutrition, 9*, 717064. DOI: 10.3389/fnut.2022.717064 PMID: 35356730

Imdad, A., Rogner, J., Sherwani, R. N., Sidhu, J., Regan, A., Haykal, M. R., Tsistinas, O., Smith, A., Chan, X. H. S., Mayo-Wilson, E., & Bhutta, Z. A. (2023). Zinc supplementation for preventing mortality, morbidity, and growth failure in children aged 6 months to 12 years. *Cochrane Database of Systematic Reviews, 2023*(3). DOI: 10.1002/14651858.CD009384.pub3

Islam, M. M., Black, R. E., Krebs, N. F., Westcott, J., Long, J., Islam, K. M., Peerson, J. M., Sthity, R. A., Khandaker, A. M., Hasan, M., El Arifeen, S., Ahmed, T., King, J. C., & McDonald, C. M. (2022). Different doses, forms, and frequencies of zinc supplementation for the prevention of diarrhea and promotion of linear growth among young Bangladeshi children: A six-arm, randomized, community-based efficacy trial. *The Journal of Nutrition*, *152*(5), 1306–1315. DOI: 10.1093/jn/nxab439 PMID: 35015856

Jin, D., Wei, X., He, Y., Zhong, L., Lu, H., Lan, J., Wei, Y., Liu, Z., & Liu, H. (2024). The nutritional roles of zinc for immune system and COVID-19 patients. *Frontiers in Nutrition*, *11*, 1385591. DOI: 10.3389/fnut.2024.1385591 PMID: 38706559

Karimi, A., Bagheri, S., Nematy, M., & Saeidi, M. (2012). Zinc deficiency in pregnancy and fetal-neonatal outcomes and impact of the supplements on pregnancy outcomes. *Iranian Journal of Neonatology IJN*, *3*(2), 77–83.

King, J. C., Brown, K. H., Gibson, R. S., Krebs, N. F., Lowe, N. M., Siekmann, J. H., & Raiten, D. J. (2016). Biomarkers of Nutrition for Development (BOND)—Zinc review. *The Journal of Nutrition*, *146*(4), 858S–885S. DOI: 10.3945/jn.115.220079 PMID: 26962190

Lin, P.-H., Sermersheim, M., Li, H., Lee, P. H. U., Steinberg, S. M., & Ma, J. (2017). Zinc in Wound Healing Modulation. *Nutrients*, *10*(1), 16. DOI: 10.3390/nu10010016 PMID: 29295546

Lindenmayer, G. W., Stoltzfus, R. J., & Prendergast, A. J. (2014). Interactions between Zinc Deficiency and Environmental Enteropathy in Developing Countries. *Advances in Nutrition*, *5*(1), 1–6. DOI: 10.3945/an.113.004838 PMID: 24425714

Liu, Y., Chen, S., Zühlke, L., Black, G. C., Choy, M., Li, N., & Keavney, B. D. (2019). Global birth prevalence of congenital heart defects 1970–2017: Updated systematic review and meta-analysis of 260 studies. *International Journal of Epidemiology*, *48*(2), 455–463. DOI: 10.1093/ije/dyz009 PMID: 30783674

Maywald, M., & Rink, L. (2022). Zinc in human health and infectious diseases. *Biomolecules*, *12*(12), 1748. DOI: 10.3390/biom12121748 PMID: 36551176

McDonald, C. M., Suchdev, P. S., Krebs, N. F., Hess, S. Y., Wessells, K. R., Ismaily, S., Rahman, S., Wieringa, F. T., Williams, A. M., Brown, K. H., & King, J. C. (2020). Adjusting plasma or serum zinc concentrations for inflammation: Biomarkers Reflecting Inflammation and Nutritional Determinants of Anemia (BRINDA) project. *The American Journal of Clinical Nutrition*, *111*(4), 927–937. DOI: 10.1093/ajcn/nqz304 PMID: 32266402

Mohammadi, H., Talebi, S., Ghavami, A., Rafiei, M., Sharifi, S., Faghihimani, Z., Ranjbar, G., Miraghajani, M., & Askari, G. (2021). Effects of zinc supplementation on inflammatory biomarkers and oxidative stress in adults: A systematic review and meta-analysis of randomized controlled trials. *Journal of Trace Elements in Medicine and Biology*, *68*, 126857. DOI: 10.1016/j.jtemb.2021.126857 PMID: 34560424

MoHFW. UNICEF. (2019). *Comprehensive National Nutrition Survey 2016–2018* [Comprehensive National Nutrition Survey (CNNS)]. Ministry of Health and Family Welfare (MoHFW), Government of India, UNICEF and Population Council. https://www.unicef.org/india/media/2646/file/CNNS-report.pdf

Murray, R. M., Davis, A. L., Shepler, L. J., Moore-Merrell, L., Troup, W. J., Allen, J. A., & Taylor, J. A. (2020). A Systematic Review of Workplace Violence Against Emergency Medical Services Responders. *New Solutions*, *29*(4), 487–503. DOI: 10.1177/1048291119893388 PMID: 31841060

Myers, S. S., Wessells, K. R., Kloog, I., Zanobetti, A., & Schwartz, J. (2015). Effect of increased concentrations of atmospheric carbon dioxide on the global threat of zinc deficiency: A modelling study. *The Lancet. Global Health*, *3*(10), e639–e645. DOI: 10.1016/S2214-109X(15)00093-5 PMID: 26189102

Nalyotov, A. V., Matsynin, A. N., & Matsynina, M. A. (2022). Zinc Availability is an Important Indicator of Human Health. *Health. Food Biotechnology*, *4*(3), 12–18.

Oh, C., Keats, E., & Bhutta, Z. (2020). Vitamin and Mineral Supplementation During Pregnancy on Maternal, Birth, Child Health and Development Outcomes in Low- and Middle-Income Countries: A Systematic Review and Meta-Analysis. *Nutrients*, *12*(2), 491. DOI: 10.3390/nu12020491 PMID: 32075071

Palacios, A. M., Hurley, K. M., De-Ponce, S., Alfonso, V., Tilton, N., Lambden, K. B., Reinhart, G. A., Freeland-Graves, J. H., Villanueva, L. M., & Black, M. M. (2020). Zinc deficiency associated with anaemia among young children in rural Guatemala. *Maternal and Child Nutrition*, *16*(1), e12885. DOI: 10.1111/mcn.12885 PMID: 31595712

Pinzón-Rondón, Á. M., Hoyos-Martínez, A., Parra-Correa, D., Pedraza-Flechas, A. M., & Ruiz-Sternberg, Á. M. (2019). Association of nutritional support programs with zinc deficiency in Colombian children: A cross-sectional study. *BMC Nutrition*, *5*(1), 42. DOI: 10.1186/s40795-019-0305-8 PMID: 32153955

Praharaj, S., Skalicky, M., Maitra, S., Bhadra, P., Shankar, T., Brestic, M., Hejnak, V., Vachova, P., & Hossain, A. (2021). Zinc biofortification in food crops could alleviate the zinc malnutrition in human health. *Molecules (Basel, Switzerland)*, *26*(12), 3509. DOI: 10.3390/molecules26123509 PMID: 34207649

Rehman, A., Farooq, M., Ozturk, L., Asif, M., & Siddique, K. H. M. (2018). Zinc nutrition in wheat-based cropping systems. *Plant and Soil, 422*(1–2), 283–315. DOI: 10.1007/s11104-017-3507-3

Sandstead, H. H., & Freeland-Graves, J. H. (2014). Dietary phytate, zinc and hidden zinc deficiency. *Journal of Trace Elements in Medicine and Biology, 28*(4), 414–417. DOI: 10.1016/j.jtemb.2014.08.011 PMID: 25439135

Sangeetha, V. J., Dutta, S., Moses, J. A., & Anandharamakrishnan, C. (2022). Zinc nutrition and human health: Overview and implications. *eFood, 3*(5), e17. DOI: 10.1002/efd2.17

Santos, C. A., Fonseca, J., Maria, T. M. L., Carolino, E., & Guerreiro, A. S. (2017). Serum zinc evolution in dysphagic patients that underwent endoscopic gastrostomy for long term enteral feeding. *Asia Pacific Journal of Clinical Nutrition, 26*(2). Advance online publication. DOI: 10.6133/apjcn.022016.03 PMID: 28244699

Sanusi, K. O., Ibrahim, K. G., Abubakar, B., Malami, I., Bello, M. B., Imam, M. U., & Abubakar, M. B. (2021). Effect of maternal zinc deficiency on offspring health: The epigenetic impact. *Journal of Trace Elements in Medicine and Biology, 65*, 126731. DOI: 10.1016/j.jtemb.2021.126731 PMID: 33610057

Shah, D., Sachdev, H. S., Gera, T., De-Regil, L. M., & Peña-Rosas, J. P. (2016). Fortification of staple foods with zinc for improving zinc status and other health outcomes in the general population. *Cochrane Database of Systematic Reviews, 2016*(6). DOI: 10.1002/14651858.CD010697.pub2

Shubham, K., Anukiruthika, T., Dutta, S., Kashyap, A., Moses, J. A., & Anandharamakrishnan, C. (2020). Iron deficiency anemia: A comprehensive review on iron absorption, bioavailability and emerging food fortification approaches. *Trends in Food Science & Technology, 99*, 58–75. DOI: 10.1016/j.tifs.2020.02.021

Skalny, A. V., Aschner, M., & Tinkov, A. A. (2021). Zinc. In *Advances in Food and Nutrition Research* (Vol. 96, pp. 251–310). Elsevier., DOI: 10.1016/bs.afnr.2021.01.003

Stanaway, J. D., Afshin, A., Gakidou, E., Lim, S. S., Abate, D., Abate, K. H., Abbafati, C., Abbasi, N., Abbastabar, H., Abd-Allah, F., Abdela, J., Abdelalim, A., Abdollahpour, I., Abdulkader, R. S., Abebe, M., Abebe, Z., Abera, S. F., Abil, O. Z., Abraha, H. N., & Murray, C. J. L. (2018). Global, regional, and national comparative risk assessment of 84 behavioural, environmental and occupational, and metabolic risks or clusters of risks for 195 countries and territories, 1990–2017: A systematic analysis for the Global Burden of Disease Study 2017. *Lancet, 392*(10159), 1923–1994. DOI: 10.1016/S0140-6736(18)32225-6 PMID: 30496105

Stevens, G. A., Beal, T., Mbuya, M. N., Luo, H., Neufeld, L. M., Addo, O. Y., Adu-Afarwuah, S., Alayón, S., Bhutta, Z., Brown, K. H., Jefferds, M. E., Engle-Stone, R., Fawzi, W., Hess, S. Y., Johnston, R., Katz, J., Krasevec, J., McDonald, C. M., Mei, Z., & Young, M. F. (2022). Micronutrient deficiencies among preschool-aged children and women of reproductive age worldwide: A pooled analysis of individual-level data from population-representative surveys. *The Lancet. Global Health*, *10*(11), e1590–e1599. DOI: 10.1016/S2214-109X(22)00367-9 PMID: 36240826

Subhasri, D., Dutta, S., Leena, M. M., Moses, J., & Anandharamakrishnan, C. (2022). Gastronomy: An extended platform for customized nutrition. *Future Foods : a Dedicated Journal for Sustainability in Food Science*, *5*, 100147. DOI: 10.1016/j.fufo.2022.100147

Victora, C. G., Christian, P., Vidaletti, L. P., Gatica-Domínguez, G., Menon, P., & Black, R. E. (2021). Revisiting maternal and child undernutrition in low-income and middle-income countries: Variable progress towards an unfinished agenda. *Lancet*, *397*(10282), 1388–1399. DOI: 10.1016/S0140-6736(21)00394-9 PMID: 33691094

Wang, H., Hu, Y.-F., Hao, J.-H., Chen, Y.-H., Su, P.-Y., Wang, Y., Yu, Z., Fu, L., Xu, Y.-Y., Zhang, C., Tao, F.-B., & Xu, D.-X. (2015). Maternal zinc deficiency during pregnancy elevates the risks of fetal growth restriction: A population-based birth cohort study. *Scientific Reports*, *5*(1), 11262. DOI: 10.1038/srep11262 PMID: 26053136

Wegmüller, R., Tay, F., Zeder, C., Brnić, M., & Hurrell, R. F. (2014). Zinc absorption by young adults from supplemental zinc citrate is comparable with that from zinc gluconate and higher than from zinc oxide. *The Journal of Nutrition*, *144*(2), 132–136. DOI: 10.3945/jn.113.181487 PMID: 24259556

Winichagoon, P. (2008). Coexistence of micronutrient malnutrition: Implication for nutrition policy and programs in Asia. *Asia Pacific Journal of Clinical Nutrition*, •••, 17. PMID: 18296375

World Health Organization. (2006). *The international pharmacopoeia* (Vol. 1). World Health Organization.

Chapter 4
Global Health Burden of Zinc Deficiency

Suresh Gadapati
https://orcid.org/0009-0005-8227-7728
University of Hyderabad, India

ABSTRACT

Zinc deficiency has long been associated with developing countries, but it is now emerging as a significant public health concern in developed countries. This chapter delves into the underappreciated problem of zinc deficiency, looking at its prevalence, contributing factors, and long-term health consequences in this population. It emphasizes zinc importance in immune function, growth, and development and its potential role in the emergence of chronic diseases. The chapter examines the dietary habits, medical conditions, and socioeconomic disparities contributing to zinc deficiency in developed countries. It emphasizes the public health implications, such as the significant healthcare burden of zinc deficiency-related conditions. Finally, the chapter proposes a multifaceted strategy to combat this hidden hunger and ensure optimal zinc status for all populations.

1. INTRODUCTION

Zinc is a crucial trace element indispensable for various physiological functions important for human health. It participates in cellular metabolism, immunological function, reproductive health, and the regulation of several biochemical pathways. Zinc insufficiency constitutes a major public health issue(Gupta et al., 2020; Mehata et al., 2021), particularly in developing countries, impacting around 15% global population (Latin America, Africa and Asia)and resulting in heightened morbidity and death(Hussain et al., 2022a), especially among vulnerable groups. The symptoms

DOI: 10.4018/979-8-3693-5355-4.ch004

of zinc insufficiency are nonspecific, influenced by age, duration, and the existence of other underlying conditions. In children from low- and middle-income countries (LMICs), it markedly impedes growth, leading to stunting in both seemingly healthy and underprivileged youngsters. Severe zinc deficiency heightens the risk of various childhood morbidities and results in cognitive impairment, recurrent infections, diarrhoea, and delayed wound healing. In adolescents and adults, substantial zinc deficiency adversely affects reproduction.

1.1. The Crucial Roles of Zinc in Human Health

Zinc's Function in the Human Body Zinc exerts a significant and widespread impact on various physiological processes within the human body. Here is a brief overview of some of its primary functionalities: Zinc functions as a defender in the immune system(Read et al., 2019), assisting in the generation of white blood cells and antibodies that combat infections (Jin et al., 2024). It plays a crucial role in promoting growth and development at all stages of life, from enhancing bone strength to facilitating healthy cell division. This element serves as a co-factor for multiple enzymes, exerting an influence on various processes such as metabolism and wound healing (Chen et al., 2024; Lin et al., 2017). An insufficiency in this vital component disturbs this intricate equilibrium, resulting in a series of health complications (Sangeetha et al., 2022).

1.2. Global Health burden of Zinc Deficiency

Zinc insufficiency is fundamental to all three interrelated forms of malnutrition: undernutrition, micronutrient deficiencies, and overweight, obesity, and diet-related non communicable illnesses, frequently coexisting with other micronutrient deficiencies(Arndt et al., 2024; Unicef, 2019). Zinc deficiency, can lead to compromised immune function, making individuals more susceptible to infections, and it varies from region to region(2019; Palacios et al., 2020; Wessells et al., 2024). Studies have shown that a deficiency in zinc is associated with a range of health issues, including inhibited growth, diminished sexual function, a compromised immune system(Yu et al., 2021), and poor cognitive functions.(Chasapis et al., 2020).

Addressing zinc deficiency is crucial for improving health outcomes and reducing the global health burden.(Ciampo & Ciampo, 2024; Kiouri et al., 2023; Marín de Jesús et al., 2024; Maywald & Rink, 2022a; Nalyotov et al., 2022). When consumed in adequate quantities, zinc's anti-inflammatory and antioxidant properties make it a potent preventive and therapeutic agent against infectious illnesses. (Murray et al., 2020). (Fanzo et al., 2018; Skalny et al., 2021; Stanaway et al., 2018). Hess (2021) has attributed the difference in these findings to the use of different statistical approaches in the two research studies (Hess et al., 2022). The Lancet Nutrition series predicts that in some low- and middle-income countries, up to 50% of children may experience inadequate zinc levels. (Victora et al., 2021).It is crucial to maintain a sufficient consumption of zinc for excellent physical well-being and overall health. This explore the causes, effects, and strategies related to zinc deficiency in developing countries, and to propose evidence-based approaches to enhance public health.

2. AN EXPLORATION OF ZINC DEFICIENCY: AN UNRECOGNIZED MENACE IN DEVELOPING NATIONS

2.1 Trends and Disparities in Zinc Deficiency in Developing Nations

Zinc deficiency, a significant and often overlooked public health issue, is a considerable challenge, particularly in underdeveloped countries. Worldwide, around 17% of the population is at danger of insufficient zinc intake; however, the actual prevalence of deficiency, especially in specific regions, presents a considerably more concerning situation. This essay analyses the trends of zinc deficiency in emerging nations, highlighting the disparities, contributing factors, and the urgent need for targeted interventions.

Global micronutrient deficiencies, particularly of zinc, persist, with Sub-Saharan Africa demonstrating the highest prevalence(Khan et al., 2022), 51–99% of adults demonstrate inadequate dietary zinc consumption, but approximately 32–63% of children are zinc deficient(Harika et al., 2017). Zinc deficiency (ZnD) in Ethiopia affects approximately 30–51% of children(Berhe et al., 2019), 68% in Zimbabwe(Manzeke-Kangara et al., 2021) whereas a recent national estimate suggests that 72% of the population is impacted by ZnD(Belay et al., 2021). Soil ZnD is widespread, affecting more than 70% of the soils in the Ethiopian highlands(Abdu et al., 2022).

Zinc deficiency, the third most common after iron and vitamin A deficiencies, significantly contributes to diseases including diarrhoea, pneumonia, and malaria, which are major factors in Disability-Adjusted Life Years (DALYs) in the region. It undermines immunological function, affecting iron and vitamin A levels, and is exacerbated by insufficient diets, particular medical conditions, and physiological states such as pregnancy and infancy. In Sub-Saharan Africa, insufficient zinc bioavailability from plant-based diets, coupled with limited access to zinc-rich animal sources, intensifies the problem(Khan et al., 2022).

Zinc deficiency impedes growth for millions of South Asians(Stevens et al., 2022). Bangladesh, India, and Pakistan—South Asia's three most populous nations—face the greatest malnutrition issues. Around 19% to 45% of the population in these three countries lacks zinc. Early stunting, wasting, and malnutrition(Beal et al., 2021). The dense populations, poverty, and plant-based diets of South Asia contribute to vitamin insufficiency. Zinc deficiency impacts children under five years old and pregnant and lactating mothers in India, Pakistan, Bangladesh, Nepal, and Sri Lanka. Research and surveys indicate that numerous of these populations are deficient in zinc.Diarrhoea, aggravated by inadequate sanitation in Bangladesh, depletes zinc, perpetuating malnutrition and sickness. Cereal-based diets with low zinc bioavailability in India and Pakistan result in deficits(Ryckman et al., 2021).

Severe zinc insufficiency is predominantly found in South Asia and Sub-Saharan Africa. In these regions, whose staple diets primarily comprise cereals with poor zinc content and bioavailability, prevalence may reach up to 30%(Skalny et al., 2021). This nutritional shortfall, along with factors like poverty and limited access to diverse dietary options, results in a significant health burden. Zinc deficiency in these areas markedly exacerbates child mortality, amplifying the impact of infectious diseases such as diarrhoea, malaria, and pneumonia(Khan et al., 2022).

Latin America micronutrient deficiencies poorly documented(De La Cruz-Góngora et al., 2024). Sub-Saharan Africa 20–83%(Berhe et al., 2019; Dembedza et al., 2024; Quamme & Iversen, 2022) and Asia, persists in facing a considerable challenge with zinc deficiency, particularly impacting child health and development. This highlights the pervasive character of the issue, extending beyond the most severely affected regions. The ongoing prevalence of child health difficulties, despite decreased rates, signifies that the problem continues to be substantial(Khan et al., 2022).

In contrast, affluent nations like the USA, UK, and Australia In Japan, impacting 46% of men and 38.4% of women(Agedew et al., 2022; Iida et al., 2023), also experience zinc deficiency, though in different forms. This issue mostly affects specific at-risk populations, including women, children, and the elderly, sometimes linked to eating habits that fail to meet zinc requirements. This highlights that while the problem is markedly more acute in developing nations, it persists as a global issue(Ghandilyan et al., 2012; Vreugdenhil et al., 2021).

Research reveals that impoverished nations generally exhibit prevalence rates ranging from 30% to 40%, while low- and middle-income countries (LMICs) frequently report rates exceeding 20% based on plasma zinc concentration data(Skalny et al., 2023). This underscores the significant effect of micronutrient deficiencies, particularly zinc, on the overall disease burden in disadvantaged regions(Gupta et al., 2020; Hall & King, 2022). Country-specific examples, such as Pakistan, where 22.1% of the population(Rehman et al., 2020), mainly women and children under five, are affected, and Ethiopia, where 30.26% of pregnant women demonstrate zinc deficiency, illustrate the severity of the problem(Zhang et al., 2020).

Moreover, demographic-specific data provides a more nuanced understanding of the circumstances. In Ethiopia, a concerning 72% of the population exhibits zinc deficiency, highlighting the imperative for targeted interventions to address spatial inequities. An extensive evaluation of research in Ethiopia revealed a cumulative prevalence of 59.9% among pregnant women and 38%(Berhe et al., 2019) among children(Belay et al., 2021; Skalny et al., 2023).

The 2019 Comprehensive National Nutrition Survey of Children (CNNSC) in India revealed that 19% of preschoolers and 32% of adolescents exhibited zinc deficiency(UNICEF, 2019). Furthermore, tribal adolescents in central India demonstrate very high rates of dietary zinc deficiency and diminished serum zinc concentrations, severely impacting their general health. The countrywide prevalence of low SZC was 31.1% among teenagers, 15.8% among school-aged children, and 17.4% among preschool children. The state-level prevalence estimates ranged from 2.4% in Mizoram to 38.8% in Himachal Pradesh(Kotnis et al., 2022; Pullakhandam et al., 2021).

In central India, tribal adolescents exhibit a significant incidence of dietary zinc deficiency (42.6% to 64.8%) and diminished serum zinc concentrations (34.4% to 57.5%), which is associated with stunting in 29% of the population(Shukla et al., 2021).18.6% in women and children Pakistan(Barman et al., 2023)

Zinc, an essential yet frequently disregarded micronutrient, plays a fundamental role in maintaining human health. It acts as a conductor in our body's functions, exerting influence over a broad spectrum of processes, including immune function and cell division. However, in developing countries, a considerable segment of the population is confronted with a hidden danger: zinc deficiency.

2.2. Factors Contributing to Zinc Deficiency: An Intricate Network

Zinc deficiency in developing countries results from a complex interaction of factors, primarily categorized as dietary, environmental, and socio-economic.

Table 1.

Category	Specific Causes	Detailed Explanation
1. Dietary Factors	Inadequate Dietary Intake of Bioavailable Zinc	Limited consumption of animal-derived foods (meat, poultry, and seafood, dairy) due to cost and availability. Reliance on plant-based diets lacking sufficient bioavailable zinc(Bakaloudi et al., 2021; Kondaiah et al., 2019; Wessells et al., 2024).
	Increased Phytate Concentrations in Diets	Phytates in grains, legumes, and nuts chelate zinc, hindering absorption. Staple foods often have high phytate levels(Lu et al., 2023).
	Limited Consumption of Animal Protein	Animal protein enhances zinc absorption. Reduced intake of meat, fish, and dairy decreases bioavailability(Ryckman et al., 2021).
	Food Processing and Preparation	Inconsistent use of traditional methods (fermentation, soaking) that reduce phytates. Inadequate food preparation and storage lead to nutrient loss(Manzoor et al., 2024).
2. Environmental Factors	Soil Zinc Shortage	Soils deficient in zinc, leading to low zinc concentrations in crops. Prevalent in alkaline soils, high rainfall, or intensive agriculture. Directly affects zinc in staple foods(Eckardt et al., 2023; Tessema et al., 2019).
	Water Quality	Contaminated water leads to diarrheal diseases, aggravating zinc deficiency. Poor sanitation and hygiene spread diseases(Li et al., 2021).
3.Socio-Economic Factors	Economic Deprivation	Limited access to nutritious foods, especially zinc-rich sources, due to poverty(Agedew et al., 2022).
	Food Insecurity	Reliance on affordable staple foods with low bioavailable zinc(Lowe et al., 2024).
	Lack of Education and Awareness	Poor dietary choices due to lack of nutrition knowledge. Lack of understanding of food preparation methods to enhance zinc absorption(Khan et al., 2022).
	Infectious Diseases	Recurrent infections (diarrheal, parasitic) increase zinc depletion and reduce absorption, creating a cycle of infection and malnutrition(Kumari et al., 2024).
	Inadequate Sanitation and Hygiene	Promotes the spread of diseases, exacerbating zinc deficiency(Gupta et al., 2020; Lowe et al., 2024).
	Limited Access to Healthcare	Hinders detection and management of zinc deficiency. Limited prenatal care impacts pregnant women and children(Quamme & Iversen, 2022).
	Cultural Practices	Dietary preferences/restrictions limit zinc-rich food consumption. Neonatal feeding practices may negatively impact zinc levels(Gupta et al., 2020).

Biochemical Mechanisms Associated with Zinc Deficiency:

Zinc functions as a cofactor for over 300 enzymes; hence, its deficiency impacts several activities. The primary mechanisms include:

Impaired Protein Synthesis: Zinc is crucial for RNA and DNA synthesis, affecting cellular growth and repair. Deficiency leads to reduced protein synthesis, negatively affecting growth, immune function, and wound healing(Costa et al., 2023).

Oxidative Stress: Zinc is a constituent of superoxide dismutase (SOD), an enzyme antioxidant. A deficit increases oxidative stress, damaging cells and worsening chronic diseases.

Zinc is crucial for the operation of T-cells and B-cells, affecting both innate and adaptive immune responses. A deficit undermines the immune system, increasing susceptibility to infections(Kim & Lee, 2021).

Zinc is essential for the optimal operation of the thymus gland, which is vital for T-cell maturation(Kido et al., 2022).

Impaired Growth and Development: Zinc is essential for cellular division and the efficacy of growth hormones. Deficiency leads to stunted growth, delayed sexual maturation, and impaired cognitive development(Carducci et al., 2021).

Impaired Vitamin A Metabolism: Zinc is crucial for the conversion of retinol to retinal, influencing vision and epithelial integrity. A deficit may lead to night blindness and increased susceptibility to infections(Division of Postharvest Management, ICAR-Central Institute for Sub-tropical Horticulture, Lucknow-226 101, India et al., 2024).

Zinc influences the senses of taste and smell. A deficiency may lead to hypogeusia (reduced taste) and hyposmia (reduced smell)(Younes, 2024).

2.3. Dietary Disparity

Although Staple foods like cereals, contain calories, they often lack bioavailable zinc, which is the form that the body can easily absorbed. Dependence on these foods leads to a deficiency in zinc, which has a particularly negative impact on vulnerable groups such as children and pregnant women(Rawat et al., 2023).

2.3.1. The Role of Phytates in Impeding Absorption

Plant-based diets, commonly consumed in numerous developing nations, frequently include phytates, which have the ability to attach to zinc and impede its assimilation (Bel-Serrat et al., 2014; Sandstead & Freeland-Graves, 2014).

2.3.2. Additional Contributing Factors

Chronic diarrhea, infectious diseases, and poverty can worsen zinc deficiency by increasing the amount of zinc lost or restricting access to a variety of foods that are rich in zinc (Carla Adriana Santos et al., 2017; Imdad et al., 2023).

2.4. Assessing Zinc Deficiency: Revealing the Subtle Menace

Identifying zinc deficiency can pose difficulties. Blood tests may not always provide a reliable indicator, as he body's depleted zinc stores can maintain stable zinc levels in the blood. Nevertheless, certain indications and manifestations, such as protracted wound healing, recurring infections, and impaired growth, can offer valuable insights (King et al., 2016; McDonald et al., 2020).

To address the issue of zinc deficiency in the developing world, it is important to comprehend the underlying causes and the difficulties associated with assessing it. This understanding will enable us to develop and implement effective strategies to combat this widespread public health problem.

3. ZINC DEFICIENCY'S IMPACT ON PUBLIC HEALTH: HINDERING DEVELOPMENT

Zinc deficiency is not simply a deficiency of a single nutrient; it is a covert crisis with extensive repercussions, especially in developing countries. This section examines the profound consequences of zinc deficiency on public health, emphasizing its wide-ranging repercussions on individuals, communities, and entire healthcare systems(Hussain et al., 2022b).

The economic ramifications of zinc scarcity are intricate, extending beyond immediate healthcare costs. Primarily, it exerts significant strain on healthcare systems. Increased susceptibility to infectious diseases due to impaired immunity leads to higher rates of hospitalizations, outpatient visits, and medication expenses. In resource-constrained settings, where healthcare infrastructure is already fragile, this added burden can be crippling. Moreover, zinc deficiency impedes the advancement of human capital(Maywald & Rink, 2022b). Impeded growth and cognitive impairments in children lead to reduced academic performance and lower future earning potential. The reduction in productivity, when summed throughout a population, is a significant obstacle to economic growth. Furthermore, the impact extends to the agricultural sector. Soils lacking zinc lead to diminished crop yields and inferior nutritional quality, thereby impacting food security and farmers' livelihoods. The cyclical relationship between hunger and poverty is perpetuated by zinc deficiency, trapping populations in a cycle of underdevelopment(Amoadu et al., 2024).

Alongside the general economic impacts, certain at-risk populations face heightened vulnerability. Older persons experience age-related physiological changes that increase their susceptibility to zinc deficiency. Reduced gastric acid output, impaired intestinal absorption, and altered zinc metabolism all contribute to this vulnerability. Zinc deficiency in the elderly is associated with impaired immune function, leading to an increased susceptibility to diseases such as pneumonia and influenza. It also results in cognitive decline, prolonged wound healing, and sarcopenia, further compromising their quality of life and exerting pressure on healthcare resources(Norman et al., 2021).

Individuals with chronic illnesses have unique challenges. Diabetes is intricately linked to zinc metabolism. Zinc is crucial for insulin production and glucose regulation. Deficiency may exacerbate insulin resistance, increasing the likelihood of diabetes complications. The absence of zinc in cardiovascular disease significantly increases the risk due to its role in endothelial function and oxidative stress(Ahmad et al., 2024). Inflammatory bowel disease, HIV/AIDS, and chronic kidney disease are associated with zinc malabsorption and increased zinc losses, creating a harmful cycle in which the condition exacerbates the deficiency. Furthermore, the elderly and individuals with chronic illnesses sometimes utilize many medications, which may impede zinc absorption and utilization, thereby aggravating the problem(Tokuyama et al., 2021).

Addressing the economic and physiological consequences of zinc deficiency requires a comprehensive approach. Interventions must transcend basic supplementation efforts to incorporate dietary diversification strategies that promote the consumption of zinc-rich foods. Biofortification, the augmentation of crops to elevate zinc levels, offers a viable long-term remedy. Public health initiatives must focus the improvement of sanitation and hygiene to reduce the incidence of infectious diseases that result in zinc deficiency(Kiran et al., 2022).

Moreover, targeted treatments are crucial for vulnerable populations. The elderly require tailored food guidelines and supplementation strategies that include their unique physiological needs and potential drug interactions. Individuals with chronic illnesses necessitate careful monitoring of zinc levels and customized management options that address their specific conditions. Healthcare practitioners must be trained to recognize the signs and symptoms of zinc deficiency in these populations and to implement appropriate treatments(Norman et al., 2021).

The economic consequences of zinc deficiency represent a hidden barrier to growth, with the needs of vulnerable groups being overlooked. By recognizing the intricate consequences of this deficiency and implementing targeted interventions, we can use the capabilities of individuals and communities, fostering healthier and more prosperous societies. Addressing zinc deficiency goes beyond public health; it represents an investment in human capital, economic advancement, and the well-being of our most vulnerable communities(Płaczek et al., 2022).

3.1. Impaired Immunity: A Compromise in the Body's Defensive Mechanisms

An alarming consequence of inadequate zinc levels is its detrimental impact on the immune system. Zinc plays a vital role in the synthesis and operation of leukocytes, which are the body's defenders against infections(Colvin et al., 2015; El-Sayed Saad et al., 2018).

Enhanced Vulnerability to Infections: Insufficient zinc levels compromise the immune response, rendering individuals more prone to a broader spectrum of infections, ranging from ordinary colds to diarrhea. Childhood mortality is heightened in developing nations where infectious diseases are already a major concern, due to the additional risk posed by zinc deficiency(Chekol Abebe et al., 2021; Haase & Rink, 2014).

3.2. Stunted Growth and Development: The Impairment of Growth and Development

Insufficient zinc levels significantly impede a child's development. It plays a critical role in cellular division and the synthesis of proteins, both of which are necessary for optimal growth. Children suffering from zinc deficiency frequently encounter physical growth retardation, resulting in stunted growth, diminished stature, and decreased muscle mass (Das et al., 2016; Escobedo-Monge et al., 2021; Islam et al., 2022; Stevens et al., 2022).

Zinc plays a crucial role in the development of the brain, particularly in relation to cognitive function. Inadequacy can result in challenges in acquiring knowledge, issues with remembering information, and hindered mental abilities (Gondal et al., 2021; Hussain et al., 2022a; Liu et al., 2019; Mohammadi et al., 2021).

These repercussions not only impact individual well-being but also have a cascading influence on a nation's future labor force and overall progress.

3.3. Maternal and Child Health: A Complex and Potentially Problematic Issue

Pregnant women and their infants are especially susceptible to the adverse effects of zinc deficiency. Pregnancy Complications: Insufficient levels of zinc can heighten the likelihood of experiencing complications during pregnancy, including preeclampsia and preterm birth (Agedew et al., 2022; Berhe et al., 2019; Karimi et al., 2012; Wang et al., 2015).

Zinc plays a vital role in the development of the fetus, particularly in preventing low birth weight and birth defects. Inadequacy can result in infants with low birth weight, making them more vulnerable to health complications throughout their lives. These repercussions establish a harmful pattern, where the well-being of mothers affects the well-being of their offspring, thus perpetuating the burden of zinc deficiency from one generation to the next (Grieger & Clifton, 2014; Sanusi et al., 2021).

3.4. Societal Implications: A Collective Responsibility

Zinc deficiency has wide-ranging effects that extend beyond individual health, negatively affecting entire communities and healthcare systems (Chekol Abebe et al., 2021).In developing countries Overburdened healthcare systems face additional strain from increased illness rates caused by weakened immunity.

3.4.1. Decreased Productivity

Impaired cognitive function and inhibited growth result in a workforce that is less efficient, thus impeding economic progress (Okwuonu et al., 2021). By remedying zinc deficiency, we can enhance both individual well-being and pave the way for a more prosperous future for entire communities in the developing world.

4. STRATEGIES FOR DEALING WITH ZINC DEFICIENCY: PROVIDING INSIGHT INTO A PATH FORWARD

In order to address zinc deficiency in developing nations, it is crucial to implement a comprehensive approach that prioritizes enhancing dietary intake and tackling underlying causes. This section explores effective strategies to illuminate a path towards a future free from this invisible threat.

4.1. Diversifying the Range of Consumed Foods: Reevaluating Staple Food Items

4.1.1. Promoting Zinc-Rich Options

Promoting the cultivation and consumption of zinc-rich foods, such as legumes (beans, lentils), nuts, and animal products (meat, eggs), can significantly increase the zinc content in one's diet(Alcorta et al., 2021; Cakmak et al., 2017; Rehman et al., 2018).

4.1.2. Bioavailability Enhancers

Spreading information to communities about food preparation techniques that enhance the absorption of zinc, such as soaking legumes and consuming dairy products with plant-based meals, can further improve dietary strategies(Chardigny & Walrand, 2016; García-Maldonado et al., 2019; Subhasri et al., 2022).

4.2. Strengthening and Enhancing: Targeted Approaches

4.2.1. Fortifying Staple Foods

Enriching staple foods like flour with zinc can significantly increase consumption among entire populations. This approach is highly cost-effective and has the capacity to exert a substantial impact over a wide geographical region(Blanco-Rojo & Vaquero, 2019; Shah et al., 2016; Shubham et al., 2020).

Specific supplementation programs can be put in place to target the particular requirements of high-risk populations, including pregnant women, young children, and individuals with chronic illnesses, in order to guarantee adequate zinc levels(Alshaikh et al., 2022; Oh et al., 2020; Wegmüller et al., 2014).

4.3. Biofortification: A Vision for the Future

Developing crops with increased bioavailable zinc levels through selective breeding programs offers a practical and long-lasting solution for enhancing zinc content(Philipo et al., 2021). This approach ensures a consistent zinc supply without relying on external fortification(Bashir et al., 2023; Praharaj et al., 2021; Singh et al., 2023). Agronomic biofortification is the application of zinc-enriched fertilizers to crops, significantly increasing the zinc content in grains. This method has shown effective in enhancing nutritional quality and crop yield, thereby offering a sustainable and cost-effective solution for addressing zinc deficiency(Barman et al., 2023; Poudel et al., 2023; Singh et al., 2023).

4.4. Addressing Fundamental Causes: Disrupting the Recurring Pattern

Moreover, integrating biofortification into existing agricultural practices and regulations will enhance its acceptance and effectiveness in addressing global nutritional deficiencies (Bhatt et al., 2020). In order to successfully combat zinc deficiency, it is imperative to address the root causes that contribute to its occurrence. Improving sanitation and hygiene practices can effectively reduce the occurrence of diarrhea and other communicable diseases, leading to a decrease in zinc depletion(Naik et al., 2024).

4.4.1. Combating Poverty

Insufficient financial resources often limit the ability to obtain a diverse range of zinc-rich foods. Investing in poverty alleviation initiatives can result in a domino effect, ultimately leading to improved dietary decision-making(Ahsan et al., 2021; Pinzón-Rondón et al., 2019).

4.5. Collaboration and Education: An Integrated Strategy

Successful execution requires the collaboration of governments, healthcare professionals, agricultural experts, and communities. Ensuring long-term success largely depends on educational programs that foster awareness about zinc deficiency, its repercussions, and the benefits of maintaining a well-balanced diet. By implementing zinc supplementation strategies(Hassan et al., 2012), we can establish a future where the adverse effects of zinc deficiency on the health and development of millions in the developing world are eradicated. The success of this fight depends on the necessity of having a unified position, however, the potential advantages - a stronger future for future generations - validate the significance of achieving victory in this conflict(Khan et al., 2022).

5. CONCLUSION

Zinc deficiency, a seemingly uncomplicated nutritional issue, emerges as a noteworthy public health problem in developing nations. The repercussions of this situation are apparent through a compromised immune system, hindered growth, and increased rates of maternal and child mortality, indicating a distinct and concerning scenario. Nevertheless, amidst these challenging circumstances, there exists an opportunity for progress. By implementing effective strategies such as expanding the variety of foods in our diet, adding essential nutrients to food, providing supplements, enhancing the nutritional content of crops through biofortification, and addressing the underlying causes, we can create a more optimistic path for the future.

We investment in zinc deficiency remedies not only to addressing a single nutrient deficiency; but also, to unlock a healthier future for millions of individuals. Augmented immune systems lead to a decrease in childhood mortality. Increased growth and development lead to a workforce that is more productive and proficient. A plentiful population enables economic advancement and a more robust healthcare system.

In order to address zinc deficiency, it is crucial to form a unified coalition that includes governments, healthcare professionals, agricultural experts, and communities. It is crucial to implement educational programs that enhance individuals' understanding and enable them to make informed choices regarding their dietary habits. By working together, we can eliminate zinc deficiency and ensure that it no longer poses a public health concern. Let us create a path towards a future where zinc symbolizes optimal health and well-being for all individuals.

ACKNOWLEDGEMENT

Suresh Gadapati thankful to the Prof. Shamanna B R for his expertise and University of Hyderabad, Telangana, for providing resources to complete this chapter.

REFERENCES

Abdu, A. O., De Groote, H., Joy, E. J. M., Kumssa, D. B., Broadley, M. R., & Gashu, D. (2022). Zinc agronomic biofortification of staple crops may be a cost-effective strategy to alleviate zinc deficiency in Ethiopia. *Frontiers in Nutrition*, *9*, 1037161. DOI: 10.3389/fnut.2022.1037161 PMID: 36438724

Agedew, E., Tsegaye, B., Bante, A., Zerihun, E., Aklilu, A., Girma, M., Kerebih, H., Wale, M. Z., & Yirsaw, M. T. (2022). Zinc deficiency and associated factors among pregnant women's attending antenatal clinics in public health facilities of Konso Zone, Southern Ethiopia. *PLoS One*, *17*(7), e0270971. DOI: 10.1371/journal.pone.0270971 PMID: 35797387

Ahmad, R., Shaju, R., Atfi, A., & Razzaque, M. S. (2024). Zinc and Diabetes: A Connection between Micronutrient and Metabolism. *Cells*, *13*(16), 1359. DOI: 10.3390/cells13161359 PMID: 39195249

Ahsan, A. K., Tebha, S. S., Sangi, R., Kamran, A., Zaidi, Z. A., Haque, T., & Ali Hamza, M. S. (2021). Zinc Micronutrient Deficiency and Its Prevalence in Malnourished Pediatric Children as Compared to Well-Nourished Children: A Nutritional Emergency. *Global Pediatric Health*, *8*, 2333794X2110503. DOI: 10.1177/2333794X211050316

Alcorta, A., Porta, A., Tárrega, A., Alvarez, M. D., & Vaquero, M. P. (2021). Foods for Plant-Based Diets: Challenges and Innovations. *Foods*, *10*(2), 293. DOI: 10.3390/foods10020293 PMID: 33535684

Alshaikh, B., Abo Zeed, M., Yusuf, K., Guin, M., & Fenton, T. (2022). Effect of enteral zinc supplementation on growth and neurodevelopment of preterm infants: A systematic review and meta-analysis. *Journal of Perinatology*, *42*(4), 430–439. DOI: 10.1038/s41372-021-01094-7 PMID: 34006967

Amoadu, M., Abraham, S. A., Adams, A. K., Akoto-Buabeng, W., Obeng, P., & Hagan, J. E.Jr. (2024). Risk Factors of Malnutrition among In-School Children and Adolescents in Developing Countries: A Scoping Review. *Children (Basel, Switzerland)*, *11*(4), 476. DOI: 10.3390/children11040476 PMID: 38671693

Arndt, M. B., Abate, Y. H., Abbasi-Kangevari, M., Abd ElHafeez, S., Abdelmasseh, M., Abd-Elsalam, S., Abdulah, D. M., Abdulkader, R. S., Abidi, H., Abiodun, O., Aboagye, R. G., Abolhassani, H., Abtew, Y. D., Abu-Gharbieh, E., Abu-Rmeileh, N. M., Acuna, J. M., Adamu, K., Adane, D. E., Addo, I. Y., & Reiner, R. C.Jr. (2024). Global, regional, and national progress towards the 2030 global nutrition targets and forecasts to 2050: A systematic analysis for the Global Burden of Disease Study 2021. *Lancet*, *404*(10471), 2543–2583. DOI: 10.1016/S0140-6736(24)01821-X PMID: 39667386

Bakaloudi, D. R., Halloran, A., Rippin, H. L., Oikonomidou, A. C., Dardavesis, T. I., Williams, J., Wickramasinghe, K., Breda, J., & Chourdakis, M. (2021). Intake and adequacy of the vegan diet. A systematic review of the evidence. *Clinical Nutrition (Edinburgh, Lothian)*, *40*(5), 3503–3521. DOI: 10.1016/j.clnu.2020.11.035 PMID: 33341313

Barman, A., Bera, A., Saha, P., Tiwari, H., Dey, S., Kumar, S., Patel, S., & Meena, D. K. (2023). Agronomic Zn Biofortification of Cereal Crops a Sustainable Way to Ensuring Nutritional Security: A Review. *International Journal of Environment and Climate Change*, *13*(3), 151–168. DOI: 10.9734/ijecc/2023/v13i31693

Bashir, A., Khan, Q. U., Alem, A., Hendi, A. A., Zaman, U., Khan, S. U., Rehman, K., Khan, A. A., Ullah, I., Anwar, Y., & Abdelrahman, E. A. (2023). Zinc and potassium fertilizer synergizes plant nutrient availability and affects growth, yield, and quality of wheat genotypes. *Plants*, *12*(12), 2241. DOI: 10.3390/plants12122241 PMID: 37375867

Beal, T., White, J. M., Arsenault, J. E., Okronipa, H., Hinnouho, G.-M., Murira, Z., Torlesse, H., & Garg, A. (2021). Micronutrient gaps during the complementary feeding period in South Asia: A Comprehensive Nutrient Gap Assessment. *Nutrition Reviews*, *79*(Supplement_1), 26–34. DOI: 10.1093/nutrit/nuaa144 PMID: 33693912

Beer, K., Singh, A., Ravi, S. C., Gupta, A. K., Kumar, A., & Sharma, M. M.Division of Postharvest Management. (2024). A comprehensive review on the role of Vitamin A on human health and nutrition. *Journal of Environmental Biology*, *45*(6), 645–653. DOI: 10.22438/jeb/45/6/MRN-5339

Bel-Serrat, S., Stammers, A.-L., Warthon-Medina, M., Moran, V. H., Iglesia-Altaba, I., Hermoso, M., Moreno, L. A., & Lowe, N. M. (2014). Factors that affect zinc bioavailability and losses in adult and elderly populations. *Nutrition Reviews*, *72*(5), 334–352. DOI: 10.1111/nure.12105 PMID: 24739133

Belay, A., Gashu, D., Joy, E. J. M., Lark, R. M., Chagumaira, C., Likoswe, B. H., Zerfu, D., Ander, E. L., Young, S. D., Bailey, E. H., & Broadley, M. R. (2021). Zinc deficiency is highly prevalent and spatially dependent over short distances in Ethiopia. *Scientific Reports*, *11*(1), 6510. DOI: 10.1038/s41598-021-85977-x PMID: 33753836

Berhe, K., Gebrearegay, F., & Gebremariam, H. (2019). Prevalence and associated factors of zinc deficiency among pregnant women and children in Ethiopia: A systematic review and meta-analysis. *BMC Public Health*, *19*(1), 1–11. DOI: 10.1186/s12889-019-7979-3 PMID: 31829213

Blanco-Rojo, R., & Vaquero, M. P. (2019). Iron bioavailability from food fortification to precision nutrition. A review. *Innovative Food Science & Emerging Technologies*, *51*, 126–138. DOI: 10.1016/j.ifset.2018.04.015

Carducci, B., Keats, E. C., & Bhutta, Z. A. (2021). Zinc supplementation for improving pregnancy and infant outcome. *Cochrane Database of Systematic Reviews*, 3. PMID: 33724446

Chasapis, C. T., Ntoupa, P.-S. A., Spiliopoulou, C. A., & Stefanidou, M. E. (2020). Recent aspects of the effects of zinc on human health. *Archives of Toxicology*, *94*(5), 1443–1460. DOI: 10.1007/s00204-020-02702-9 PMID: 32394086

Chekol Abebe, E., Asmamaw Dejenie, T., Mengie Ayele, T., Dagnew Baye, N., Agegnehu Teshome, A., & Tilahun Muche, Z. (2021). The role of regulatory B cells in health and diseases: A systemic review. *Journal of Inflammation Research*, *14*, 75–84. DOI: 10.2147/JIR.S286426 PMID: 33469337

Ciampo, L. A. D., & Ciampo, I. R. L. D. (2024). Zinc: A Critical Micronutrient for Children's Health. *Archives of Current Research International*, *24*(10), 251–256. DOI: 10.9734/acri/2024/v24i10928

Costa, M. I., Sarmento-Ribeiro, A. B., & Gonçalves, A. C. (2023). Zinc: From Biological Functions to Therapeutic Potential. *International Journal of Molecular Sciences*, *24*(5), 4822. DOI: 10.3390/ijms24054822 PMID: 36902254

De La Cruz-Góngora, V., Palazuelos-González, R., & Domínguez-Flores, O. (2024). Micronutrient Deficiencies in Older Adults in Latin America: A Narrative Review. *Food and Nutrition Bulletin*, *45*(2, suppl), S26–S38. DOI: 10.1177/03795721231214587 PMID: 38146136

Dembedza, M. P., Chopera, P., & Matsungo, T. M. (2024). Risk of zinc deficiency among children aged 0–59 months in sub-Saharan Africa: A narrative review. *The South African Journal of Clinical Nutrition : SAJCN : the Official Journal of the South African Society of Parenteral and Enteral Nutrition and the Association for Dietetics in South Africa*, *37*(2), 69–76. DOI: 10.1080/16070658.2023.2275932

Eckardt, N. A., Ainsworth, E. A., Bahuguna, R. N., Broadley, M. R., Busch, W., Carpita, N. C., Castrillo, G., Chory, J., DeHaan, L. R., Duarte, C. M., Henry, A., Jagadish, S. V. K., Langdale, J. A., Leakey, A. D. B., Liao, J. C., Lu, K.-J., McCann, M. C., McKay, J. K., Odeny, D. A., & Zhang, X. (2023). Climate change challenges, plant science solutions. *The Plant Cell*, *35*(1), 24–66. DOI: 10.1093/plcell/koac303 PMID: 36222573

El-Sayed Saad, A. M., El-Gebally, E.-S. I., El-Mashad, G. M., & El-Hefnawy, S. M. (2018). Effect of zinc supplementation on serum zinc and leptin levels in children on regular hemodialysis. *Menoufia Medical Journal*, *31*(2), 664–670.

Escobedo-Monge, M. F., Torres-Hinojal, M. C., Barrado, E., Escobedo-Monge, M. A., & Marugán-Miguelsanz, J. M. (2021). Zinc nutritional status in a series of children with chronic diseases: A cross-sectional study. *Nutrients*, *13*(4), 1121. DOI: 10.3390/nu13041121 PMID: 33805416

Fanzo, J., Hawkes, C., Udomkesmalee, E., Afshin, A., Allemandi, L., Assery, O., Baker, P., Battersby, J., Bhutta, Z., & Chen, K. (2018). *2018 Global Nutrition Report: Shining a light to spur action on nutrition*. 88149.

García-Maldonado, E., Gallego-Narbón, A., & Vaquero, M. (2019). ¿ Son las dietas vegetarianas nutricionalmente adecuadas? Una revisión de la evidencia científica. *Nutrición Hospitalaria*, *36*(4), 950–961. PMID: 31232583

Gondal, A. H., Zafar, A., Zainab, D., Toor, M., Sohail, S., Ameen, S., Ijaz, A. Ch. B., Hussain, I., & Haider, S. (2021). A detailed review study of zinc involvement in animal, plant and human nutrition. *Indian Journal of Pure & Applied Biosciences*, *9*(2), 262–271. DOI: 10.18782/2582-2845.8652

Gupta, S., Brazier, A. K. M., & Lowe, N. M. (2020). Zinc deficiency in low- and middle-income countries: Prevalence and approaches for mitigation. *Journal of Human Nutrition and Dietetics*, *33*(5), 624–643. DOI: 10.1111/jhn.12791 PMID: 32627912

Hall, A. G., & King, J. C. (2022). Zinc fortification: Current trends and strategies. *Nutrients*, *14*(19), 3895. DOI: 10.3390/nu14193895 PMID: 36235548

Hess, S. Y., McLain, A. C., Lescinsky, H., Brown, K. H., Afshin, A., Atkin, R., & Osendarp, S. J. (2022). Basis for changes in the disease burden estimates related to vitamin A and zinc deficiencies in the 2017 and 2019 Global Burden of Disease Studies. *Public Health Nutrition, 25*(8), 2225–2231. DOI: 10.1017/S1368980021004821 PMID: 34889182

Hussain, A., Jiang, W., Wang, X., Shahid, S., Saba, N., Ahmad, M., Dar, A., Masood, S. U., Imran, M., & Mustafa, A. (2022a). Mechanistic Impact of Zinc Deficiency in Human Development. *Frontiers in Nutrition, 9*, 717064. DOI: 10.3389/fnut.2022.717064 PMID: 35356730

Hussain, A., Jiang, W., Wang, X., Shahid, S., Saba, N., Ahmad, M., Dar, A., Masood, S. U., Imran, M., & Mustafa, A. (2022b). Mechanistic Impact of Zinc Deficiency in Human Development. *Frontiers in Nutrition, 9*, 717064. DOI: 10.3389/fnut.2022.717064 PMID: 35356730

Iida, D., Shigemura, T., Yamamoto, Y., & Murata, Y. (2023). *Prevalence and Predictive Factors of Zinc Deficiency in Orthopaedic Inpatients.* Medicine and Pharmacology. DOI: 10.20944/preprints202312.0416.v1

Imdad, A., Rogner, J., Sherwani, R. N., Sidhu, J., Regan, A., Haykal, M. R., Tsistinas, O., Smith, A., Chan, X. H. S., Mayo-Wilson, E., & Bhutta, Z. A. (2023). Zinc supplementation for preventing mortality, morbidity, and growth failure in children aged 6 months to 12 years. *Cochrane Database of Systematic Reviews, 2023*(3). DOI: 10.1002/14651858.CD009384.pub3

Islam, M. M., Black, R. E., Krebs, N. F., Westcott, J., Long, J., Islam, K. M., Peerson, J. M., Sthity, R. A., Khandaker, A. M., Hasan, M., El Arifeen, S., Ahmed, T., King, J. C., & McDonald, C. M. (2022). Different doses, forms, and frequencies of zinc supplementation for the prevention of diarrhea and promotion of linear growth among young Bangladeshi children: A six-arm, randomized, community-based efficacy trial. *The Journal of Nutrition, 152*(5), 1306–1315. DOI: 10.1093/jn/nxab439 PMID: 35015856

Khan, S. T., Malik, A., Alwarthan, A., & Shaik, M. R. (2022). The enormity of the zinc deficiency problem and available solutions; an overview. *Arabian Journal of Chemistry, 15*(3), 103668. DOI: 10.1016/j.arabjc.2021.103668

Kido, T., Suka, M., & Yanagisawa, H. (2022). Effectiveness of interleukin-4 administration or zinc supplementation in improving zinc deficiency–associated thymic atrophy and fatty degeneration and in normalizing T cell maturation process. *Immunology, 165*(4), 445–459. DOI: 10.1111/imm.13452 PMID: 35138640

Kim, B., & Lee, W.-W. (2021). Regulatory Role of Zinc in Immune Cell Signaling. *Molecules and Cells*, *44*(5), 335–341. DOI: 10.14348/molcells.2021.0061 PMID: 33986184

Kiouri, D. P., Tsoupra, E., Peana, M., Perlepes, S. P., Stefanidou, M. E., & Chasapis, C. T. (2023). Multifunctional role of zinc in human health: An update. *EXCLI Journal*, *22*, 809. PMID: 37780941

Kiran, A., Wakeel, A., Mahmood, K., Mubaraka, R., Hafsa, , & Haefele, S. M. (2022). Biofortification of Staple Crops to Alleviate Human Malnutrition: Contributions and Potential in Developing Countries. *Agronomy (Basel)*, *12*(2), 452. DOI: 10.3390/agronomy12020452

Kondaiah, P., Yaduvanshi, P. S., Sharp, P. A., & Pullakhandam, R. (2019). Iron and zinc homeostasis and interactions: Does enteric zinc excretion cross-talk with intestinal iron absorption? *Nutrients*, *11*(8), 1885. DOI: 10.3390/nu11081885 PMID: 31412634

Kotnis, A., Bhatt, G. C., Joshi, D., Shukla, A. K., Gupta, P., Shah, D., Choudhary, B., Patil, R., Dubey, S. K., Shukla, M., Joshi, A., & Pakhare, A. P. (2022). Assessment of zinc inadequacy among tribal adolescent population of central India-A cross-sectional study. *The Indian Journal of Medical Research*, *156*(2), 339–347. DOI: 10.4103/ijmr.ijmr_3130_21 PMID: 36629194

Kumari, D., Nair, N., & Bedwal, R. (2024). Effects of dietary zinc deficiency and supplementation on prepubertal rat testes: Sulfhydryl and antioxidant status. *Indian Journal of Clinical Biochemistry : IJCB*, *39*(4), 539–547. DOI: 10.1007/s12291-023-01167-8 PMID: 39346712

Lakshmi, V., & Bandi, K. (2024). Zinc Deficiency. In Nayak, A., & Misra, S. (Eds.), *Advances in Medical Diagnosis, Treatment, and Care* (pp. 248–263). IGI Global., DOI: 10.4018/979-8-3693-2947-4.ch014

Li, L., He, Y., Song, K., Xie, F., Li, H., & Sun, F. (2021). Derivation of water quality criteria of zinc to protect aquatic life in Taihu Lake and the associated risk assessment. *Journal of Environmental Management*, *296*, 113175. DOI: 10.1016/j.jenvman.2021.113175 PMID: 34243093

Liu, Y., Chen, S., Zühlke, L., Black, G. C., Choy, M., Li, N., & Keavney, B. D. (2019). Global birth prevalence of congenital heart defects 1970–2017: Updated systematic review and meta-analysis of 260 studies. *International Journal of Epidemiology*, *48*(2), 455–463. DOI: 10.1093/ije/dyz009 PMID: 30783674

Lowe, N. M., Hall, A. G., Broadley, M. R., Foley, J., Boy, E., & Bhutta, Z. A. (2024). Preventing and Controlling Zinc Deficiency Across the Life Course: A Call to Action. *Advances in Nutrition*, *15*(3), 100181. DOI: 10.1016/j.advnut.2024.100181 PMID: 38280724

Lu, J., Zhang, H., Cao, W., Jiang, S., Fang, H., Yu, D., & Yang, L. (2023). Study on the Zinc Nutritional Status and Risk Factors of Chinese 6–18-Year-Old Children. *Nutrients*, *15*(7), 1685. DOI: 10.3390/nu15071685 PMID: 37049525

Manzeke-Kangara, M. G., Joy, E. J. M., Mtambanengwe, F., Chopera, P., Watts, M. J., Broadley, M. R., & Mapfumo, P. (2021). Good soil management can reduce dietary zinc deficiency in Zimbabwe. *CABI Agriculture and Bioscience*, *2*(1), 36. DOI: 10.1186/s43170-021-00057-4

Manzoor, M. F., Ali, A., Ain, H. B. U., Kausar, S., Khalil, A. A., Aadil, R. M., & Zeng, X.-A. (2024). Bioaccessibility mechanisms, fortification strategies, processing impact on bioavailability, and therapeutic potentials of minerals in cereals. *Future Foods : a Dedicated Journal for Sustainability in Food Science*, *10*, 100425. DOI: 10.1016/j.fufo.2024.100425

Maywald, M., & Rink, L. (2022a). Zinc in human health and infectious diseases. *Biomolecules*, *12*(12), 1748. DOI: 10.3390/biom12121748 PMID: 36551176

Maywald, M., & Rink, L. (2022b). Zinc in Human Health and Infectious Diseases. *Biomolecules*, *12*(12), 1748. DOI: 10.3390/biom12121748 PMID: 36551176

McDonald, C. M., Suchdev, P. S., Krebs, N. F., Hess, S. Y., Wessells, K. R., Ismaily, S., Rahman, S., Wieringa, F. T., Williams, A. M., Brown, K. H., & King, J. C. (2020). Adjusting plasma or serum zinc concentrations for inflammation: Biomarkers Reflecting Inflammation and Nutritional Determinants of Anemia (BRINDA) project. *The American Journal of Clinical Nutrition*, *111*(4), 927–937. DOI: 10.1093/ajcn/nqz304 PMID: 32266402

Mehata, S., Tamang, M. K., Parajuli, K. R., Rayamajhee, B., Yadav, U. N., Mehta, R. K., & Singh, D. R. (2021). Serum zinc status is a matter of concern among children and non-pregnant women in a nationwide survey of Nepal. *Scientific Reports*, *11*(1), 14904. DOI: 10.1038/s41598-021-94344-9 PMID: 34290324

Mohammadi, H., Talebi, S., Ghavami, A., Rafiei, M., Sharifi, S., Faghihimani, Z., Ranjbar, G., Miraghajani, M., & Askari, G. (2021). Effects of zinc supplementation on inflammatory biomarkers and oxidative stress in adults: A systematic review and meta-analysis of randomized controlled trials. *Journal of Trace Elements in Medicine and Biology*, *68*, 126857. DOI: 10.1016/j.jtemb.2021.126857 PMID: 34560424

MoHFW. UNICEF. (2019). *Comprehensive National Nutrition Survey 2016–2018* [Comprehensive National Nutrition Survey (CNNS)]. Ministry of Health and Family Welfare (MoHFW), Government of India, UNICEF and Population Council. https://www.unicef.org/india/media/2646/file/CNNS-report.pdf

Murray, R. M., Davis, A. L., Shepler, L. J., Moore-Merrell, L., Troup, W. J., Allen, J. A., & Taylor, J. A. (2020). A Systematic Review of Workplace Violence Against Emergency Medical Services Responders. *New Solutions*, *29*(4), 487–503. DOI: 10.1177/1048291119893388 PMID: 31841060

Naik, B., Kumar, V., Rizwanuddin, S., Mishra, S., Kumar, V., Saris, P. E. J., Khanduri, N., Kumar, A., Pandey, P., Gupta, A. K., Khan, J. M., & Rustagi, S. (2024). Biofortification as a solution for addressing nutrient deficiencies and malnutrition. *Heliyon*, *10*(9), e30595. DOI: 10.1016/j.heliyon.2024.e30595 PMID: 38726166

Nalyotov, A. V., Matsynin, A. N., & Matsynina, M. A. (2022). Zinc Availability is an Important Indicator of Human Health. *Health. Food Biotechnology*, *4*(3), 12–18.

Norman, K., Haß, U., & Pirlich, M. (2021). Malnutrition in Older Adults—Recent Advances and Remaining Challenges. *Nutrients*, *13*(8), 2764. DOI: 10.3390/nu13082764 PMID: 34444924

Oh, C., Keats, E., & Bhutta, Z. (2020). Vitamin and Mineral Supplementation During Pregnancy on Maternal, Birth, Child Health and Development Outcomes in Low- and Middle-Income Countries: A Systematic Review and Meta-Analysis. *Nutrients*, *12*(2), 491. DOI: 10.3390/nu12020491 PMID: 32075071

Palacios, A. M., Hurley, K. M., De-Ponce, S., Alfonso, V., Tilton, N., Lambden, K. B., Reinhart, G. A., Freeland-Graves, J. H., Villanueva, L. M., & Black, M. M. (2020). Zinc deficiency associated with anaemia among young children in rural Guatemala. *Maternal and Child Nutrition*, *16*(1), e12885. DOI: 10.1111/mcn.12885 PMID: 31595712

Philipo, M., Ndakidemi, P. A., & Mbega, E. R. (2021). Importance of common bean genetic zinc biofortification in alleviating human zinc deficiency in sub-Saharan Africa. *Cogent Food & Agriculture*, *7*(1), 1907954. DOI: 10.1080/23311932.2021.1907954

Pinzón-Rondón, Á. M., Hoyos-Martínez, A., Parra-Correa, D., Pedraza-Flechas, A. M., & Ruiz-Sternberg, Á. M. (2019). Association of nutritional support programs with zinc deficiency in Colombian children: A cross-sectional study. *BMC Nutrition*, *5*(1), 42. DOI: 10.1186/s40795-019-0305-8 PMID: 32153955

Płaczek, A., Machaj, D., Białas, F., Cyboran, K., & Kuc, M. (2022). Consequences of zinc deficiency in selected diseases—Literature review. *Journal of Education, Health and Sport, 12*(7), 775–779. DOI: 10.12775/JEHS.2022.12.07.076

Poudel, P., Di Gioia, F., Lambert, J. D., & Connolly, E. L. (2023). Zinc biofortification through seed nutri-priming using alternative zinc sources and concentration levels in pea and sunflower microgreens. *Frontiers in Plant Science, 14*, 1177844. DOI: 10.3389/fpls.2023.1177844 PMID: 37139105

Praharaj, S., Skalicky, M., Maitra, S., Bhadra, P., Shankar, T., Brestic, M., Hejnak, V., Vachova, P., & Hossain, A. (2021). Zinc biofortification in food crops could alleviate the zinc malnutrition in human health. *Molecules (Basel, Switzerland), 26*(12), 3509. DOI: 10.3390/molecules26123509 PMID: 34207649

Pullakhandam, R., Agrawal, P. K., Peter, R., Ghosh, S., Reddy, G. B., Kulkarni, B., Thomas, T., Kurpad, A. V., Sachdev, H. S., Porwal, A., Khan, N., Ramesh, S., Acharya, R., Sarna, A., Kapil, U., Rajkumar, H., De Wagt, A., Deb, S., & Johnston, R. (2021). Prevalence of low serum zinc concentrations in Indian children and adolescents: Findings from the Comprehensive National Nutrition Survey 2016–18. *The American Journal of Clinical Nutrition, 114*(2), 638–648. DOI: 10.1093/ajcn/nqab066 PMID: 33831945

Quamme, S. H., & Iversen, P. O. (2022). Prevalence of child stunting in Sub-Saharan Africa and its risk factors. *Clinical Nutrition Open Science, 42*, 49–61. DOI: 10.1016/j.nutos.2022.01.009

Rawat, M., Varshney, A., Rai, M., Chikara, A., Pohty, A. L., Joshi, A., Binjola, A., Singh, C. P., Rawat, K., Rather, M. A., & Gupta, A. K. (2023). A comprehensive review on nutraceutical potential of underutilized cereals and cereal-based products. *Journal of Agriculture and Food Research, 12*, 100619. DOI: 10.1016/j.jafr.2023.100619

Read, S. A., Obeid, S., Ahlenstiel, C., & Ahlenstiel, G. (2019). The role of zinc in antiviral immunity. *Advances in Nutrition, 10*(4), 696–710. DOI: 10.1093/advances/nmz013 PMID: 31305906

Rehman, A., Farooq, M., Ozturk, L., Asif, M., & Siddique, K. H. M. (2018). Zinc nutrition in wheat-based cropping systems. *Plant and Soil, 422*(1–2), 283–315. DOI: 10.1007/s11104-017-3507-3

Rehman, A., Farooq, M., Ullah, A., Nadeem, F., Im, S. Y., Park, S. K., & Lee, D.-J. (2020). Agronomic Biofortification of Zinc in Pakistan: Status, Benefits, and Constraints. *Frontiers in Sustainable Food Systems, 4*, 591722. DOI: 10.3389/fsufs.2020.591722

Ryckman, T., Beal, T., Nordhagen, S., Murira, Z., & Torlesse, H. (2021). Affordability of nutritious foods for complementary feeding in South Asia. *Nutrition Reviews*, *79*(Supplement_1), 52–68. DOI: 10.1093/nutrit/nuaa139 PMID: 33693914

Sanusi, K. O., Ibrahim, K. G., Abubakar, B., Malami, I., Bello, M. B., Imam, M. U., & Abubakar, M. B. (2021). Effect of maternal zinc deficiency on offspring health: The epigenetic impact. *Journal of Trace Elements in Medicine and Biology*, *65*, 126731. DOI: 10.1016/j.jtemb.2021.126731 PMID: 33610057

Shubham, K., Anukiruthika, T., Dutta, S., Kashyap, A., Moses, J. A., & Anandharamakrishnan, C. (2020). Iron deficiency anemia: A comprehensive review on iron absorption, bioavailability and emerging food fortification approaches. *Trends in Food Science & Technology*, *99*, 58–75. DOI: 10.1016/j.tifs.2020.02.021

Shukla, A. K., Behera, S. K., Prakash, C., Tripathi, A., Patra, A. K., Dwivedi, B. S., Trivedi, V., Rao, Ch. S., Chaudhari, S. K., Das, S., & Singh, A. K. (2021). Deficiency of phyto-available sulphur, zinc, boron, iron, copper and manganese in soils of India. *Scientific Reports*, *11*(1), 19760. DOI: 10.1038/s41598-021-99040-2 PMID: 34611190

Singh, S., Kaur, J., Ram, H., Singh, J., & Kaur, S. (2023). Agronomic bio-fortification of wheat (Triticum aestivum L.) to alleviate zinc deficiency in human being. *Reviews in Environmental Science and Biotechnology*, *22*(2), 505–526. DOI: 10.1007/s11157-023-09653-4 PMID: 37234132

Skalny, A. V., Aschner, M., & Tinkov, A. A. (2021). Zinc. In *Advances in Food and Nutrition Research* (Vol. 96, pp. 251–310). Elsevier., DOI: 10.1016/bs.afnr.2021.01.003

Skalny, A. V., Sotnikova, T. I., Korobeynikova, T. V., & Tinkov, A. A. (2023). Significance of zinc deficiency correction for practical medicine: A review. *Sechenov Medical Journal*, *13*(4), 4–17. DOI: 10.47093/2218-7332.2022.13.4.4-17

Stanaway, J. D., Afshin, A., Gakidou, E., Lim, S. S., Abate, D., Abate, K. H., Abbafati, C., Abbasi, N., Abbastabar, H., Abd-Allah, F., Abdela, J., Abdelalim, A., Abdollahpour, I., Abdulkader, R. S., Abebe, M., Abebe, Z., Abera, S. F., Abil, O. Z., Abraha, H. N., & Murray, C. J. L. (2018). Global, regional, and national comparative risk assessment of 84 behavioural, environmental and occupational, and metabolic risks or clusters of risks for 195 countries and territories, 1990–2017: A systematic analysis for the Global Burden of Disease Study 2017. *Lancet*, *392*(10159), 1923–1994. DOI: 10.1016/S0140-6736(18)32225-6 PMID: 30496105

Stevens, G. A., Beal, T., Mbuya, M. N., Luo, H., Neufeld, L. M., Addo, O. Y., Adu-Afarwuah, S., Alayón, S., Bhutta, Z., Brown, K. H., Jefferds, M. E., Engle-Stone, R., Fawzi, W., Hess, S. Y., Johnston, R., Katz, J., Krasevec, J., McDonald, C. M., Mei, Z., & Young, M. F. (2022). Micronutrient deficiencies among preschool-aged children and women of reproductive age worldwide: A pooled analysis of individual-level data from population-representative surveys. *The Lancet. Global Health*, *10*(11), e1590–e1599. DOI: 10.1016/S2214-109X(22)00367-9 PMID: 36240826

Subhasri, D., Dutta, S., Leena, M. M., Moses, J., & Anandharamakrishnan, C. (2022). Gastronomy: An extended platform for customized nutrition. *Future Foods : a Dedicated Journal for Sustainability in Food Science*, *5*, 100147. DOI: 10.1016/j.fufo.2022.100147

Tessema, M., De Groote, H., & Brouwer, D., I., JM Feskens, E., Belachew, T., Zerfu, D., ... & S. Gunaratna, N. (2019). Soil zinc is associated with serum zinc but not with linear growth of children in Ethiopia. *Nutrients*, *11*(2), 221.

Tokuyama, A., Kanda, E., Itano, S., Kondo, M., Wada, Y., Kadoya, H., Kidokoro, K., Nagasu, H., Sasaki, T., & Kashihara, N. (2021). Effect of zinc deficiency on chronic kidney disease progression and effect modification by hypoalbuminemia. *PLoS One*, *16*(5), e0251554. DOI: 10.1371/journal.pone.0251554 PMID: 33974681

UNICEF, M. (2019). *Comprehensive National Nutrition Survey (CNNS) 2016-2018*.

Victora, C. G., Christian, P., Vidaletti, L. P., Gatica-Domínguez, G., Menon, P., & Black, R. E. (2021). Revisiting maternal and child undernutrition in low-income and middle-income countries: Variable progress towards an unfinished agenda. *Lancet*, *397*(10282), 1388–1399. DOI: 10.1016/S0140-6736(21)00394-9 PMID: 33691094

Vreugdenhil, M., Akkermans, M. D., Van Der Merwe, L. F., Van Elburg, R. M., Van Goudoever, J. B., & Brus, F. (2021). Prevalence of Zinc Deficiency in Healthy 1–3-Year-Old Children from Three Western European Countries. *Nutrients*, *13*(11), 3713. DOI: 10.3390/nu13113713 PMID: 34835970

Wessells, K. R., Manger, M. S., Tsang, B. L., Brown, K. H., & McDonald, C. M. (2024). Mandatory large-scale food fortification programmes can reduce the estimated prevalence of inadequate zinc intake by up to 50% globally. *Nature Food*, *5*(7), 625–637. DOI: 10.1038/s43016-024-00997-w PMID: 38898330

Younes, S. (2024). The impact of micronutrients on the sense of taste. *Human Nutrition & Metabolism*, *35*, 200231. DOI: 10.1016/j.hnm.2023.200231

Yu, B.-G., Liu, Y.-M., Chen, X.-X., Cao, W.-Q., Ding, T.-B., & Zou, C.-Q. (2021). Foliar zinc application to wheat may lessen the zinc deficiency burden in rural Quzhou, China. *Frontiers in Nutrition*, *8*, 697817. DOI: 10.3389/fnut.2021.697817 PMID: 34262927

Zhang, X., Wang, C., Zhao, D., Chen, X., Zhang, C., Zheng, J., & Liu, X. (2020). Zinc deficiency induces abnormal development of the myocardium by promoting SENP5 overexpression. *PLoS One*, *15*(11), e0242606. DOI: 10.1371/journal.pone.0242606 PMID: 33211757

Chapter 5
Confronting Zinc Deficiency:
A Public Health Challenge in the Developing World

Anuradha Singh
https://orcid.org/0000-0002-8145-1369
University of Allahabad, India

Anjali Maurya
University of Allahabad, India

ABSTRACT

This chapter highlights the significance of zinc deficiency as a pressing public health issue in developing countries. It explores the root causes, including inadequate dietary intake, frequent infectious diseases, and overall malnutrition. Furthermore, the review examines various strategies to combat zinc deficiency and manage its consequences. These strategies include promoting dietary diversification, fortifying staple foods with zinc, developing biofortified crops with higher inherent zinc content, implementing targeted zinc supplementation programs, and launching educational initiatives. The review emphasizes the need for a multi-faceted approach that tackles both dietary and non-dietary factors. This comprehensive strategy holds promise for achieving sustainable improvements in zinc nutrition and public health outcomes in developing countries.

DOI: 10.4018/979-8-3693-5355-4.ch005

1. BACKGROUND

The essential trace element zinc exerts pleiotropic effects on human physiology. Functioning as a co-factor for over 300 enzymes, zinc is indispensable for diverse cellular metabolic processes including protein, carbohydrate, and fat metabolism, thereby impacting energy production and nutrient utilization (Pajarillo et al., 2021). Furthermore, zinc bolsters the immune system and is critical for growth and development throughout the lifespan. During childhood and adolescence, it facilitates cell division, DNA synthesis, and tissue maturation, particularly in skeletal and reproductive systems (Ozturk et al., 2023). Additionally, zinc promotes wound healing via collagen production. Its role in taste perception underscores its broader impact on sensory function (Maywald & Rink, 2022). In conclusion, zinc's extensive involvement in enzymatic activity and cellular processes highlights its essential role for maintaining optimal health across various physiological systems (Hussain et al., 2022; Cunha et al., 2022). The multifaceted role of zinc in human physiology, coupled with the potential detrimental effects of deficiency, underscore the importance of maintaining adequate zinc status as shown in **Table 1**. Without enough zinc, our bodies can suffer negative consequences. These consequences include:

- **Weakened Immune System:** A zinc deficiency makes us more susceptible to illnesses (Skalny et al., 2021).
- **Stunted Growth and Development in Children:** Low zinc intake can hinder growth, delay sexual maturity, and impair cognitive development (Ahsan et al.,2021).
- **Slow Wound Healing:** Zinc helps produce collagen, a crucial component for tissue repair. When zinc is deficient, wounds may take longer to heal (Yu & Yu 2023).
- **Diarrhea and a Vicious Cycle:** Zinc deficiency can cause diarrhea, which can further deplete zinc stores, creating a self-perpetuating issue (Siddiqui et al.,2021).
- **Skin and Hair Problems:** Dermatitis and hair loss can be signs of zinc deficiency (Searle et al., 2022).

Table 1. Recommended Zn intakes, key benefits and deficiency symptoms by age group

Life Stages	RDA (in mg/day)	Symptoms of Zinc Deficiency	Key Benefits of Zinc Intake
Pregnancy & Lactation	~12-13	• Prenatal complications and infertility • Fetal growth retardation • Susceptible to infections • Inadequate breastfeeding • Increased mortality • Immuno-compromised health	• Supports fetal development • Reduces risk of preterm birth • Less susceptible to infections • Lesser prenatal complications
Infancy & Childhood	~2-5	• Frequent infections • Delayed wound healing • Hair loss • Diarrhea • Loss of appetite • Decreased taste and smell	• Promotes healthy growth • Strengthens immune system • Less susceptible to infections
Adolescence	~8-10	• Same as infancy & childhood • Stunted growth • Delayed sexual development • Lesser chances of mood disorders • Less prone to skin diseases	• Supports sexual maturation cognitive development • Reduces mental health problems
Adulthood	~10-11	• Frequent infections • Delayed wound healing • Hair loss • Loss of appetite • Decreased taste and smell • Elevated levels of blood ammonia • Hypogonadism	• Maintains wound healing • Supports immune function • Reduces elevated levels of blood ammonia
Older Adults	~11	• Frequent infections • Delayed wound healing • Hair loss • Loss of appetite • Decreased taste and smell • Elevated levels of blood ammonia	• Increase immunity • May improve cognitive function • Reduce age-related muscular degeneration risk • No behavioral anomaly

Note: RDA (Recommended Dietary Allowances)-This value represents the average daily intake sufficient to meet the nutrient requirements of nearly all (97–98%) healthy individuals. It serves as a cornerstone for planning nutritionally adequate diets on an individual basis.

Zinc is primarily absorbed in the small intestine during digestion. However, the efficiency of this absorption process is influenced by several factors. Liquid zinc supplements consumed on an empty stomach boast a high absorption rate, reaching around 60-70%. Conversely, zinc absorption from solid foods is less efficient and varies depending on the inherent zinc content and the overall dietary composition. Notably, smaller dietary zinc intakes are absorbed more efficiently by the body compared to larger quantities (Katimba et al.,2024). Furthermore, the bio-availability of zinc plays a crucial role in absorption. Plant-based sources of zinc generally offer lower bio-availability compared to animal sources due to the presence of phytates in plants, which act as chelators and inhibit zinc absorption (Singh and Prasad 2023).

Following absorption, zinc concentrates primarily within skeletal muscle and bone tissues, comprising over 85% of the total body content, estimated at 2-3 grams. Unlike other essential elements, the human body doesn't possess a dedicated long-term storage system for zinc. Therefore, consistent dietary intake is critical for maintaining steady state zinc levels (Chen et al.,2024; Duan et al.,2023).

Zinc excretion primarily occurs through feces, with daily losses ranging from less than 1 mg on a zinc-depleted diet to exceeding 5 mg on a zinc-rich diet. Urinary excretion accounts for a much smaller percentage, typically less than 10% of total zinc elimination. However, certain conditions can increase urinary zinc losses, such as starvation, muscle breakdown (catabolism), rigorous exercise, and high ambient temperatures, all of which can lead to increased zinc excretion through sweat (Katimba et al., 2024).

Zinc deficiency (ZnD) constitutes a major global public health threat, particularly impacting low- and middle-income countries (LMICs). It disproportionately affects a significant portion of their populations, hindering overall well-being and posing a substantial risk to child development, immune function, and reproductive health (Patil et al.2023). ZnD manifests through a cascade of adverse outcomes, including increased childhood mortality (Prashanth et al. 2023), impaired linear growth (Brion et al. 2020), and heightened susceptibility to infections (Seifi et al. 2024). Furthermore, ZnD, alongside other micro-nutrient deficiencies, incurs a substantial economic burden on healthcare systems and national economies through increased morbidity and mortality (Djoumessi et al. 2022). Staple food sources in LMICs often have low bio-available zinc, further exacerbated by poverty-restricted access to diverse diets rich in natural zinc sources like legumes, animal products, and nuts (Gupta et al.2020; Knez & Stangoulis 2021). Beyond dietary limitations, prevalent infectious diseases in LMICs significantly contribute to ZnD. Diarrheal illnesses and parasitic infections lead to increased zinc loss and impaired intestinal absorption, creating a vicious cycle. ZnD itself worsens malnutrition by hindering nutrient utilization and weakening the immune system, increasing susceptibility to infections that exacerbate ZnD (Prashanth and Hegde, 2023).

Given the multifaceted nature of ZnD and its severe impact on public health in LMICs, a comprehensive approach is crucial. This background section lays the groundwork for exploring the far-reaching public health significance of ZnD in LMICs, delving into the underlying dietary and non-dietary causes, and outlining various strategies for effective intervention and long-term management. By implementing a multi-pronged approach that tackles both dietary and non-dietary factors, we can strive for sustainable improvements in zinc nutrition and public health outcomes in developing countries.

2. INTRODUCTION

Zinc deficiency (ZnD) represents a significant, yet under-recognized, global public health challenge. Accounting for one of the most prevalent forms of micronutrient malnutrition, ZnD affects an estimated 17% of the global population with inadequate zinc intake. This translates to over 2 billion individuals worldwide impacted by ZnD, with a disproportionate burden borne by populations in low- and middle-income countries (LMICs). Furthermore, ZnD ranks among the ten leading risk factors contributing to the disease burden in developing countries (Knez & Stangoulis, 2021; Lowe et al., 2024).

This widespread deficiency is not simply a matter of dietary inadequacy; it represents a significant public health threat with far-reaching consequences. In these nations, where infectious diseases already strain healthcare resources considerably, ZnD further amplifies morbidity and mortality rates. This disparity reflects the complex interplay of socioeconomic factors, dietary limitations, and public health challenges prevalent in many developing regions. The frequency of zinc insufficiency is significantly greater in rural than urban regions, but it is found in both. Zinc deficiency is of particular concern in newborns, children, and women of reproductive age, but it also occurs in teenagers and older people.

The consequences of ZnD in the developing world are far-reaching and have the potential to derail human development. Clinical manifestations of zinc deficiency (ZnD) are often nonspecific, with severity influenced by age, duration of deficiency, and the presence of co-morbidities (Wessels et al., 2022). In children from LMICs, ZnD emerges as a significant growth-limiting factor, contributing to stunting in both seemingly healthy and malnourished children (Pujiastuti et al 2018). Beyond increasing susceptibility to various childhood illnesses, severe ZnD is associated with recurrent infections and diarrhea and delayed wound healing (Abolurin et al., 2020). In adolescents and adults, overt ZnD can impair reproductive function (Mertens et al., 2023). Furthermore, it may hinder cognitive growth, reducing learning ability and memory function. This translates into long-term ramifications for these youngsters, possibly hurting their school performance and future economic potential (Ahsan et al., 2021).

Pregnant women are another demographic group especially prone to ZnD. Zinc is vital for prenatal development, regulating placental function and foetal growth. ZnD during pregnancy may cause several problems, including intrauterine growth restriction (IUGR), premature delivery, and low birth weight. These issues not only influence the immediate health of the infant but also raise the risk of chronic illnesses like diabetes and cardiovascular disease later in life (Han et al.,2023). Additionally, ZnD in pregnant women might influence maternal health outcomes, increasing the risk of postpartum infections and delaying wound healing after delivery (Agedew et al., 2022).

The impact of ZnD extends beyond the individual, affecting families and communities. Increased child illness can place a significant strain on healthcare systems already stretched thin in developing countries. Reduced work capacity due to ZnD can further impact household income and economic development. Understanding the complex interplay of dietary and non-dietary factors that contribute to the widespread prevalence of ZnD in LMICs is crucial for designing effective mitigation strategies (Skalny et al., 2022).

This review comprehensively analyses zinc deficiency, a critical public health challenge in developing countries. It sheds light on the far-reaching consequences of zinc scarcity, elucidating its detrimental impacts on immune function, growth and development trajectories, and maternal and infant health outcomes. Following this analysis, it shows the fundamental causes of zinc insufficiency in these regions, including dietary limitations characterized by low bio available zinc in staple crops, frequent infectious diseases that exacerbate zinc loss, and the synergistic relationship with malnutrition. Shifting the focus towards solutions, the review proposes a multifaceted approach to combat zinc deficiency and manage its associated public health burden. By emphasizing the need to address both dietary and non-dietary factors that contribute to zinc deficiency, this review also emphasizes the significance of a comprehensive approach to attaining sustainable improvements in zinc nutrition and public health outcomes in developing countries.

3. PUBLIC HEALTH SIGNIFICANCE OF ZD IN DEVELOPING COUNTRIES

Once disregarded as a global health threat following its initial identification in the 1960s (Prasad, 2013), ZnD is now recognized as a critical public health challenge, particularly in LMICs. The World Health Organization (WHO) emphasizes its significance, ranking ZnD as the fifth leading risk factor for disease burden in LMICs and the eleventh globally (Knez & Stangoulis, 2021). This alarming ranking underscores the urgency of addressing ZnD as a widespread nutritional issue.

Estimating the magnitude of ZnD relies on a multi-pronged approach. National Stunting Prevalence Data (accessed through the WHO Global Database on Child Growth and Malnutrition and UNICEF's State of the World's Children Report) provides insights into the prevalence of stunting, a condition often associated with ZnD. Additionally, the Food and Agriculture Organization's food balance sheets offer information on zinc content in national food supplies. Finally, national surveys that measure plasma zinc concentrations help assess the prevalence of Zn inadequacy.

Integrating data from these various sources suggests that ZnD affects an estimated 17-20% of the global population (Gupta et al., 2015).

The burden of ZnD exhibits significant geographic disparities that reflects the complex interplay of socioeconomic factors, dietary limitations, and public health challenges prevalent in many developing regions. Populations in Southeast Asia, Central America, and South America face a heightened risk due to their predominantly plant-based diets (Lowe et al., 2024). These regions typically have limited access to animal-source foods, a rich source of bio-available zinc. Populations in Asia and Sub-Saharan Africa exhibit a higher vulnerability to insufficient zinc absorption compared to developed nations. This elevated ZnD burden aligns with the concerning prevalence of childhood stunting in Africa and Asia, with an estimated 155 million stunted children under-five concentrated in these regions. Intriguingly, the recognition of ZnD is on the rise in developed countries as well. This underscores the necessity for comprehensive public health interventions to tackle this global challenge. **Figure 1** highlights the significant disparity between developed and developing countries. Data from the World Health Organization (WHO) shows a considerably higher ZnD prevalence in developing regions, reaching up to 40%, compared to a range of 10-30% observed in developed nations (Lowe et al., 2024).

Figure 1. Prevalence of zinc deficiency by region

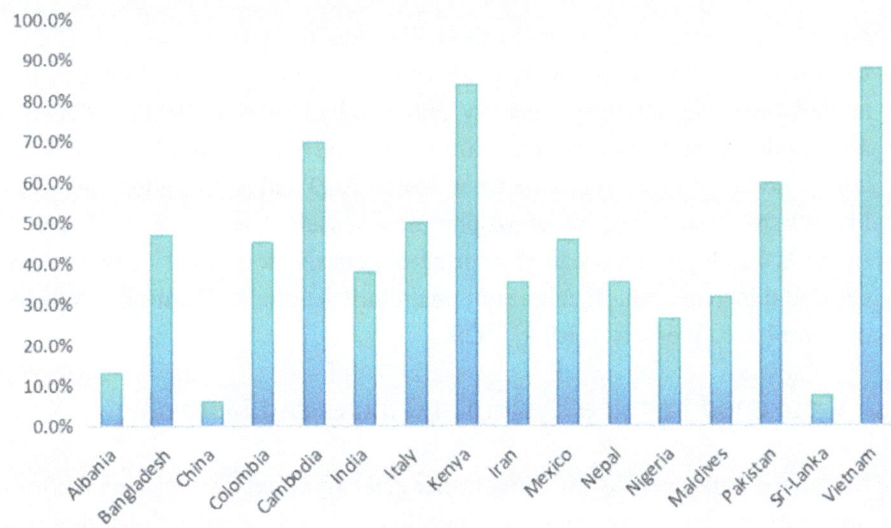

Socioeconomic factors further exacerbate ZnD in LMICs (Abolurin et al., 2020) demonstrates a statistically significant association ($p=0.013$) between low socioeconomic status (SES) and a substantially higher prevalence of ZnD. Ahsan et al. (2021) reinforces this link, highlighting the increased risk of ZnD in LMIC children and its potential to lead to physical and neurological impairments. The consequences of ZnD are far-reaching, with Skalny et al. (2021) emphasizing its connection to increased mortality and disability-adjusted life years (DALYs). This data underscores the significant public health burden ZnD poses in LMICs.

3.1. Consequences of Zinc Scarcity

ZnD, posing a major obstacle to human development. This invisible enemy disrupts various aspects of human growth and well-being, leaving a lasting impact on individuals and communities. Here, we explore the multifaceted consequences of ZnD on human development in developing countries:

3.1.1. Impaired Growth and Development

- **Stunted Growth**: Due to its involvement in enzymes essential for protein synthesis and DNA replication, Zn plays a vital role in growth and development. It also regulates hormones like growth hormone and insulin-like growth factor 1 (IGF-1) crucial for linear growth and tissue development. ZnD hinders linear growth, leading to stunting, a condition characterized by low height for age. This not only affects physical stature but also reduces muscle mass and bone density, impacting future health and productivity (Hussain et al., 2022).
- **Cognitive Decline**: ZnD can negatively impact cognitive development, potentially affecting learning, memory, and problem-solving abilities. This can hinder educational attainment and limit future earning potential (Ahsan et al., 2021). Studies suggest a link between severe ZnD and neurological disorders like autism, depression, and schizophrenia (Wessels & Rink, 2020). Research suggests Zn deprivation can disrupt neurogenesis (formation of new nerve cells) and increase neural cell death, potentially leading to learning and memory problems (Wessels & Rink, 2020).

3.1.2. Weakened Immune System and Increased Morbidity

- **Increased Vulnerability to Infections:** ZnD significantly weakens the host immune system, increasing susceptibility to various infectious diseases caused by bacteria, viruses, and parasites (Chen et al., 2021). Children with ZnD demonstrate heightened vulnerability to respiratory illnesses such as pneumonia and diarrhoeal episodes (Kinash et al., 2021). ZnD is estimated to significantly contribute to child mortality from infectious diseases, including pneumonia and diarrhea (Chasapis et al., 2020). Mechanistically, ZnD disrupts the delicate balance of the inflammatory response, hindering the body's ability to effectively combat infections (Chen et al., 2021). Zn plays a critical role in both innate and adaptive immunity in children, influencing crucial processes like enzyme activity, gene regulation, and immune cell function (Kinash et al., 2021). ZnD can severely compromise these functions, especially in young children, rendering them more susceptible to recurrent infections. The high prevalence of malnutrition in developing countries contributes significantly to ZnD, creating a cascade of immunological problems and increased susceptibility to infectious diseases (Maywald & Rink, 2022).

During infectious episodes, the body up-regulates the production of metallothionein, an inflammatory protein with a high affinity for zinc (Aziz et al., 2021). This sequestration limits the availability of free zinc for other essential functions within the immune system. Conversely, zinc deficiency weakens the immune response, increasing susceptibility to infections (Baarz & Rink, 2022). This creates a vicious cycle, as infections further deplete zinc stores. Children are particularly vulnerable due to their developing immune systems and higher zinc requirements for growth and development (Prasad, 2020). Chronic zinc deficiency can manifest as stunting, a marker of undernutrition in children under five (Goyena et al., 2021). This association suggests that inadequate dietary zinc intake or limited bio-availability of zinc in the diet can contribute to stunting.

Additionally, the elderly population appears particularly susceptible to both infections and Zn deficiency. This vulnerability might be attributed to age-related decline in immune function, potentially increasing the incidence of cancer, infections, and autoimmune diseases (Kloubert et al. 2021). Furthermore, Kloubert et al. (2021) suggests that zinc influences cytokine production and T cell subsets in this age group.

- **Delayed Wound Healing:** ZnD can impair wound healing, hindering recovery from injuries and surgeries (Abolurin et al., 2020). In vitro studies suggest a link between zinc deficiency and altered thrombosis. Lopes-Pires et al. (2021) demonstrated that Zn deficiency inhibited agonist-stimulated reactive oxygen species (ROS) production by platelets, while also decreasing glutathione levels and glutathione peroxidase activity. These findings suggest that Zn deficiency may influence thrombus formation.

3.1.3. Adverse Maternal and Child Health Outcomes

- **Pregnancy Complications:** ZnD during pregnancy increases the risk of complications like pre-eclampsia, preterm birth, and low birth weight (Gohari et al., 2023). These complications can have a lifelong impact on both mother and child.

- **Intergenerational Effects:** Maternal ZnD may lead to epigenetic modifications in offspring, potentially increasing their risk of chronic diseases like diabetes and heart disease later in life (Sanusi et al., 2021). This creates a vicious cycle of health disparities across generations.

3.1.4. Socioeconomic Burden

Zinc deficiency (ZnD) has adverse consequences not only on human health but also on the economic situation of poor nations (Bhatt, 2020). The association between zinc deficiency (ZnD) and heightened susceptibility to sickness results in a wide range of economic hardships (Freeland-Graves, 2020). The analysis of these challenges are as follows:

- **Decreased Productivity:** ZnD results in reduced productivity because people are away from work due to sickness. This not only impacts personal earnings but also disrupts the smooth flow of workers, possibly impeding productivity and economic performance (Kottala, 2023).
- **Increased healthcare expenditures:** Healthcare expenditures increase as the demand for treatment of ZnD-associated disorders grows (Hatch & Smith, 2023). This imposes pressure on already limited healthcare resources in underdeveloped nations. We should better allocate these resources to preventative measures or the treatment of other significant health conditions (Ahsan et al., 2021).
- **Reduced Earning potential:** Impaired cognitive development in youngsters suffering from ZnD may have long-term economic effects (Chitekwe et al., 2022). These youngsters may encounter constraints in their educational achievement and future earning potential, reducing their capacity to fully participate in the workforce. This creates a cycle of poverty because people may struggle to provide for themselves and their families (Madjdianet al., 2018).
- **Intergenerational Impact:** ZnD's economic effects may be inter-generational. Mothers with ZnD are more likely to encounter problems during pregnancy, perhaps resulting in low-birth-weight children. These children may also suffer from ZnD, repeating the cycle of disease, low productivity, and restricted economic possibilities (Skalny et al., 2021).

Beyond ZnD, deficiencies in other essential micro-nutrients, particularly prevalent in developing countries, contribute substantially to economic losses (Sangeetha et al., 2022). These deficiencies collectively reduce workforce productivity, increase healthcare costs associated with treating preventable illnesses, and ultimately hinder the gross domestic product (GDP) of these nations. Addressing micro-nutrient deficiencies, including ZnD, presents a strategic opportunity to improve public health and economic outcomes in developing countries.

3.2. Underlying Causes of Zinc Deficiency

ZD is a prevalent global health concern, affecting people of all ages and socio-economic backgrounds. This section explores the various underlying causes of zinc deficiency, highlighting factors that contribute to inadequate zinc intake or absorption.

Dietary Deficiency

- **Low Dietary Zinc Content**

Zinc, an essential trace element, cannot be synthesized by the human body and relies solely on dietary intake (Stiles et al., 2024). Inadequate dietary intake stands as the primary cause of zinc deficiency, particularly prevalent in LMICs. Staple foods in developing countries, like refined cereals, are often low in bio-available zinc, the form readily absorbed by the body (Duan et al., 2023; Hoque et al., 2023).

- **Limited Access to Animal-Source Protein**

Diets high in refined grains, fruits, and vegetables, while providing essential nutrients, generally offer lower zinc content compared to those rich in animal protein, shellfish, legumes, nuts, and seeds (**Table 2**). Poverty further restricts access to a diversified diet rich in these bio-available sources (Khan et al., 2022). This imbalance leads to a scenario where individuals might consume adequate total zinc, but their bodies struggle to utilize it effectively due to limited absorption (Hall & King, 2022).

Table 2. Key dietary sources of bioavailable zinc

Food Group	Examples
Nuts & Seeds	Hemp seeds (9.9 mg, 90%); Sesem seeds (7.75 mg, 70%); Pine nuts (4-5mg, 41%); Cashew nuts (5.78mg, 53%); Chia seeds (4.6mg, 42%); Pecan nuts (4.5mg, 41%); Flaxseeds (4.3mg, 39%); Brazil nuts (4.06mg, 37%); Almonds (3.12mg, 28%); Walnuts (3.09mg, 28%); Hazelnuts (2.45mg, 22%); Pistachio (2.22mg, 20%)
Legumes	Soy flour (3.92mg, 36%); Peanuts (3.27mg, 30%); Cooked Hyacinth beans (2.85mg, 26%); Chickpea flour (2.81mg, 26%)
Cereal grains	Rye flour (5.04mg, 46%); Oats (3.97mg, 36%); Whole wheat flour (3.24mg, 29%); Millet flour (2.63mg, 24%)
Fruits and Vegetable	Shiitake mushrooms (5mg, 43%); Green peas (2.8mg, 26%); Spinach (6.6mg, 60%); Lima beans (1.3mg, 12%); Lentil sprouts (2.8mg, 26%); Asparagus (5.5mg, 50%); Beet greens (3.7mg, 34%); Broccoli (2.6mg, 23%); Okra (3.9mg, 36%); Sweet corn (1.1mg, 10%)
Animal products	Beef (12mg, 105%); Chicken leg (2mg, 20%); Firm tofu (2mg, 20%); Lean pork chops (2mg, 19%); Beef patty (6.6mg, 60%); Cooked buffalo sirloin steak (6mg, 54%); Ostrich steak (6mg, 54%)
Sea food	Oyster (155mg,1405%); Alaskan king crab (15.7mg, 143%); Cooked spiny lobster (10.2mg, 92%); Cooked Cuttle fish (4.4mg, 40%); Cray fish (4.3mg, 39%); Canned shrimp (3.9mg, 36%)

Note. (serving size 100 g or equivalent); % daily values based on 2000 cal. Diet Source: USDA Food data Central (https://fdc.nal.usda.gov/fdc-app.html#/food-search?component=1095)

- **Poor Dietary Diversity**

Poor dietary diversity, characterized by a limited intake of various food groups, presents a significant risk factor for ZnD. This is particularly concerning in developing countries where food insecurity and limited access to fresh produce are prevalent. When individuals consume primarily a few staple foods, their overall nutrient intake becomes skewed. Staple crops like refined grains, while providing calories, often lack bioavailable zinc, the form readily absorbed by the body (Li et al., 2020). Furthermore, these diets might be high in phytates (found in legumes and whole grains), which can bind to zinc, hindering its absorption. This imbalanced intake reduces the total zinc available for the body's needs, increasing the risk of ZnD (Goyena et al., 2021).

- **Food Processing Techniques:**

Staple crops like wheat, rice, and corn are often subjected to various processing techniques to improve shelf life, enhance texture, and create convenient food products. However, these seemingly beneficial processes can have an unintended consequence: exacerbating zinc deficiency (ZnD), particularly in developing countries. The bran and germ fractions of cereal grains, often removed during processing, are the richest sources of bio-available zinc. Bioavailable zinc refers to the form of zinc readily absorbed by the human body. When these fractions are discarded, the remaining endosperm, which forms the bulk of refined grains, is significantly lower in zinc content (Zaman et al., 2018).

Milling, a cornerstone of grain processing, removes the nutrient-rich outer layers – the bran and germ – to create finer flours. While this produces a smoother texture and extends shelf life, it also removes up to 80% of the total zinc content present in the whole grain (Mendoza et al., 2017). Further processing, like polishing rice to remove bran layers, can further reduce zinc levels. The resulting polished rice is visually appealing but significantly lower in zinc compared to brown rice, which retains the bran. Apart from zinc, milling and polishing also remove other essential nutrients like dietary fiber, iron, and B vitamins. This depletion necessitates fortification – the addition of synthetic nutrients – to enriched flour or polished rice. However, fortification might not always fully compensate for the loss of naturally occurring, bio-available forms of these nutrients (Praharaj et al., 2021).

- **Dietary Interactions:**

Dietary composition plays a significant role in zinc (Zn) absorption. Anti-nutrients like phytates (abundant in legumes, seeds, and whole grains) and oxalates (found in spinach, nuts, and tea) can chelate Zn, reducing its bio-availability. Iron supplementation, particularly in high doses and without food, can also hinder Zn absorption. Conversely, iron-fortified foods have minimal impact. To optimize absorption, it's recommended to separate iron and Zn supplements and consume them with meals. Interestingly, excessive Zn intake (>50mg/day for extended periods) can limit copper absorption. Similarly, certain dietary sources of phosphorus, including phytates and milk casein, may pose challenges for Zn bio-availability. The relationship between Zn and folate is complex. While low Zn intake might decrease folate absorption, the impact of folate supplementation on Zn status remains under investigation. Understanding these intricate dietary interactions is crucial for formulating effective strategies to optimize Zn absorption, particularly for populations with limited access to animal-source foods (Singh & Prasad, 2023; Singh & Prasad, 2023).

Non-Dietary Causes:

- **Breastfeeding practices:**

Although breast-milk offers the ideal source of nourishment for infants, prolonged exclusive breastfeeding (beyond 6 months of age) without introducing complementary zinc supplementation can trigger deficiency. This risk is particularly pronounced in mothers with borderline zinc status themselves. The limited zinc stores in breastmilk coupled with the increasing zinc requirements of a growing infant create a scenario where dietary diversification and potential zinc supplementation become crucial to ensure adequate zinc homeostasis and prevent deficiency in both mother and child (Dumrongwongsiri et al., 2021; Gohari et al., 2023).

- **Chronic Diseases:**

Beyond the well-established dietary factors influencing zinc (Zn) status, underlying chronic illnesses can further exacerbate Zn deficiency (ZnD). Conditions like sickle cell disease and inflammatory bowel disease (IBD) disrupt the intricate processes of Zn absorption and utilization within the body. Sickle cell disease, characterized by abnormal hemoglobin structure, can lead to increased gastrointestinal losses of Zn, while chronic inflammation associated with IBD disrupts intestinal Zn absorption mechanisms. (Ahsan et al., 2021).

- **Frequent Infectious Diseases and Zinc Loss**

The burden of infectious diseases, another hallmark of developing countries, creates a double-edged sword for zinc status (Mao et al., 2024). A vicious cycle links zinc deficiency (ZnD) with diarrhoeal and parasitic infections, particularly prevalent in low- and middle-income countries (LMICs) (Abolurin et al., 2020). ZnD weakens the immune system, increasing susceptibility to these very infections (Gupta et al., 2020). Conversely, these infections trigger significant zinc losses through increased faecal excretion. While the precise source of this lost zinc (dietary or endogenous stores) remains under investigation (Abolurin et al., 2020), the overall effect is a depletion of zinc stores. This negative cycle is particularly concerning for children in LMICs, where both ZnD and diarrhoeal diseases are highly prevalent. Chronic ZnD and its associated health complications can be the consequence of this persistent depletion.

● Malnutrition and its Link to Zinc Deficiency

Zinc deficiency rarely exists in isolation. It often intertwines with other micronutrient deficiencies, creating a complex web of malnutrition. (Yaqob, 2019). In particular, vulnerable populations, such as the elderly in western countries and children in developing countries, are often affected. The sufficient zinc intake and homeostasis is essential for a healthy life, as it is known that zinc deficiency is associated with a multitude of immune disorders such as metabolic and chronic diseases, as well as infectious diseases such as respiratory infections, malaria, HIV, or tuberculosis. (Maywald & Rink, 2022). On the one hand, a deficiency of one micro-nutrient is often accompanied by a deficiency of another micro-nutrient, or even by a general micro-nutrient deficiency, as occurs particularly in the elderly or in people on a plant-based diet, often due to malnutrition. (Berendsen, 2019). Protein-energy malnutrition, a common issue in developing countries, further impedes zinc absorption and utilization. The body prioritizes using available zinc for protein synthesis during protein deficiency, leaving less for other essential functions. Severely malnourished children or those with protein-energy malnutrition produce retinol-binding protein at a diminished rate and have lower serum retinol and zinc concentrations. (Goyena, 2021) Additionally, deficiencies in iron and vitamin A, frequently co-occurring with zinc deficiency, can further exacerbate the overall health impact. This tangled web of deficiencies creates a synergistic effect, worsening the consequences of each individual deficiency. For example, iron deficiency can worsen the effects of zinc deficiency on anaemia, while vitamin A deficiency can hinder immune function, already compromised by zinc deficiency. Despite daily zinc supplementation for ≥7 months, high rates of maternal hypozincaemia were observed. The association of hypozincaemia with impaired fatal growth suggests widespread zinc deficiency in these settings. (Kemp, 2024). In addition to nutritional causes (undernutrition, malnutrition, veganism, geophagy, a phytate-rich diet, low-Zn parenteral nutrition), conditioned Zn deficiency has been observed in association with many diseases and inflammatory reactions. (Mcdonald, 2020; Wessels & Rink, 2020).

4. STRATEGIES FOR ALLEVIATING ZINC DEFICIENCY AND MANAGING CONSEQUENCES

Zinc deficiency (ZnD) casts a long shadow on global public health particularly for children in low-resource settings. It demonstrably hinders growth, development, and immune function, leading to a cascade of adverse health outcomes. This widespread deficiency necessitates a multifaceted approach that tackles both dietary and non-dietary factors to achieve lasting improvements in zinc status. Fortunately, there are several effective strategies that can be implemented to mitigate ZnD and manage its consequences for this vulnerable population. This section will explore these strategies, including dietary modifications, supplementation programs, and public health initiatives.

4.1. Dietary Strategies to Enhance Zinc Intake

Zinc (Zn) is an essential nutrient for maintaining good health, and dietary diversity is crucial for achieving adequate intake (Weyh et al., 2022). Restricting dietary choices to a limited range of foods increases the risk of Zn deficiency. Conversely, a varied diet rich in bioavailable zinc sources, as exemplified in **Table 2**, promotes optimal Zn absorption (Nolla et al., 2021). Bioavailability refers to the proportion of dietary Zn that the body can absorb and utilize. Optimizing Zn intake plays a significant role in overall health. Following key dietary strategies can improve Zn status, particularly for populations at risk of deficiency:

- **Consuming Animal-Source Protein:**

Animal-source foods like red meat, poultry, seafood, and eggs are premier sources of bio-available zinc (Zn), readily absorbed by the human body (Pellinen et al., 2022). Regular consumption of these protein sources is a straightforward strategy to optimize dietary zinc intake. Notably, shellfish, particularly oysters, stand out for their exceptionally high zinc content (Nolla et al., 2021). Enhancing Absorption from Plant Sources: Combining plant-based zinc sources (legumes, nuts) with animal protein in a single meal can further improve zinc absorption. Animal proteins contain sulfur-containing amino acids that act as chelators, facilitating zinc uptake in the intestines (Bouranis & Chorianopoulou, 2023).

- **Diversifying Plant-Based Sources:**

While generally lower in bio-available Zn compared to animal products, specific plant-based foods can contribute significantly. Legumes (lentils, beans), nuts, and seeds are good sources. They provide a valuable source of plant-based protein, complex carbohydrates, fiber, and various minerals, including zinc (Aiqing et al., 2022; Semba et al., 2021). However, phytates, naturally occurring in legumes, can hinder zinc absorption (Zhang et al., 2022).

- **Balancing Whole Grains with Refining Processes:**

Encouraging the consumption of whole grains, which retain the bran and germ layers, can contribute to higher zinc intake and bio-availability (Aiqing, et al.,2022). While grains contain zinc, they are also rich in phytates. Refining processes like those used for polished rice and white flour significantly decrease zinc content (Gowda et al., 2022). Individuals relying heavily on refined grains are at increased risk of Zn deficiency. Therefore, encouraging whole grain consumption while promoting diversity in dietary sources of zinc is crucial.

- **Bio-availability Enhancement:**

Several dietary practices can improve the bio-availability of zinc (Zn) from staple foods like legumes and grains (Arafsha et al., 2023). These strategies primarily target the reduction of phytates, anti-nutrients that hinder zinc absorption.

Pre-processing Techniques:

Pre-processing techniques like soaking, sprouting, and fermentation can significantly improve the bio-availability of zinc in legumes. These traditional food preparation methods effectively decrease phytate content in legumes. Soaking legumes overnight, followed by discarding the soaking water, significantly reduces phytates. Sprouting further enhances Zn bio-availability by breaking down complex carbohydrates and phytates. Fermentation, a microbial process used for some legume products like tempeh, also reduces phytates while enriching the nutritional profile with beneficial bacteria (Singh & Prasad, 2023; Jindal, 2023).

Dietary Pairing for Improved Absorption:

Consuming legumes alongside fruits and vegetables rich in vitamin C, like citrus fruits and bell peppers, can promote Zn absorption (Bhantana et al., 2021). Vitamin C forms a complex with phytate, improving zinc solubility and facilitating its uptake in the intestines.

- **Food Fortification: Enhancing Staple Foods with Zinc**

Food fortification, the strategic addition of micro-nutrients to staple foods, emerges as a cost-effective and sustainable approach to address ZD (Rai et al., 2024; Semba et al., 2021). This approach involves enriching staple foods like wheat, rice, salt, and sugar with bio-available zinc compounds during processing (Singh et al., 2023). The selection of zinc fortificants depends on several factors, including cost, stability during processing and storage, and potential interactions with other food components. Zinc sulfate and zinc oxide are the most common fortificants used due to their affordability and stability. This method offers a sustainable and cost-effective solution as it doesn't necessitate significant dietary modifications from individuals. Consequently, fortification ensures a continuous intake of zinc for vulnerable groups who may not have consistent access to a varied diet, ultimately contributing to improved public health outcomes (Tarini et al., 2021).

- **Engineering Crops with Higher Zinc Content**

Biofortification offers a sustainable strategy to address micro-nutrient deficiencies by increasing the inherent content of essential nutrients in staple food crops. This approach utilizes traditional breeding or advanced biotechnology to "bio-engineer" crops for enhanced nutritional value (Almendros et al., 2022). Notably, bio-fortification does not require significant changes in dietary patterns. Individuals consuming their customary staple foods can significantly improve their micro-nutrient intake when these staples are bio-fortified.

Several agricultural strategies are employed in bio-fortification:

- **Selective Breeding:** This traditional method involves breeding crops with naturally higher levels of specific nutrients (Kumar et al., 2023).
- **Agronomic Approach:** This strategy utilizes optimized fertilization practices and other soil amendments to enhance nutrient uptake by crops (Lagoriya et al., 2023).
- **Transgenic Approach:** Genetic engineering techniques can be used to introduce genes for increased production of desired micro-nutrients (Hina et al., 2023).

Some engineering crops with higher zinc content have been shown in **Table 3**. In addition to cost savings from development to distribution and synergies through aggregated health effects, multi-nutrient bio-fortification can result in significantly higher market coverage by preventing competition between numerous single-nutrient bio-fortified varieties (Van Der Straeten et al., 2020). Enhancing dietary zinc content and bio-availability by zinc bio-fortification is an inclusive nutrition solution that may assist the most disadvantaged persons and groups impacted by insufficient diets to the greatest extent (Lowe et al., 2024).

Table 3. Engineering crops with higher zinc content

Crop	Engineering Technique	Increase in Zinc Content	Current Development Stage	Potential Benefits	Potential Challenges	References
Rice	Genome editing *via* (CRISPR)/CRISPR- (Cas9), focusing on the OsNAS2 promoter	Higher than Control	Field Trial	Reduced zinc deficiency	Zinc uptake not accumulated in the grain or edible plant parts	*Ludwig et al., (2024)*
Rice	Overexpression of Transporter genes: OsZIP11 and OsNRAMP1	Higher than Control	Field trial	Higher accumulation of Zinc in Rice grains	Plants greatly influenced by environmental factors	*Dhanyalakshmi et al., (2024)*
Rice	Yeast vector mediated Zinc transporter OsZIP9 incorporation in rice plant	Higher than Control	Field trial	Enhanced zinc uptake by plants	expression of OsZIP9 did not affect, accumulation of Fe, Mn and Cu	*Yang et al., (2020)*
Rice	Upregulation of OsZIP3 gene	Higher than Control	Field trial	Content of zinc ions in the leaves.	Leaf senescence	*Ma et al., (2023)*
Rice	OsZIP5) and (OsZIP9)	Higher than Control	Field trial	enhanced Zn levels in the aboveground tissues and brown rice	Enhanced Cd Bioavailability	*Tan et al., (2020)*
Rice	Expression of metallothionein genes, OsMT2b and OsMT2c	Higher than Control	Field trial	Subsequent transport of Zn in the phloem in rice	Highly expressed in the node only	*Lei et al., (2021)*
Rice	OsZIP9 expression *via* Yeast vector at root epidermis	Higher than Control	Field trial	Enhanced zinc uptake in the roots throughout all growth stages	--	*Huang et al., (2020)*
Wheat	Overexpression of wheat vacuolar iron transporter gene TaVIT2-D	Higher than Control	Field trial	Enhanced zinc uptake	Increased Iron uptake in combination	*Harrington et al., (2023)*
Wheat	Genome editing *via* CRISPR -Cas9 by disrupting IPK1 gene	Higher than Control	Research stage	Enhanced zinc uptake by plants	Increased Fe and Zn accumulation in wheat grains,	*Ibrahim et al., (2021)*
Wheat	Gene silencing of eTdABCC13 proteins *via* TdMRP3 transporters TaMRP3-A1 and TaMRP3-B1	Higher than Control	Commercially available as "Durum Wheat"	Higher accumulation of Zinc in wheat kernels	Zinc concentration was reduced in the TdMRP3-B1- genotype	*Frittelli et al., (2023)*
Maize	Overexpression of *ZmZIP* genes in roots	Higher than Control	Field trial	Enhanced zinc uptake	Zinc uptake more in roots than shoots	*Xu et al., (2021)*

(CRISPR)/CRISPR- (Cas9)- clustered regularly interspaced short palindromic repeats (CRISPR)/CRISPR-associated protein 9 (Cas9); OsNAS2- Rice ni OsZIP11 – Zinc transporter; OsNRAMP1-plasma membrane-localized protein; OsZIP9- Zinc transporter; OsMT2b and OsMT2c- type 2 metallothionein g Vacuolar Iron Transporter; eTdABCC13 – Electron transfer dissociation protein; TdMRP3 – Multi drug resistant protein transporter

- **Targeted Supplementation Programs for Vulnerable Populations**

Supplementation programs can be particularly beneficial for specific populations (Loechl et al., 2023). Children in developing regions, often at risk of deficiency due to limited dietary diversity, can see significant health improvements with zinc (Lowe et al., 2024). Supplementation during pregnancy can improve maternal and child health outcomes (Obeagu et al., 2023). Additionally, individuals with chronic conditions like diarrhoea or inflammatory bowel disease may lose zinc through their illnesses. For these individuals, zinc supplementation can help replenish lost stores and promote healing. Incorporating zinc supplementation strategies for at-risk populations has the potential to improve overall health and well-being (Bloom et al., 2021).

- **Educational Initiatives: Empowering Communities**

ZnD remains a critical public health issue in LMICs. It negatively impacts child development, immune function, and overall health in these populations. While interventions like fortification and supplementation are crucial, educational initiatives offer immense potential. Effective knowledge dissemination is paramount. Educational materials should communicate the diverse roles zinc plays in the body, emphasizing its involvement in critical processes. Clear messaging can be delivered through community outreach, pamphlets, and school curriculum. Additionally, mass media can reach wider audiences. Empowering informed dietary choices is essential (Dsouza, 2023). Educational materials should highlight various zinc-rich food sources, categorized by local accessibility and affordability (Rizwan et al., 2022).

Animal products like red meat, poultry, seafood, and dairy should be emphasized due to their high bio-availability. However, recognizing limitations in LMICs, the focus should extend to plant-based sources like legumes, nuts, and seeds (Mariotti, 2023). Techniques to improve zinc absorption from these sources, such as soaking and sprouting, can be included . Educational initiatives should not solely focus on identifying zinc-rich foods but also aim to promote dietary diversification (Berti & Socha, 2023). Communities can be empowered to cultivate home gardens or participate in Community Supported Agriculture practices to increase access to a wider array of fresh produce, potentially contributing to a more balanced and zinc-sufficient diet. The success of these initiatives relies on empowering change agents within communities, such as health workers or educators. These individuals can be trained to translate scientific knowledge into locally relevant messages for behaviour modification. Educational initiatives can create a sustainable future for ZnD management in LMICs.

- **Non-Dietary Strategies for Enhanced Zinc Intake**

Control of Diarrhoeal Diseases

Frequent diarrhoea, a common issue in developing regions, can significantly hinder zinc absorption. Implementing strategies to improve sanitation, hygiene practices, and access to clean water can reduce diarrhoea episodes and improve zinc status.

Management of Underlying Medical Conditions

Certain medical conditions, such as chronic inflammatory bowel disease and sickle cell disease, can impair zinc absorption. Effective management of these conditions can improve zinc utilization.

Alcohol Dependence

Excessive alcohol consumption can interfere with zinc absorption and increase its excretion. Addressing alcohol dependence can be crucial for improving zinc status in affected individuals (Tadokoro et al., 2023).

Improving Maternal and Child Health Practices

Promoting exclusive breastfeeding for the first 6 months of life, followed by the introduction of zinc-rich complementary foods, is essential for ensuring adequate zinc intake in infants and young children (Berti & Socha, 2023).

5. KNOWLEDGE GAP AND PUBLIC HEALTH NEED

While the public health burden of zinc deficiency (ZnD) in developing countries is clear (Mao et al., 2024), several key knowledge gaps limit the development of efficient interventions:

- **Sub-population Vulnerability:** We know children, pregnant women, and those with chronic illnesses are at high risk. However, more precise data on ZnD prevalence across demographics and socioeconomic groups is crucial for targeted treatments (Mao et al., 2024).
- **Beyond Food Intake:** Factors influencing ZnD beyond diet, such as enteric infections and genetic variations in zinc absorption, need further investigation (Palmer et al., 2024).
- **Intervention Effectiveness:** Dietary diversification with bio-available zinc sources (animal protein, nuts, legumes) is a cornerstone strategy. However, research is needed on its practicality and sustainability in resource-limited settings.

Existing interventions, such as dietary diversification and supplementation programs, have shown promise in mitigating ZnD. However, their effectiveness can be limited by factors like poverty, access to diverse foods, and underlying health conditions (McClements et al., 2023). This highlights the need for a comprehensive approach that tackles ZnD from multiple angles.

6. FUTURE PERSPECTIVE AND CHALLENGES

The fight against zinc deficiency (ZnD) in developing countries requires a forward-looking approach that anticipates future challenges and harnesses emerging opportunities. While significant progress has been made in understanding the causes and consequences of ZnD, several key areas warrant further exploration and action.

Technological Advancements: The advent of innovative technologies like CRISPR-Cas9 gene editing holds immense promise for developing biofortified crops with enhanced zinc content and bioavailability. By precisely targeting and modifying genes involved in zinc uptake and transport within plants, scientists can create staple food crops that deliver higher levels of absorbable zinc to consumers. This approach offers a sustainable and scalable solution to address dietary zinc inadequacy, particularly in regions where access to diverse food sources is limited. Additionally, nanotechnology presents exciting possibilities for developing novel zinc delivery systems that improve absorption and utilization. Nanoparticles can encapsulate zinc, protecting it from degradation in the digestive tract and enhancing its uptake in the intestines. This targeted delivery approach could improve the efficacy of zinc supplementation programs and reduce the required dosage, making them more cost-effective and accessible.

Stakeholder Collaboration: The fight against ZnD necessitates a concerted effort from various stakeholders, including governments, international organizations, NGOs, and the private sector. Governments play a crucial role in creating an enabling environment for addressing ZnD through policy development and resource allocation. International organizations like the World Health Organization and UNICEF can provide technical expertise, advocacy, and financial support for ZnD interventions. NGOs can play a vital role in community engagement, education, and program implementation at the grassroots level. The private sector, including food manufacturers and agricultural companies, can contribute to ZnD mitigation through fortification initiatives and the development of innovative food products with enhanced zinc content. Effective collaboration and coordination among these stakeholders are essential to ensure the successful implementation and scaling up of ZnD interventions.

Policy Interventions: Policy changes are crucial to create a supportive framework for addressing ZnD. Governments need to strengthen food fortification programs by mandating the addition of zinc to staple foods like wheat flour, rice, and salt. Regulations should also be established to ensure the quality and safety of zinc supplements, particularly in informal markets. Promoting dietary diversification through agricultural policies and nutrition education campaigns can further contribute to improving zinc intake. These policies should focus on increasing the production and accessibility of zinc-rich foods, such as animal-source protein, legumes, nuts, and seeds.

Addressing Challenges and Barriers: Despite the promising potential of various interventions, several challenges and barriers hinder the effective mitigation of ZnD. Limited resources, logistical constraints, cultural barriers, and lack of political will can impede the implementation and scaling up of ZnD programs. Addressing these challenges requires innovative approaches and sustained commitment from all stakeholders. Community-based interventions that empower local communities to take ownership of ZnD mitigation efforts can be particularly effective. Leveraging existing healthcare and social welfare programs to integrate ZnD interventions can also enhance their reach and sustainability.

7. CONCLUSION

In conclusion, the future of ZnD mitigation lies in a multi-pronged approach that combines technological advancements, stakeholder collaboration, policy interventions, and community engagement. By addressing the challenges and harnessing the opportunities, we can strive towards a future where ZnD is no longer a major public health concern in developing countries. This will require a sustained commitment from all stakeholders to prioritize ZnD prevention and treatment, invest in research and innovation, and create an enabling environment for sustainable solutions. The ultimate goal is to ensure that every individual, regardless of their socioeconomic status or geographic location, has access to adequate zinc nutrition, leading to improved health, well-being, and human development.

ACKNOWLEDGMENT

The authors gratefully acknowledge DST-CURIE, Department of Science and Technology, New Delhi for financial support through sanction number DST/CURIE-PG/2022/10 (G).

REFERENCES

Abolurin, O. O., Oyelami, O. A., & Oseni, S. B. (2020). A comparative study of the prevalence of zinc deficiency among children with acute diarrhoea in SouthWestern Nigeria. *African Health Sciences, 20*(1), 406–412. DOI: 10.4314/ahs.v20i1.47 PMID: 33402929

Agedew, E., Tsegaye, B., Bante, A., Zerihun, E., Aklilu, A., Girma, M., Kerebih, H., Wale, M. Z., & Yirsaw, M. T. (2022). Zinc deficiency and associated factors among pregnant women's attending antenatal clinics in public health facilities of Konso Zone, Southern Ethiopia. *PLoS ONE, 17*(7 July), 1–12. https://doi.org/.DOI: 10.1371/journal.pone.0270971

Ahsan, A. K., Tebha, S. S., Sangi, R., Kamran, A., Zaidi, Z. A., Haque, T., & Ali Hamza, M. S. (2021). Zinc Micronutrient Deficiency and Its Prevalence in Malnourished Pediatric Children as Compared to Well-Nourished Children: A Nutritional Emergency. *Global Pediatric Health, 8*, 22–23. DOI: 10.1177/2333794X211050316 PMID: 34660849

Aiqing, Z., Zhang, L., Ning, P., Chen, Q., Wang, B., Zhang, F., Yang, X., & Zhang, Y. (2022). Zinc in cereal grains: Concentration, distribution, speciation, bioavailability, and barriers to transport from roots to grains in wheat. *Critical Reviews in Food Science and Nutrition, 62*(28), 7917–7928. DOI: 10.1080/10408398.2021.1920883 PMID: 34224281

Almendros, P., González, D., Fernández, M. D., García-Gomez, C., & Obrador, A. (2022). Both Zn biofortification and nutrient distribution pattern in cherry tomato plants are influenced by the application of ZnO nanofertilizer. *Heliyon, 8*(3), e09130. Advance online publication. DOI: 10.1016/j.heliyon.2022.e09130 PMID: 35846478

Arafsha, S. M., Aslam, M. F., Ellis, P. R., Latunde-Dada, G. O., & Sharp, P. A. (2023). Strategies to increase the bio-accessibility and bio-availability of iron and zinc from cereal products. *Proceedings of the Nutrition Society,* 1-7. DOI: 10.1017/S0029665123003543

Aziz, J., Rahman, M. T., & Vaithilingam, R. D. (2021). Dysregulation of metallothionein and zinc aggravates periodontal diseases. *Journal of Trace Elements in Medicine and Biology, 66*, 126754. DOI: 10.1016/j.jtemb.2021.126754 PMID: 33831799

Baarz, B. R., & Rink, L. (2022). Rebalancing the unbalanced aged immune system–A special focus on zinc. *Ageing Research Reviews, 74*, 101541. DOI: 10.1016/j.arr.2021.101541 PMID: 34915196

Berendsen, A. A. M., Kramer, C. S., & de Groot, L. C. P. G. M. (2019). The Newly Developed Elderly Nutrient-Rich Food Score Is a Useful Tool to Assess Nutrient Density in European Older Adults. *Frontiers in Nutrition, 6*(August), 1–14. DOI: 10.3389/fnut.2019.00119 PMID: 31457017

Berti, C., & Socha, P. (2023). Infant and Young Child Feeding Practices and Health. *Nutrients, 15*(5), 1184. DOI: 10.3390/nu15051184 PMID: 36904182

Bhantana, P., Moussa, M. G., Malla, R., Khadka, D., Vista, S. P., Shrestha, R. K., & Hu, C. X. (2022). Foliar versus soil biofortification of Zn in citrus (citrus reticulata Blanco) effect on mineral nutrition and fruit yield and quality. *Biomedical Journal of Scientific & Technical Research, 41*(3), 32755–32568. DOI: 10.26717/BJSTR.2022.41.006612

Bloom, A., Bloom, S., Silva, H., Nicoll, A. J., & Sawhney, R. (2021). Zinc supplementation and its benefits in the management of chronic liver disease: An in-depth literature review. *Annals of Hepatology, 25*, 100549. DOI: 10.1016/j.aohep.2021.100549 PMID: 34614431

Bouranis, D. L., & Chorianopoulou, S. N. (2023). Foliar Application of Sulfur-Containing Compounds—Pros and Cons. *Plants, 12*(22), 3794. DOI: 10.3390/plants12223794 PMID: 38005690

Brion, L. P., Heyne, R., Steven Brown, L., Lair, C. S., Edwards, A., Burchfield, P. J., & Caraig, M. (2020). Zinc deficiency limiting head growth to discharge in extremely low gestational age infants with insufficient linear growth: A cohort study. *Journal of Perinatology, 40*(11), 1694–1704. DOI: 10.1038/s41372-020-00778-w PMID: 32788617

Chen, B., Yu, P., Chan, W. N., Xie, F., Zhang, Y., Liang, L., Leung, K. T., Lo, K. W., Yu, J., Tse, G. M. K., Kang, W., & To, K. F. (2024). Cellular zinc metabolism and zinc signaling: From biological functions to diseases and therapeutic targets. *Signal Transduction and Targeted Therapy, 9*(1), 6. DOI: 10.1038/s41392-023-01679-y PMID: 38169461

Chitekwe, S., Parajuli, K. R., Paudyal, N., Haag, K. C., Renzaho, A., Issaka, A., & Agho, K. (2022). Individual, household and national factors associated with iron, vitamin A and zinc deficiencies among children aged 6–59 months in Nepal. *Maternal and Child Nutrition, 18*(S1), 1–11. DOI: 10.1111/mcn.13305 PMID: 34897980

Cunha, T. A., Vermeulen-Serpa, K. M., Grilo, E. C., Leite-Lais, L., Brandão-Neto, J., & Vale, S. H. (2022). Association between zinc and body composition: An integrative review. *Journal of Trace Elements in Medicine and Biology, 71*, 126940. DOI: 10.1016/j.jtemb.2022.126940 PMID: 35121408

Dhanyalakshmi, K. H., Mohan, R., Behera, S., Jha, U. C., Moharana, D., Behera, A., & Beena, R. (2024). Next Generation Nutrition: Genomic and Molecular Breeding Innovations for Iron and Zinc Biofortification in Rice. *Rice Science, 31*(5), 526–544. Advance online publication. DOI: 10.1016/j.rsci.2024.04.008

Djoumessi, Y. F. (2022). The impact of malnutrition on infant mortality and life expectancy in Africa. *Nutrition (Burbank, Los Angeles County, Calif.), 103*, 111760. DOI: 10.1016/j.nut.2022.111760 PMID: 35843043

Dsouza, M. B. P.Mrs Barthalomea Prathibha Dsouza. (2023). A Study On The Health And Nutrition Education For Teenagers. [IJMR]. *EPRA International Journal of Multidisciplinary Research, 9*(9), 68–71. DOI: 10.36713/epra14326

Duan, M., Li, T., Liu, B., Yin, S., Zang, J., Lv, C., Zhao, G., & Zhang, T. (2023). Zinc nutrition and dietary zinc supplements. *Critical Reviews in Food Science and Nutrition, 63*(9), 1277–1292. DOI: 10.1080/10408398.2021.1963664 PMID: 34382897

Dumrongwongsiri, O., Chongviriyaphan, N., Chatvutinun, S., Phoonlabdacha, P., Sangcakul, A., Siripinyanond, A., & Suthutvoravut, U. (2021). Dietary intake and milk micro-nutrient levels in lactating women with full and partial breastfeeding. *Maternal and Child Health Journal, 25*(6), 991–997. DOI: 10.1007/s10995-020-03049-4 PMID: 33230681

Frittelli, A., Botticella, E., Palombieri, S., Masci, S., Celletti, S., Fontanella, M. C., Astolfi, S., De Vita, P., Volpato, M., & Sestili, F. (2023). The suppression of TdMRP3 genes reduces the phytic acid and increases the nutrient accumulation in durum wheat grain. *Frontiers in Plant Science, 14*, 1079559. DOI: 10.3389/fpls.2023.1079559 PMID: 36743506

Gohari, H., Khajavian, N., Mahmoudian, A., & Bilandi, R. R. (2023). Copper and zinc deficiency to the risk of preterm labor in pregnant women: A case-control study. *BMC Pregnancy and Childbirth, 23*(1), 366. DOI: 10.1186/s12884-023-05625-2 PMID: 37208743

Gowda, N. N., Siliveru, K., Prasad, P. V., Bhatt, Y., Netravati, B. P., & Gurikar, C. (2022). Modern processing of Indian millets: A perspective on changes in nutritional properties. *Foods*, *11*(4), 499. DOI: 10.3390/foods11040499 PMID: 35205975

Goyena, E. A., Maniego, M. L. V., Ducay, A. J. D., Musa, M. C. A., & Angeles-Agdeppa, I. (2021). Dietary zinc intake and the underlying factors of serum zinc deficiency among preschool children in the Philippines. *Philippine Journal of Science*, *150*(3), 799–812. DOI: 10.56899/150.03.16

Gupta, S., Brazier, A. K. M., & Lowe, N. M. (2020). Zinc deficiency in low-and middle-income countries: Prevalence and approaches for mitigation. *Journal of Human Nutrition and Dietetics*, *33*(5), 624–643. DOI: 10.1111/jhn.12791 PMID: 32627912

Hall, A. G., & King, J. C. (2022). Zinc Fortification: Current Trends and Strategies. *Nutrients*, *14*(19), 1–16. DOI: 10.3390/nu14193895 PMID: 36235548

Han, S. M., Devaraj, S., Derraik, J. G., Vickers, M. H., Huang, F., Dubascoux, S., Godfrey, K. M., Chan, S.-Y., Pang, W. W., Thakkar, S. K., & Cutfield, W. S. (2023). A nutritional supplement containing zinc during preconception and pregnancy increases human milk zinc concentrations. *Frontiers in Nutrition*, *9*, 1034828. DOI: 10.3389/fnut.2022.1034828 PMID: 36704795

Harrington, S. A., Connorton, J. M., Nyangoma, N. I., McNelly, R., Morgan, Y. M., Aslam, M. F., Sharp, P. A., Johnson, A. A. T., Uauy, C., & Balk, J. (2023). A two-gene strategy increases iron and zinc concentrations in wheat flour, improving mineral bioaccessibility. *Plant Physiology*, *191*(1), 528–541. DOI: 10.1093/plphys/kiac499 PMID: 36308454

Hatch-McChesney, A., & Smith, T. J. (2023). Nutrition, immune function, and infectious disease in military personnel: A narrative review. *Nutrients*, *15*(23), 4999. DOI: 10.3390/nu15234999 PMID: 38068857

Hina, A., Abbasi, A., Imtiaz, S., Ul Haq, I., Ul Hassan, A., & Chaudhry, A. (2023). General Aspects of Genetic Improvement (Traditional and Transgenic Methods) Aiming to Food Biofortification. In *Legumes Biofortification* (pp. 73–109). Springer International Publishing., DOI: 10.1007/978-3-031-33957-8_4

Hoque, M., Emon, K., Malo, P. C., Hossain, M. H., Tannu, S. I., & Roshed, M. M. (2023). Comprehensive guide to vitamin and mineral sources with their requirements. *Indiana Journal of Agriculture and Life Sciences*, *3*(6), 23–31. DOI: 10.5281/zenodo.10284736

Huang, S., Sasaki, A., Yamaji, N., Okada, H., Mitani-Ueno, N., & Ma, J. F. (2020). The ZIP transporter family member OsZIP9 contributes to root zinc uptake in rice under zinc-limited conditions. *Plant Physiology*, *183*(3), 1224–1234. DOI: 10.1104/pp.20.00125 PMID: 32371522

Hussain, A., Jiang, W., Wang, X., Shahid, S., Saba, N., Ahmad, M., Dar, A., Masood, S. U., Imran, M., & Mustafa, A. (2022, March 9). 11 Wang X, Shahid S, Saba N, Ahmad M, Dar A, Masood SU, Imran M, Mustafa A. Mechanistic impact of zinc deficiency in human development. *Frontiers in Nutrition*, *9*, 717064. DOI: 10.3389/fnut.2022.717064 PMID: 35356730

Ibrahim, S., Saleem, B., Rehman, N., Zafar, S. A., Naeem, M. K., & Khan, M. R. (2022). CRISPR/Cas9 mediated disruption of Inositol Pentakisphosphate 2-Kinase 1 (TaIPK1) reduces phytic acid and improves iron and zinc accumulation in wheat grains. *Journal of Advanced Research*, *37*, 33–41. DOI: 10.1016/j.jare.2021.07.006 PMID: 35499048

Jindal, A. (2023). Zinc enrichment strategies in legumes and cereals: Assessing current advancements and future prospects. *The Pharma Innovation Journal*, *12*(8), 935–944.

Katimba, H. A., Wang, R., Cheng, C., Zhang, Y., Lu, W., & Ma, Y. (2024). Zinc Absorption & Homeostasis in the Human Body: A General Overview. *Food Reviews International*, *40*(2), 715–739. DOI: 10.1080/87559129.2023.2195188

Kemp, J. F., Hambidge, K. M., Westcott, J. L., Ali, S. A., Saleem, S., Garcés, A., Figueroa, L., Somannavar, M. S., Goudar, S. S., Long, J. M., Hendricks, A. E., Krebs, N. F., Dhaded, S. M., Vernekar, S. S., Herekar, V. R., Yogeshkumar, S., McClure, E. M., Das, A., Thorsten, V. R., & Koso-Thomas, M. W. (2024). Zinc supplementation initiated prior to or during pregnancy modestly impacted maternal status and high prevalence of hypozincemia in pregnancy and lactation: The Women First Preconception Maternal Nutrition Trial. *The Journal of Nutrition*, *154*(6), 1917–1926. Advance online publication. DOI: 10.1016/j.tjnut.2024.04.018 PMID: 38621624

Khan, S. T., Malik, A., Alwarthan, A., & Shaik, M. R. (2022). The enormity of the zinc deficiency problem and available solutions; an overview. *Arabian Journal of Chemistry*, *15*(3), 103668. DOI: 10.1016/j.arabjc.2021.103668

Kloubert, V., Wessels, I., Wolf, J., Blaabjerg, K., Janssens, V., Hapala, J., Wagner, W., & Rink, L. (2021). Zinc deficiency leads to reduced interleukin-2 production by active gene silencing due to enhanced CREMα expression in T cells. *Clinical Nutrition (Edinburgh, Lothian)*, *40*(5), 3263–3278. DOI: 10.1016/j.clnu.2020.10.052 PMID: 33183881

Knez, M., & Stangoulis, J. C. (2023). Dietary Zn deficiency, the current situation and potential solutions. *Nutrition Research Reviews*, *36*(2), 199–215. DOI: 10.1017/S0954422421000342 PMID: 37062532

Kottala, S. Y., & Sahu, A. K. (2023). Evaluating ergonomics and financial distress in manufacturing organization behavior: Resiliency framework from operations and strategic management. *The Learning Organization*. Advance online publication. DOI: 10.1108/TLO-03-2023-0041

Kumar, A., Kerketta, A., Dewali, S., Sharma, N., Kumari Panda, A., & Singh Bisht, S. (2023). Tackling Hidden Hunger: Understanding Micronutrient Deficiency and Effective Mitigation Strategies. In *Emerging Solutions in Sustainable Food and Nutrition Security* (pp. 305–319). Springer International Publishing., DOI: 10.1007/978-3-031-40908-0_12

Lei, G. J., Yamaji, N., & Ma, J. F. (2021). Two metallothionein genes highly expressed in rice nodes are involved in distribution of Zn to the grain. *The New Phytologist*, *229*(2), 1007–1020. DOI: 10.1111/nph.16860 PMID: 32772382

Li, X., Yadav, R., & Siddique, K. H. (2020). Neglected and underutilized crop species: The key to improving dietary diversity and fighting hunger and malnutrition in Asia and the Pacific. *Frontiers in Nutrition*, *7*, 593711. DOI: 10.3389/fnut.2020.593711 PMID: 33330593

Loechl, C. U., Datta-Mitra, A., Fenlason, L., Green, R., Hackl, L., Itzkowitz, L., Koso-Thomas, M., Moorthy, D., Owino, V. O., Pachón, H., Stoffel, N., Zimmerman, M. B., & Raiten, D. J. (2023). Approaches to address the anemia challenge. *The Journal of Nutrition*, *153*, S42–S59. DOI: 10.1016/j.tjnut.2023.07.017 PMID: 37714779

Lopes-Pires, M. E., Ahmed, N. S., Vara, D., Gibbins, J. M., Pula, G., & Pugh, N. (2021). Zinc regulates reactive oxygen species generation in platelets. *Platelets*, *32*(3), 368–377. DOI: 10.1080/09537104.2020.1742311 PMID: 32248725

Lowe, N. M., Hall, A. G., Broadley, M. R., Foley, J., Boy, E., & Bhutta, Z. A. (2024). Preventing and controlling zinc deficiency across the life course: A call to action. *Advances in Nutrition*, *100181*(3), 100181. Advance online publication. DOI: 10.1016/j.advnut.2024.100181 PMID: 38280724

Ludwig, Y., Dueñas, C.Jr, Arcillas, E., Macalalad-Cabral, R. J., Kohli, A., Reinke, R., & Slamet-Loedin, I. H. (2024). CRISPR-mediated promoter editing of a cis-regulatory element of OsNAS2 increases Zn uptake/translocation and plant yield in rice. *Frontiers in Genome Editing*, *5*, 1308228. DOI: 10.3389/fgeed.2023.1308228 PMID: 38322756

Ma, Y., Wen, Y., Wang, C., Wu, Z., Yuan, X., Xiong, Y., Chen, K., He, L., Zhang, Y., Wang, Z., Li, L., Yang, Z., Sun, Y., Chen, Z., & Ma, J. (2023). ZIP genes are involved in the retransfer of zinc ions during the senescence of zinc-deficient rice leaves. *International Journal of Molecular Sciences*, *24*(18), 13989. DOI: 10.3390/ijms241813989 PMID: 37762290

Mao, C., Shen, Z., Long, D., Liu, M., Xu, X., Gao, X., Lin, Y., & Wang, X. (2024). Epidemiological study of paediatric nutritional deficiencies: An analysis from the global burden of disease study 2019. *Nutrition Journal*, *23*(1), 44. DOI: 10.1186/s12937-024-00945-1 PMID: 38637763

Mariotti, F. (2023). Nutritional and health benefits and risks of plant-based substitute foods. *Proceedings of the Nutrition Society*, 1-14.DOI: 10.1017/S0029665123004767

Maywald, M., & Rink, L. (2022). Zinc in Human Health and Infectious Diseases. *Biomolecules*, *12*(12), 1748. Advance online publication. DOI: 10.3390/biom12121748 PMID: 36551176

Mcdonald, C. M., Suchdev, P. S., Krebs, N. F., Hess, S. Y., Wessells, K. R., Ismaily, S., Rahman, S., Wieringa, F. T., Williams, A. M., Brown, K. H., & King, J. C. (2020). Adjusting plasma or serum zinc concentrations for inflammation: Biomarkers Reflecting Inflammation and Nutritional Determinants of Anaemia (BRINDA) project. *The American Journal of Clinical Nutrition*, *111*(4), 927–937. DOI: 10.1093/ajcn/nqz304 PMID: 32266402

Mertens, A., Benjamin-Chung, J., Colford, J. M.Jr, Coyle, J., Van der Laan, M. J., Hubbard, A. E., & Arnold, B. F. (2023). Causes and consequences of child growth faltering in low-resource settings. *Nature*, *621*(7979), 568–576. DOI: 10.1038/s41586-023-06501-x PMID: 37704722

Nolla, N. P., Sop, M. M. K., Mananga, M. J., & Gouado, I. (2021). Nutrition Education of Mothers and Zinc Supplementation among Children in the Rural Community, Cameroon. *European Journal of Nutrition & Food Safety*, *13*(1), 59–69. DOI: 10.9734/ejnfs/2021/v13i130348

Obeagu, E. I., Ubosi, N. I., & Uzoma, G. (2023). Antioxidant Supplementation in Pregnancy: Effects on Maternal and Infant Health. *Int. J. Adv. Multidiscip. Res*, *10*(11), 60–70.

Ozturk, H., Niazi, P., Mansoor, M., Monib, A. W., Alikhail, M., & Azizi, A. (2023). The function of zinc in animal, plant, and human nutrition. *Journal for Research in Applied Sciences and Biotechnology*, *2*(2), 35–43. DOI: 10.55544/jrasb.2.2.6

Pajarillo, E. A. B., Lee, E., & Kang, D. K. (2021). Trace metals and animal health: Interplay of the gut microbiota with iron, manganese, zinc, and copper. *Animal Nutrition*, *7*(3), 750–761. DOI: 10.1016/j.aninu.2021.03.005 PMID: 34466679

Palmer, A. C., Bedsaul-Fryer, J. R., & Stephensen, C. B. (2024). Interactions of Nutrition and Infection: The Role of Micronutrient Deficiencies in the Immune Response to Pathogens and Implications for Child Health. *Annual Review of Nutrition*, *44*(1), 99–124. Advance online publication. DOI: 10.1146/annurev-nutr-062122-014910 PMID: 38724105

Patil, R., Sontakke, T., Biradar, A., & Nalage, D. (2023). Zinc: An essential trace element for human health and beyond. *Food Health*, *5*(3), 13. DOI: 10.53388/FH2023013

Pellinen, T., Päivärinta, E., Isotalo, J., Lehtovirta, M., Itkonen, S. T., Korkalo, L., & Pajari, A. M. (2022). Replacing dietary animal-source proteins with plant-source proteins changes dietary intake and status of vitamins and minerals in healthy adults: A 12-week randomized controlled trial. *European Journal of Nutrition*, •••, 1–14. PMID: 34837522

Praharaj, S., Skalicky, M., Maitra, S., Bhadra, P., Shankar, T., Brestic, M., Hejnak, V., Vachova, P., & Hossain, A. (2021). Zinc biofortification in food crops could alleviate the zinc malnutrition in human health. *Molecules (Basel, Switzerland)*, *26*(12), 3509. DOI: 10.3390/molecules26123509 PMID: 34207649

Prasad, A. S. (2013). Discovery of human zinc deficiency: Its impact on human health and disease. *Advances in Nutrition*, *4*(2), 176–190. DOI: 10.3945/an.112.003210 PMID: 23493534

Prasad, A. S. (2020). Lessons learned from experimental human model of zinc deficiency. *Journal of Immunology Research*, *2020*, 1–12. Advance online publication. DOI: 10.1155/2020/9207279 PMID: 32411807

Prashanth, G. P., & Hegde, D. G. (2023). Zinc Prophylaxis to Reduce Mortality and Morbidity in Under-5 Children: Clinical and Global Health Points of View. Global Pediatric Health, 10, 2333794X231156043. https://doi.org/DOI: 10.1177/2333794X23115604

Pujiastuti, I. T., Deliana, M., Mutiara, E., & Lubis, M. (2018). Effect of zinc supplementation on linear growth velocity of children with short stature. In *Stem Cell Oncology* (pp. 321–324). CRC Press. DOI: 10.1201/9781351190152-68

Rai, D., Chaudhary, C., Khatak, A., & Banyal, S. (2024). A Sustainable Approach to Combat Micronutrient Deficiencies and Ensure Global Food Security through Biofortification. *European Journal of Nutrition & Food Safety*, *16*(4), 15–30. DOI: 10.9734/ejnfs/2024/v16i41404

Rizwan, M., Abbas, A., Xu, H., Ahmed, U. I., Qing, P., He, P., Iqbal, M. A., & Shahzad, M. A. (2022). Role of nutrition information in acceptance and willingness to pay for biofortified cereal food: Implications for better health and sustainable diet. *Nutrients*, *14*(16), 3352. DOI: 10.3390/nu14163352 PMID: 36014858

Sangeetha, V. J., Dutta, S., Moses, J. A., & Anandharamakrishnan, C. (2022). Zinc nutrition and human health: Overview and implications. *eFood*, *3*(5), e17. Advance online publication. DOI: 10.1002/efd2.17

Sanusi, K. O., Ibrahim, K. G., Abubakar, B., Malami, I., Bello, M. B., Imam, M. U., & Abubakar, M. B. (2021). Effect of maternal zinc deficiency on offspring health: The epigenetic impact. Journal of Trace Elements in Medicine and Biology, 65(October 2020), 126731. .DOI: 10.1016/j.jtemb.2021.126731

Searle, T., Ali, F. R., & Al-Niaimi, F. (2022). Zinc in dermatology. *The Journal of Dermatological Treatment*, *33*(5), 2455–2458. DOI: 10.1080/09546634.2022.2062282 PMID: 35437093

Seifi, N., Bahari, H., Ghiasi Hafezi, S., Ghotbani, F., Afzalinia, A., Ferns, G. A., Farkhani, E. M., & Ghayour-mobarhan, M. (2024). Dietary mineral intakes predict Coronavirus-disease 2019 (COVID-19) incidence and hospitalization in older adults. *BMC Nutrition*, *10*(1), 1–8. DOI: 10.1186/s40795-024-00821-5 PMID: 38439106

Semba, R. D., Ramsing, R., Rahman, N., Kraemer, K., & Bloem, M. W. (2021). Legumes as a sustainable source of protein in human diets. Global Food Security, 28(June 2020), 100520. DOI: 10.1016/j.gfs.2021.100520

Shankar, A. H. (2020). Mineral deficiencies. In *Hunter's Tropical Medicine and Emerging Infectious Diseases* (pp. 1048–1054). Elsevier., DOI: 10.1016/B978-0-323-55512-8.00145-9

Siddiqui, F. J., Belayneh, G., & Bhutta, Z. A. (2021). Nutrition and diarrheal disease and enteric pathogens. *Nutrition and infectious diseases: Shifting the clinical paradigm*, 219-241..DOI: 10.1007/978-3-030-56913-6_8

Singh, A., Rajput, V. D., Pandey, D., Sharma, R., Ghazaryan, K., & Minkina, T. (2023). Nano Zinc-Enabled Strategies in Crops for Combatting Zinc Malnutrition in Human Health. *Frontiers in Bioscience (Landmark Edition)*, *28*(8), 158. DOI: 10.31083/j.fbl2808158 PMID: 37664935

Singh, P., & Prasad, S. (2023). A review on iron, zinc and calcium biological significance and factors affecting their absorption and bioavailability. *Journal of Food Composition and Analysis, 123*, 105529. DOI: 10.1016/j.jfca.2023.105529

Singh, P., & Prasad, S. (2023). A review on iron, zinc and calcium biological significance and factors affecting their absorption and bioavailability. *Journal of Food Composition and Analysis, 105529*, 105529. Advance online publication. DOI: 10.1016/j.jfca.2023.105529

Skalny, A. V., Aschner, M., & Tinkov, A. A. (2021). Zinc. *Advances in Food and Nutrition Research, 96*, 251–310. DOI: 10.1016/bs.afnr.2021.01.003 PMID: 34112355

Skalny, A. V., Sotnikova, T. I., Korobeynikova, T. V., & Tinkov, A. A. (2022). Significance of zinc deficiency correction for practical medicine: A review. *Sechenov Medical Journal, 13*(4), 4–17. DOI: 10.47093/2218-7332.2022.13.4.4-17

Stiles, L. I., Ferrao, K., & Mehta, K. J. (2024). Role of zinc in health and disease. *Clinical and Experimental Medicine, 24*(1), 38. Advance online publication. DOI: 10.1007/s10238-024-01302-6 PMID: 38367035

Tadokoro, T., Morishita, A., Himoto, T., & Masaki, T. (2023). Nutritional support for alcoholic liver disease. *Nutrients, 15*(6), 1360. DOI: 10.3390/nu15061360 PMID: 36986091

Tan, L., Qu, M., Zhu, Y., Peng, C., Wang, J., Gao, D., & Chen, C. (2020). ZINC TRANSPORTER5 and ZINC TRANSPORTER9 function synergistically in zinc/cadmium uptake. *Plant Physiology, 183*(3), 1235–1249. DOI: 10.1104/pp.19.01569 PMID: 32341004

Tarini, A., Manger, M. S., Brown, K. H., Mbuya, M. N., Rowe, L. A., Grant, F., Black, R. E., & McDonald, C. M. (2021). Enablers and barriers of zinc fortification; experience from 10 low-and middle-income countries with mandatory large-scale food fortification. *Nutrients, 13*(6), 2051. DOI: 10.3390/nu13062051 PMID: 34203987

TRIPATHI. P. (2024). Food Nutrition in Human Science. Blue Rose Publishers.

USDA Food data Central. https://fdc.nal.usda.gov/fdc-app.html#/food-search?component=1095

Van Der Straeten, D., Bhullar, N. K., De Steur, H., Gruissem, W., MacKenzie, D., Pfeiffer, W., Qaim, M., Slamet-Loedin, I., Strobbe, S., Tohme, J., Trijatmiko, K. R., Vanderschuren, H., Van Montagu, M., Zhang, C., & Bouis, H. (2020). Multiplying the efficiency and impact of biofortification through metabolic engineering. *Nature Communications, 11*(1), 1–10. DOI: 10.1038/s41467-020-19020-4 PMID: 33060603

Wessels, I., & Rink, L. (2020). Micronutrients in autoimmune diseases: Possible therapeutic benefits of zinc and vitamin D. *The Journal of Nutritional Biochemistry*, *77*, 108240. DOI: 10.1016/j.jnutbio.2019.108240 PMID: 31841960

Weyh, C., Krüger, K., Peeling, P., & Castell, L. (2022). The role of minerals in the optimal functioning of the immune system. *Nutrients*, *14*(3), 644. DOI: 10.3390/nu14030644 PMID: 35277003

Xu, J., Wang, X., Zhu, H., & Yu, F. (2021). Maize genotypes with different zinc efficiency in response to low zinc stress and heterogeneous zinc supply. *Frontiers in Plant Science*, *12*, 736658. DOI: 10.3389/fpls.2021.736658 PMID: 34691112

Yang, M., Li, Y., Liu, Z., Tian, J., Liang, L., Qiu, Y., Wang, G., Du, Q., Cheng, D., Cai, H., Shi, L., Xu, F., & Lian, X. (2020). A high activity zinc transporter OsZIP9 mediates zinc uptake in rice. *The Plant Journal*, *103*(5), 1695–1709. DOI: 10.1111/tpj.14855 PMID: 32449251

Yaqob, K. S. (2019). ZINC The Friendly and Forgotten Micronutrient. *Global Journal of Pediatrics & Neonatal Care*, *1*(3). Advance online publication. DOI: 10.33552/GJPNC.2019.01.000512

Yu, S. M., & Yu, M. M. (2023). Molecular mechanisms of wound healing: The role of zinc as an essential microelement. *Research Results in Pharmacology*, *9*(1), 25–40. DOI: 10.18413/rrpharmacology.9.10003

Zaman, Q. U., Aslam, Z., Yaseen, M., Ihsan, M. Z., Khaliq, A., Fahad, S., Bashir, S., Ramzani, P. M. A., & Naeem, M. (2018). Zinc biofortification in rice: Leveraging agriculture to moderate hidden hunger in developing countries. *Archives of Agronomy and Soil Science*, *64*(2), 147–161. DOI: 10.1080/03650340.2017.1338343

Zhang, Y. Y., Stockmann, R., Ng, K., & Ajlouni, S. (2022). Revisiting phytate-element interactions: Implications for iron, zinc and calcium bioavailability, with emphasis on legumes. *Critical Reviews in Food Science and Nutrition*, *62*(6), 1696–1712. DOI: 10.1080/10408398.2020.1846014 PMID: 33190514

Chapter 6
Zinc Supplementation: A Preventive Measure for Zinc Deficiency

Hrithik Dey
https://orcid.org/0009-0000-6196-1911
Lloyd Institute of Management and Technology, India

Surovi Paul
https://orcid.org/0009-0000-6972-331X
Lloyd Institute of Management and Technology, India

Meenakshi Kaira
Lloyd Institute of Management and Technology, India

ABSTRACT

Zinc, vital for growth, immunity, wound healing, and DNA synthesis, faces global deficiency issues, especially in regions with limited dietary diversity. About 17.3% of the world is at risk, with vulnerable groups including pregnant women and the elderly. Deficiency leads to growth impairment, weakened immunity, and increased infection susceptibility, affecting both physical and cognitive health. Supplementation, in forms like zinc gluconate and zinc citrate, is crucial, with dosages tailored to age groups. It aids growth, reduces respiratory infections' severity, and may alleviate common cold symptoms if taken early. In acute diarrhea, zinc can shorten illness duration, while in conditions like age-related macular degeneration (AMD) and Wilson's disease, it plays a vital role in management. However, excessive intake may cause adverse effects like gastrointestinal discomfort and copper deficiency. Zinc supplementation is essential for public health strategies to prevent deficiency and ensure overall well-being, particularly in high-risk populations.

DOI: 10.4018/979-8-3693-5355-4.ch006

INTRODUCTION

Zinc is an essential trace mineral that plays a fundamental role in numerous physiological processes within the human body. (Mozaffar et al., 2023) It is vital for overall health and well-being, participating in functions ranging from immune system support to DNA synthesis and wound healing. (Patil et al., 2023) Zinc is found in every cell and tissue in the body and is involved in the activity of over 300 enzymes, making it indispensable for various biochemical reactions. (S. R. Lee, 2018) Zinc deficiency can lead to a wide range of health issues affecting different physiological systems (Mozaffar et al., 2023) (as shown in *Figure 1*). Among these effects, immune system malfunction is the most common. It makes people more prone to bacterial, viral, and fungal infections, which frequently result in extended illness and a hampered recovery. (Read et al., 2019) Moreover, zinc deficiency hampers growth and development, especially during crucial stages like infancy and adolescence, when it can lead to growth retardation, developmental delays, and cognitive impairments. (El Din et al., 2019; Farias et al., 2020) Zinc deficiency is associated with impaired wound healing, which is characterized by delayed closure, increased risk of infection, and chronic wounds. This highlights the critical role zinc plays in collagen synthesis and tissue repair. (Molenda & Kolmas, 2023; Mozaffar et al., 2023) Dermatological manifestations include dermatitis, eczema, and acne, (Dhaliwal et al., 2020) alongside compromised vision marked by night blindness and impaired dark adaptation. (Serhan et al., 2022) The extensive effects of zinc deficiency are altered taste and smell perception, (Sevryugin et al., 2021) mental health disorders, (Shayganfard, 2022) bone health issues, (Amin et al., 2020) reproductive health issues, (Vickram et al., 2021), and links to chronic diseases like diabetes, (X. Wang et al., 2019) age-related macular degeneration, (Blasiak et al., 2020) and cardiovascular disease. (Mozaffar et al., 2023) Zinc supplements play a crucial role in addressing a myriad of health problems associated with zinc deficiency. (Takeda et al., 2018) Supporting immune function, zinc can help combat infections by ensuring optimal zinc levels in the body. For growth retardation and developmental delay, zinc facilitates healthy growth and cell proliferation. (Scrimgeour et al., 2011) Accelerating wound healing, zinc promotes tissue repair and collagen synthesis. (Jones & Williams, 2004) In managing dermatological issues, like dermatitis or acne, zinc regulates sebum production and reduces inflammation. (M. Gupta et al., 2014) For vision impairment, zinc supports retinal function and visual adaptation. (Bartlett & Eperjesi, 2003) Restoring taste and smell perception, zinc addresses sensory impairments. (Finzi & Harrington, 2021) Supporting mental health, zinc aids neurotransmitter regulation and cognitive function. (Cummings & Kovacic, 2009) Enhancing bone health, zinc citrate or zinc amino acid chelate promotes bone density and mineralization. (Upadhaya & Kim, 2020) Supporting reproductive health, zinc aids hormonal balance and fertility. (Allouche-Fitoussi & Breitbart, 2020) In managing chronic diseases like cardiovascular disease or diabetes, zinc mitigates disease progression by regulating inflammation and oxidative stress. (Foster & Samman, 2010) However, individual factors such as dosage, duration, and health status should be considered, and consultation with a healthcare professional is advisable for personalized supplementation recommendations (Walke et al., 2023).

Figure 1. Zinc deficiency symptoms

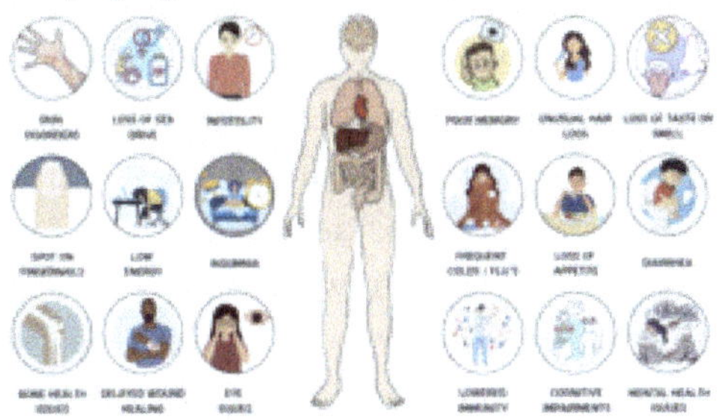

(Classen et al., 2011; Prasad, 2004)

Epidemiology Of Zinc Deficiency

Zinc is an essential trace element crucial for various physiological functions, including immune response, cellular growth, and DNA synthesis. (Stefanidou et al., 2006) Zinc deficiency is a significant public health issue, particularly in developing countries, (Hambidge & Krebs, 2007) and affects a wide range of populations due to various factors including dietary inadequacies, malabsorption, and increased physiological needs. (Mozaffar et al., 2023)

Prevalence and Global Distribution

Zinc deficiency is a significant global health issue, affecting millions of people across various regions and demographics. (Mozaffar et al., 2023) It is a widespread nutritional issue affecting various populations across the globe, with significant differences observed among countries and demographic groups. (Caulfield & Black, 2004) In India, from 2016 to 2018, the prevalence of zinc deficiency varied among different age groups: 18.9% in children aged 1-4 years, 16.8% in children aged 5-9 years, 28.4% in adolescent girls aged 10-19 years, and 35.1% in adolescent boys of the same age group. In Bangladesh, the data from 2011 to 2012 reveal extremely high prevalence rates, with 44.6% of children aged 6-59 months and

57.3% of non-pregnant, non-lactating women aged 15-49 years suffering from zinc deficiency. South Africa, in 2005, reported a 51% prevalence rate among children aged 1-3 years. Nigeria's 2001 data show that 20% of children under 60 months and 28.1% of mothers of these participating children are affected by zinc deficiency. In Pakistan, the 2011 data indicate that 36.5% of children aged 6-59 months, 41.6% of non-pregnant women aged 15-49 years, and 48.3% of pregnant women in the same age group suffer from zinc deficiency. In Mexico, 2006 data reveal varied prevalence rates: 26.6% among children aged 1-11 years, 33.8% in women over 20 years, 42.6% in men over 20 years, 28.1% in adolescent girls aged 12-19 years, and 24.5% in adolescent boys of the same age group. In Sri Lanka, 2012 data show a lower prevalence rate of 5.1% among children aged 6-59 months, while China, in 2013, reported a 4% prevalence among children aged 36-72 months. Kenya's 2011 data reveal alarmingly high rates of zinc deficiency: 81.6% among children aged 6-59 months, 79.9% among non-pregnant women aged 15-49 years, 67.9% among pregnant women in the same age group, and 77.4% among men aged 15-54 years. These statistics highlight the critical need for effective interventions to combat zinc deficiency worldwide (Mozaffar et al., 2023) (as shown in *Figure 2*).

Table 1. Prevalence rates of zinc deficiency in various population groups of various countries

Country	Year	Gender, Age group, Special population	% Prevalence
India	2016 - 2018	• Children (1-4 years) • Children (5-9 years) • Adolescent girls (10-19 years) • Adolescent boys (10-19 years)	18.9 16.8 28.4 35.1
Bangladesh	2011 – 2012	• Children (6-59 months) • Non-pregnant women (15-49 years)	44.6 57.3
South Africa	2005	• Children (1-3 years)	51
Nigeria	2001	• Children (<60 months) • Mother of participating children	20 28.1
Pakistan	2011	• Children (6-59 months) • Non-pregnant women (15-49 years) • Pregnant women (15-49 years)	36.5 41.6 48.3
Mexico	2006	• Children (1-11 years) • Women (>20 years) • Men (>20 years) • Adolescent girls (12-19 years) • Adolescent boys (12-19 years)	26.6 33.8 42.6 28.1 24.5
Sri-Lanka	2012	• Children (6-59 months)	5.1

continued on following page

Table 1. Continued

Country	Year	Gender, Age group, Special population	% Prevalence
China	2013	• Children (36-72 months)	4
Kenya	2011	• Children (6-59 months) • Non-pregnant women (15-49 years) • Pregnant women (15-49 years) • Men (15-54 years)	81.6 79.9 67.9 77.4

(Mozaffar et al., 2023)

Figure 2. Global distribution of zinc deficiency around the world 1990 v/s 2005

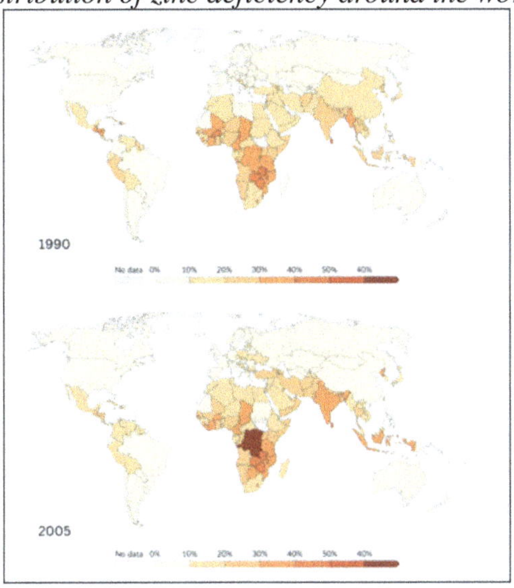

(Wessells & Brown, 2012)

Population Groups at Risk

Zinc deficiency is a prevalent nutritional issue affecting various population groups differently based on physiological, dietary, and socioeconomic factors. (Mozaffar et al., 2023) The groups most at risk include infants and young children, (Mozaffar et al., 2023) pregnant and lactating women, (Mozaffar et al., 2023) the elderly, (Kvamme et al., 2015) individuals with malabsorption syndromes, (Wapnir, 2000) populations with high-phytate diets, (Sandstead & Freeland-Graves, 2014) and those with chronic illnesses or specific lifestyles. (Kaur et al., 2014)

1. INFANTS AND YOUNG CHILDREN

Infants and young children are particularly vulnerable to zinc deficiency due to several interrelated factors. (Mozaffar et al., 2023) Rapid growth and development during infancy and early childhood significantly increase zinc requirements, making adequate intake crucial. (Mozaffar et al., 2023) During the first six months of life, infants rely heavily on breast milk for their zinc supply; (Butte et al., 2002) however, the concentration of zinc in breast milk decreases over time, especially if the mother's zinc status is marginal. (Dumrongwongsiri et al., 2015) As infants transition to solid foods, commonly used complementary foods such as cereals and plant-based purees often lack sufficient zinc and are high in phytates, compounds that inhibit zinc absorption. (Gibbs, 2010) This dietary inadequacy is further compounded by frequent infections like diarrhea, which not only increase zinc loss but also reduce zinc absorption. (Mozaffar et al., 2023) The health impacts of zinc deficiency in infants and young children are profound and multifaceted. (Hotz & Brown, 2004) Zinc is essential for immune function, and its deficiency can lead to a weakened immune system, making children more susceptible to infections such as pneumonia and diarrhea, which are major causes of morbidity and mortality in this age group. (Gombart et al., 2020) Moreover, zinc deficiency can impair growth, leading to stunted growth and reduced physical development. (Mozaffar et al., 2023) It also affects cognitive development, potentially resulting in delayed motor skills and cognitive impairments. (S. Bhatnagar & Taneja, 2001) Overall, zinc deficiency in early childhood can have lasting effects on health and development, emphasizing the importance of ensuring adequate zinc intake through appropriate dietary practices and public health interventions. (Gibson, 2006)

2. PREGNANT AND LACTATING WOMEN

Pregnant and lactating women are at heightened risk of zinc deficiency due to increased physiological demands and various dietary challenges. (Khayat et al., 2017) During pregnancy, the body's requirement for zinc escalates to support the rapid cell growth, immune function, and overall development of the fetus. (Grzeszczak et al., 2020) This increased demand continues into lactation, as zinc is crucial for milk production and maintaining the health of both mother and child. (Ackland & Michalczyk, 2016) Often, pregnant women may experience dietary restrictions due to nausea or cultural dietary practices, which can limit their intake of zinc-rich foods like meat, seafood, and dairy. (Zand et al., 2015) Additionally, zinc absorption can be impaired by high-phytate diets, common in many parts of the world where cereals and legumes are staples. (Gibson et al., 2018) The health impacts of zinc deficiency in pregnant and lactating women are significant. Insufficient zinc levels can lead to complications such as prolonged labor, preterm delivery, and low birth weight, which are associated with higher infant mortality and morbidity rates. (Kumari et al., 2022) For the mother, zinc deficiency can impair immune function, increasing susceptibility to infections (Calder & Jackson, 2000) and delaying wound healing postpartum. (Prasad, 1996) During lactation, inadequate zinc can affect the quality of breast milk, potentially compromising the infant's growth and immune development. (Erick, 2018; Krebs, 2013)

3. ELDERLY

Elderly individuals are particularly at risk for zinc deficiency due to a combination of dietary, physiological, and health-related factors. (Hotz & Brown, 2004) As people age, their dietary intake often decreases due to factors such as reduced appetite, difficulty chewing, and changes in taste and smell, which can lead to insufficient consumption of zinc-rich foods like meat, dairy, and seafood. (Deshpande et al., 2013) Additionally, the aging process affects gastrointestinal function, including decreased gastric acid production and impaired intestinal absorption, both of which can reduce zinc bioavailability. (Bel-Serrat et al., 2014) Chronic health conditions, which are more common in the elderly, can also impact zinc status. Diseases such as diabetes, kidney disease, and gastrointestinal disorders can increase zinc loss or interfere with its absorption. (Aggett & Harries, 1979) Furthermore, medications frequently prescribed to older adults, including diuretics and proton pump inhibitors, can adversely affect zinc metabolism. (Mohn et al., 2018) The health impacts of zinc deficiency in the elderly are substantial and wide-ranging. Zinc plays a crucial role in immune function, and its deficiency can lead to a weakened immune system, making older adults more susceptible to infections and slower to recover from illnesses. (Maggini et al., 2018) Zinc is also vital for skin health and wound healing, so a deficiency can result in delayed wound healing and an increased risk of pressure ulcers. (Lin et al., 2017) Additionally, zinc is important for cognitive function, and its deficiency has been associated with cognitive decline and an increased risk of neurodegenerative diseases such as Alzheimer's. (Szewczyk, 2013)

4. INDIVIDUALS WITH MALABSORPTION SYNDROMES

Individuals with malabsorption syndromes are at significant risk of zinc deficiency due to their impaired ability to absorb nutrients effectively from the gastrointestinal tract. (Wapnir, 2000) Conditions such as Crohn's disease, celiac disease, and short bowel syndrome compromise the intestinal lining, reducing its capacity to absorb zinc and other essential nutrients. (Montoro-Huguet et al., 2021) Surgical interventions like gastric bypass or bowel resection further exacerbate this issue by decreasing the surface area available for nutrient absorption. (Shikora et al., 2007) Chronic diarrhea, often associated with these disorders, leads to increased zinc loss and further diminishes zinc levels in the body. (Hassan et al., 2020) Additionally, inflammation and the altered gut microbiota common in malabsorption syndromes can interfere with zinc metabolism. (Scarpellini et al., 2022) Zinc is crucial for immune function, and its deficiency can result in a compromised immune system, making individuals more susceptible to infections and slower to recover. (Gombart et al., 2020) Zinc is also essential for cellular growth and repair, and its deficiency can impair wound healing and exacerbate symptoms like dermatitis and alopecia. (Ogawa et al., 2018) In children, chronic zinc deficiency can lead to growth retardation and delayed sexual maturation. (Prasad, 1988) Moreover, zinc plays a role in neurological function, and its deficiency can contribute to cognitive impairments and mood disorders. (Prakash et al., 2015) Overall, managing zinc deficiency in individuals with malabsorption syndromes involves careful dietary planning, possible supplementation, and ongoing monitoring to prevent these severe health consequences. (King et al., 2016)

5. POPULATIONS WITH HIGH-PHYTATE DIETS

Populations with high phytate diets are at substantial risk for zinc deficiency due to the inhibitory effects of phytates on zinc absorption. (Gibson et al., 2018) Phytates, which are found in high concentrations in staple foods such as cereals, legumes, nuts, and seeds, bind to zinc in the digestive tract and form insoluble complexes that the body cannot absorb. (R. K. Gupta et al., 2015) Additionally, traditional food preparation methods, such as fermentation and soaking, which can reduce phytate levels, are not always practiced consistently, further increasing the risk of deficiency. (Samtiya et al., 2020) Addressing zinc deficiency in these populations requires strategies such as dietary diversification, food fortification, and public health initiatives to promote the use of phytate-reducing food preparation methods, thereby improving zinc bioavailability and overall nutritional status. (Gibson, 2015)

6. INDIVIDUALS WITH CHRONIC ILLNESSES

Individuals with chronic illnesses are at heightened risk for zinc deficiency due to several interrelated factors that affect zinc metabolism and absorption. (Prasad, 2013) Chronic conditions such as diabetes, chronic kidney disease, liver disease, and gastrointestinal disorders can disrupt zinc homeostasis. (Barman & Srinivasan, 2022) For example, diabetes can lead to increased urinary zinc excretion, while chronic kidney disease can impair zinc reabsorption and utilization. (Damianaki et al., 2020) Liver diseases like cirrhosis affect zinc storage and metabolism, further contributing to deficiency. (Himoto & Masaki, 2018) Gastrointestinal disorders, such as inflammatory bowel disease and celiac disease, damage the intestinal lining, reducing the absorption of zinc. (Wan & Zhang, 2022) Additionally, chronic inflammation, common in these conditions, can alter zinc metabolism by increasing the body's demand for zinc in immune responses and tissue repair. (Haase & Rink, 2014) Medications commonly used to manage chronic illnesses, such as diuretics, proton pump inhibitors, and ACE inhibitors, can also interfere with zinc absorption and increase its excretion. (Mohn et al., 2018)

Zinc Supplementation for Health Issues Associated with Zinc Deficiency

Skin Conditions

Zinc supplementation is a promising intervention for managing skin conditions associated with zinc deficiency, such as dermatitis, eczema, and acne. (Dhaliwal et al., 2020) Zinc plays a crucial role in maintaining skin health by supporting wound healing, reducing inflammation, and regulating sebum production. (Schwartz et al., 2005) Studies have shown that zinc supplementation can reduce the severity and frequency of dermatitis and eczema flare-ups, as well as decrease acne lesions. (Reynolds, 2018) Zinc supplements are available in various forms, including zinc gluconate, zinc sulfate, and zinc oxide, with oral supplementation being the most common route of administration. (Wegmüller et al., 2014) Topical zinc preparations, such as zinc oxide creams and ointments, are also available for localized skin conditions. (M. Gupta et al., 2014) However, it is essential to consult with a healthcare professional before starting zinc supplementation, as excessive zinc intake can have adverse effects and interactions with medications. (Plum et al., 2010) Additionally, addressing underlying dietary factors and ensuring a balanced diet rich in zinc-containing foods can complement supplementation efforts for optimal skin health. (King et al., 2016)

Hair Loss

Zinc supplementation can potentially help with hair loss by addressing underlying zinc deficiencies, which play a crucial role in maintaining healthy hair growth and follicle function. (Almohanna et al., 2019) Deficiencies in zinc levels can disrupt the hair growth cycle and impair follicle function, leading to hair thinning and loss. (Rajput, 2018) By supplementing with zinc, individuals may replenish depleted zinc stores, supporting optimal hair growth and reducing hair loss. (Rushton, 2002) Additionally, zinc has anti-inflammatory properties that may help alleviate scalp inflammation, a common factor in certain types of hair loss, such as alopecia areata. (M. Gupta et al., 2014) While research on the effectiveness of zinc supplementation for hair loss is ongoing, preliminary evidence suggests that correcting zinc deficiencies may lead to improvements in hair growth and reduction in hair shedding. (Ruiz-Tagle et al., 2018)

Neurological Disorders

Zinc supplementation has shown promise as a potential intervention for neurological disorders associated with zinc deficiency, as zinc plays a crucial role in neurotransmitter function, neuronal signaling, and overall brain health. (Cummings & Kovacic, 2009; Liu et al., 2021; Squitti et al., 2020) Zinc deficiency has been implicated in various neurological conditions, including depression, anxiety, cognitive impairment, and neurodegenerative diseases such as Alzheimer's and Parkinson's. (Prakash et al., 2015; B. Wang et al., 2023) Zinc is essential for the regulation of neurotransmitters like dopamine, serotonin, and glutamate, which are involved in mood regulation, cognition, and memory. (Petrilli et al., 2017; Swardfager et al., 2013) Additionally, zinc acts as an antioxidant, protecting against oxidative stress and neuroinflammation, both of which are implicated in the pathogenesis of neurodegenerative diseases. (Mezzaroba et al., 2019) Supplementing with zinc can help correct deficiencies, potentially alleviating symptoms and improving neurological function. (M Grabrucker et al., 2011)

Reproductive Health

Zinc supplementation is recognized as a valuable intervention for addressing reproductive health issues associated with zinc deficiency, given zinc's critical role in reproductive processes and hormone regulation. (Baltaci et al., 2019; Garner et al., 2021) Zinc deficiency has been linked to various reproductive problems, including infertility, menstrual irregularities, and pregnancy complications. (Uriu-Adams & Keen, 2010) In men, zinc is essential for sperm production, motility, and overall sperm quality, and deficiency can lead to decreased sperm count and impaired fertility. (Fallah et al., 2018; Mirnamniha et al., 2019) In women, zinc plays a role in menstrual cycle regulation, ovulation, and fetal development during pregnancy. (Garner et al., 2021; Kapper et al., 2024) Supplementing with zinc can help correct deficiencies, potentially improving fertility outcomes and reducing the risk of pregnancy complications such as preterm birth and low birth weight. (Birhanie et al., 2020; Schaefer & Nock, 2019)

Olfactory and Gustatory Dysfunction

Zinc supplementation may help improve olfactory and gustatory dysfunction by addressing underlying zinc deficiencies, which can contribute to alterations in taste and smell perception. (J. Lee et al., 2015) Zinc plays a crucial role in the function of taste and smell receptors, as well as in the maintenance of the olfactory epithelium and taste buds. (Henkin, 1984) Deficiencies in zinc levels can disrupt the structure and function of these sensory organs, leading to changes in taste and smell sensitivity. (Ackerman & Kasbekar, 1997) By supplementing with zinc, individuals may replenish depleted zinc stores, potentially restoring normal function to taste and smell receptors. (Cummings & Kovacic, 2009)

Bone Health

Zinc supplementation can contribute to bone health through various mechanisms. Zinc plays a crucial role in bone metabolism and mineralization, making it essential for maintaining optimal bone density and strength. (Gaffney-Stomberg, 2019; Molenda & Kolmas, 2023) One way zinc supports bone health is by stimulating osteoblast activity, the cells responsible for bone formation. (Yamaguchi, 2007) Zinc enhances the synthesis of collagen, a key component of bone tissue, and promotes the deposition of calcium and other minerals into the bone matrix, thus aiding in bone mineralization. (Yamaguchi, 1998) Additionally, zinc has anti-inflammatory properties that help regulate bone remodeling processes by inhibiting the activity of osteoclasts, the cells responsible for bone resorption. (Yamaguchi & Weitzmann, 2011) By modulating the balance between bone formation and resorption, zinc supplementation may help prevent bone loss and reduce the risk of osteoporosis and fractures. (Qi et al., 2020)

Gastrointestinal Disorders

Zinc supplements can potentially help alleviate gastrointestinal disorders by addressing underlying zinc deficiencies and exerting beneficial effects on gut health. (Skalny et al., 2021) Zinc plays a critical role in maintaining the integrity of the gastrointestinal mucosa, which serves as a protective barrier against harmful substances and pathogens. (Wan & Zhang, 2022) Zinc deficiency can compromise the integrity of the gut lining, leading to increased permeability (leaky gut) and susceptibility to inflammation and digestive disorders such as inflammatory bowel disease (IBD), celiac disease, and gastritis. (Chao, 2023; Wierdsma et al., 2013) By supplementing with zinc, individuals may replenish depleted zinc stores, supporting the repair and regeneration of the gut lining. (X. Wang et al., 2013)

Eye Health

Zinc supplements can support eye health through various mechanisms. Zinc is essential for maintaining the health of the eyes, particularly the retina, which is the light-sensitive tissue located at the back of the eye. (Álvarez-Barrios et al., 2021; Khadamy, n.d.) The retina contains high concentrations of zinc, which plays a vital role in visual function and protects against oxidative stress. (Ugarte & Osborne, 2001) Zinc is involved in the metabolism of vitamin A, an essential nutrient for vision, and helps transport vitamin A from the liver to the retina, where it is converted into rhodopsin, a pigment necessary for low-light vision. (Carazo et al., 2021) Additionally, zinc has antioxidant properties that help protect the eyes from oxidative damage caused by free radicals, which can contribute to age-related macular degeneration (AMD), cataracts, and other eye conditions. (Khoo et al., 2019; McCusker et al., 2016) Studies have suggested that zinc supplementation may help reduce the risk of AMD progression and slow the development of cataracts. (Hobbs & Bernstein, 2014)

Zinc Supplementation

Zinc supplementation is a targeted approach to address zinc deficiency, involving the provision of zinc in the form of pills, tablets, capsules, or liquid formulations. This method is particularly effective for individuals or populations at high risk of zinc deficiency or those already exhibiting symptoms. (Penny, 2013)

Indications for Zinc Supplementation

Infants and young children, particularly in regions with high rates of malnutrition, require zinc supplementation for growth and immune function. (Allai et al., 2022; Salgueiro et al., 2002) Pregnant and lactating women have increased zinc requirements, necessitating supplementation to support both maternal health and fetal development. (Ladipo, 2000; Oh et al., 2020) Elderly individuals may need supplementation due to age-related declines in zinc absorption and utilization. (Mocchegiani et al., 2013) Individuals with chronic illnesses, such as chronic kidney disease, diabetes, and gastrointestinal disorders, often experience impaired zinc absorption and increased requirements. (Gembillo et al., 2022; Jankowska et al., 2017; Wapnir, 2000) Vegetarians and vegans, who primarily consume plant-based diets with less bioavailable zinc, also benefit from supplementation to meet their dietary needs. (Neufingerl & Eilander, 2021)

Forms of Zinc Supplements

Various forms of zinc supplements offer distinct advantages and are utilized for different purposes. Zinc gluconate, renowned for its high bioavailability, is commonly found in lozenges, tablets, and syrups. (Mossad, 1996) Zinc picolinate, known for good absorption, is available in capsules and tablets. (Chinnasamy et al., 2019) Zinc sulfate, often used in liquid form for addressing zinc deficiency and diarrhea, is also found in tablets and solutions. (Bajait & Thawani, 2011; Lamberti et al., 2013) Zinc acetate, effective for colds and respiratory infections, is typically used in lozenges and tablets. (Hemilä & Chalker, 2015) Zinc orotate, claimed to have high bioavailability, is present in tablets and capsules. ("Orotic Acid Salts as Sources of Orotic Acid and Various Minerals Added for Nutritional Purposes to Food Supplements," n.d.) Zinc citrate, well-absorbed and gentle on the stomach, is commonly available in tablets and capsules. (Severe, n.d.) While zinc oxide is primarily used in topical applications, it's also found in oral supplements. (Schwartz et al., 2005)

Dosage and Administration

Zinc supplementation dosages vary depending on age, gender, and specific health needs. The Recommended Daily Allowance (RDA) for infants typically ranges from 2 to 3 mg/day, while children may require 5 to 10 mg/day depending on their age. (Ackland & Michalczyk, 2016) For adults, the RDA is set at 8 mg/day for women and 11 mg/day for men. (Moser-Veillon, 1990) Pregnant and lactating women have higher requirements, with recommended intakes of 11 to 12 mg/day and 12 to 13 mg/day, respectively. (Naem et al., 2014) In therapeutic contexts, such as addressing acute diarrhea, dosage ranges from 10 to 20 mg/day for a duration of 10 to 14 days. (Barffour et al., 2020) For immune support and managing common colds, dosages may range from 80 to 92 mg/day. (Hemilä, 2017)

Table 2. Recommended dietary allowances (RDA) for zinc

Age	Male	Female	Pregnancy	Lactation
0-6 months	2mg	2mg	-	-
7-12 months	3mg	3mg	-	-
1-3 years	3mg	3mg	-	-
4-8 years	5mg	5mg	-	-
9-13 years	8mg	8mg	-	-
14-18 years	11mg	9mg	12mg	13mg
19+ years	11mg	8mg	11mg	12mg

(P. Bhatnagar & Suman, 2020)

Safety and Side Effects

While zinc supplementation offers numerous health benefits, it's crucial to be aware of potential side effects and safety considerations. Common side effects may include nausea, vomiting, diarrhea, and stomach cramps, particularly at higher doses. (Nriagu, 2007) Prolonged use of high doses can result in copper deficiency and other imbalances, underscoring the importance of moderation. (Hoffman II et al., 1988; Osredkar & Sustar, 2011) Additionally, individuals undergoing long-term zinc supplementation may require regular monitoring to prevent potential adverse effects, emphasizing the need for ongoing oversight and adjustment as needed to ensure safety and efficacy. (Livingstone, 2015)

Implementation Strategies

Integrating zinc supplementation into healthcare practices is vital for promoting overall health and addressing deficiencies effectively. This includes routine incorporation of zinc supplements in prenatal and pediatric care to support maternal and child health. (Garcia-Casal et al., 2018) Screening and supplementation programs within healthcare settings, particularly in high-risk regions, can help identify and address deficiencies early on. (Bruins et al., 2018) Public health programs play a crucial role through community initiatives that distribute zinc supplements and educational campaigns emphasizing the importance of zinc and proper supplementation practices. (Larson et al., 2012) Moreover, policy and regulation are essential for establishing guidelines and standards for zinc supplementation, ensuring accessibility and affordability of supplements to maximize their impact on public health. (Faber et al., 2014; Penny, 2013) Its implementation requires careful consideration of dosages, forms, and potential side effects, along with robust public health strategies to ensure widespread access and adherence. By addressing zinc deficiency through supplementation, significant improvements in public health and individual well-being can be achieved. (D. N. Gupta et al., 2007; Penny, 2013)

Zinc Supplements Over Other Preventive Measures

Zinc supplements offer distinct advantages over other preventive measures like zinc fortification, and dietary strategies in addressing zinc deficiency and promoting overall health. (Caulfield & Black, 2004) One significant advantage lies in their targeted and precise dosing capabilities. (Hambidge et al., 2010) Unlike dietary interventions, which rely on the consumption of specific foods rich in zinc, supplements provide a concentrated source of zinc, allowing for precise control over dosage levels. (Mocchegiani et al., 2013) This is particularly beneficial in populations where zinc intake may be inadequate or where higher doses are required to meet increased nutritional demands, such as during pregnancy or in individuals with certain medical conditions. (Roohani et al., 2013) Moreover, zinc supplements offer a convenient and accessible means of supplementation. (Penny, 2013) While dietary strategies may require significant changes to eating habits or access to specific foods, supplements can be easily incorporated into daily routines and are readily available over the counter or through healthcare providers. (Gibson & Ferguson, 1998) Another key advantage of zinc supplements is their consistency and reliability in delivering the desired dosage. (Heyland et al., 2008) Unlike dietary sources of zinc, which may vary in their zinc content due to factors like soil quality, processing methods, or cooking techniques, supplements provide a standardized and consistent amount of zinc per serving. (Gibson, 1994, 2012) Furthermore, zinc supplements often boast enhanced bioavailability, meaning that the zinc is more easily absorbed and utilized by the body compared to certain dietary sources. (Li et al., 2022; Singh & Prasad, 2023) This is particularly advantageous for individuals with conditions that may impair zinc absorption, such as gastrointestinal disorders or aging-related changes in digestive function. (Lovat, 1996) Zinc supplements are generally safe and well-tolerated when taken as directed. (Saper & Rash, 2009) While other preventive measures, such as zinc fortification of foods or dietary modifications, may pose challenges related to taste preferences, food availability, or potential interactions with other nutrients, supplements offer a straightforward and controlled approach to zinc supplementation. (Sangeetha et al., 2022) Overall, the targeted dosing, convenience, reliability, bioavailability, and safety profile of zinc supplements make them a valuable tool in addressing zinc deficiency and supporting optimal health outcomes. Whether used as a primary preventive measure or as part of a comprehensive approach to nutritional health, supplements offer an effective and accessible means of meeting the body's zinc requirements. (Duan et al., 2023)

CONCLUSION

Zinc supplementation is essential in combating zinc deficiency, a common nutritional issue with significant health impacts. Zinc deficiency is widespread globally, affecting vulnerable groups such as children, pregnant women, and the elderly. Supplementation is crucial to prevent and treat health problems related to low zinc levels, including impaired immunity and growth issues. Various strategies have been explored, but zinc supplementation is particularly effective. Indications for its use are well-documented, and the forms, dosages, and administration methods are designed to ensure safety and efficacy. Proper implementation of supplementation programs, integrated into healthcare services, can significantly improve accessibility and adherence. Compared to other preventive measures, zinc supplements provide a direct and potent intervention, especially for those unable to meet their zinc needs through diet alone. Overall, targeted zinc supplementation can greatly reduce the prevalence of zinc deficiency and enhance health outcomes.

REFERENCES

Ackerman, B. H., & Kasbekar, N. (1997). Disturbances of Taste and Smell Induced by Drugs. *Pharmacotherapy, 17*(3), 482–496. DOI: 10.1002/j.1875-9114.1997.tb03058.x PMID: 9165552

Ackland, M. L., & Michalczyk, A. A. (2016). Zinc and infant nutrition. *Archives of Biochemistry and Biophysics, 611*, 51–57. DOI: 10.1016/j.abb.2016.06.011 PMID: 27317042

Aggett, P. J., & Harries, J. T. (1979). Current status of zinc in health and disease states. *Archives of Disease in Childhood, 54*(12), 909–917. DOI: 10.1136/adc.54.12.909 PMID: 119488

Allai, F. M., Gul, K., Zahoor, I., Ganaie, T. A., Nasir, G., & Azad, Z. R. A. A. (2022). Malnutrition: Impact of Zinc on Child Development. In Khan, S. T., & Malik, A. (Eds.), *Microbial Biofertilizers and Micronutrient Availability* (pp. 83–100). Springer International Publishing., DOI: 10.1007/978-3-030-76609-2_4

Allouche-Fitoussi, D., & Breitbart, H. (2020). The role of zinc in male fertility. *International Journal of Molecular Sciences, 21*(20), 7796. DOI: 10.3390/ijms21207796 PMID: 33096823

Almohanna, H. M., Ahmed, A. A., Tsatalis, J. P., & Tosti, A. (2019). The Role of Vitamins and Minerals in Hair Loss: A Review. *Dermatology and Therapy, 9*(1), 51–70. DOI: 10.1007/s13555-018-0278-6 PMID: 30547302

Álvarez-Barrios, A., Álvarez, L., García, M., Artime, E., Pereiro, R., & González-Iglesias, H. (2021). Antioxidant defenses in the human eye: A focus on metallothioneins. *Antioxidants, 10*(1), 89. DOI: 10.3390/antiox10010089 PMID: 33440661

Amin, N., Clark, C. C. T., Taghizadeh, M., & Djafarnejad, S. (2020). Zinc supplements and bone health: The role of the RANKL-RANK axis as a therapeutic target. *Journal of Trace Elements in Medicine and Biology, 57*, 126417. DOI: 10.1016/j.jtemb.2019.126417 PMID: 31653549

Bajait, C., & Thawani, V. (2011). Role of zinc in pediatric diarrhea. *Indian Journal of Pharmacology, 43*(3), 232–235. DOI: 10.4103/0253-7613.81495 PMID: 21713083

Baltaci, A. K., Mogulkoc, R., & Baltaci, S. B. (2019). The role of zinc in the endocrine system. *Pakistan Journal of Pharmaceutical Sciences, 32*(1). https://www.researchgate.net/profile/Saltuk-Baltaci/publication/331438506_Review_The_role_of_zinc_in_the_endocrine_system/links/5e1ffc32458515ba208a861e/Review-The-role-of-zinc-in-the-endocrine-system.pdf PMID: 30772815

Barffour, M. A., Hinnouho, G.-M., Wessells, K. R., Kounnavong, S., Ratsavong, K., Sitthideth, D., Bounheuang, B., Sengnam, K., Chanhthavong, B., Arnold, C. D., Brown, K. H., Larson, C. P., & Hess, S. Y. (2020). Effects of therapeutic zinc supplementation for diarrhea and two preventive zinc supplementation regimens on the incidence and duration of diarrhea and acute respiratory tract infections in rural Laotian children: A randomized controlled trial. *Journal of Global Health*, *10*(1), 010424. DOI: 10.7189/jogh.10.010424 PMID: 32612816

Barman, S., & Srinivasan, K. (2022). Diabetes and zinc dyshomeostasis: Can zinc supplementation mitigate diabetic complications? *Critical Reviews in Food Science and Nutrition*, *62*(4), 1046–1061. DOI: 10.1080/10408398.2020.1833178 PMID: 33938330

Bartlett, H., & Eperjesi, F. (2003). Age-related macular degeneration and nutritional supplementation: A review of randomised controlled trials. *Ophthalmic & Physiological Optics*, *23*(5), 383–399. DOI: 10.1046/j.1475-1313.2003.00130.x PMID: 12950886

Bel-Serrat, S., Stammers, A.-L., Warthon-Medina, M., Moran, V. H., Iglesia-Altaba, I., Hermoso, M., Moreno, L. A., & Lowe, N. M.EURRECA Network. (2014). Factors that affect zinc bioavailability and losses in adult and elderly populations. *Nutrition Reviews*, *72*(5), 334–352. DOI: 10.1111/nure.12105 PMID: 24739133

Bhatnagar, P., & Suman, M. (2020). *A review on role of zinc deficiency in humans and its rectification through Horti-agro food supplements*. 447–451.

Bhatnagar, S., & Taneja, S. (2001). Zinc and cognitive development. *British Journal of Nutrition*, *85*(S2), S139–S145. DOI: 10.1079/BJN2000306 PMID: 11509102

Birhanie, M. W., Adekunle, A. O., Arowojolu, A. O., Dugul, T. T., & Mebiratie, A. L. (2020). Micronutrients Deficiency and Their Associations with Pregnancy Outcomes: A Review. *Nutrition and Dietary Supplements*, *12*(Supplements), 237–254. DOI: 10.2147/NDS.S274646

Blasiak, J., Pawlowska, E., Chojnacki, J., Szczepanska, J., Chojnacki, C., & Kaarniranta, K. (2020). Zinc and Autophagy in Age-Related Macular Degeneration. *International Journal of Molecular Sciences*, *21*(14), 4994. DOI: 10.3390/ijms21144994 PMID: 32679798

Bruins, M. J., Bird, J. K., Aebischer, C. P., & Eggersdorfer, M. (2018). Considerations for secondary prevention of nutritional deficiencies in high-risk groups in high-income countries. *Nutrients*, *10*(1), 47. DOI: 10.3390/nu10010047 PMID: 29304025

Butte, N. F., Lopez-Alarcon, M. G., & Garza, C. (2002). *Nutrient adequacy of exclusive breastfeeding for the term infant during the first six months of life*. World Health Organization. https://apps.who.int/iris/bitstream/handle/10665/42519/9241562110.pdf

Calder, P. C., & Jackson, A. A. (2000). Undernutrition, infection and immune function. *Nutrition Research Reviews*, *13*(1), 3–29. DOI: 10.1079/095442200108728981 PMID: 19087431

Carazo, A., Macáková, K., Matoušová, K., Krčmová, L. K., Protti, M., & Mladěnka, P. (2021). Vitamin A update: Forms, sources, kinetics, detection, function, deficiency, therapeutic use and toxicity. *Nutrients*, *13*(5), 1703. DOI: 10.3390/nu13051703 PMID: 34069881

Caulfield, L. E., & Black, R. E. (2004). Zinc deficiency. *Comparative Quantification of Health Risks: Global and Regional Burden of Disease Attributable to Selected Major Risk Factors*, *1*, 257–280. PMID: 15100497

Chao, H.-C. (2023). Zinc Deficiency and Therapeutic Value of Zinc Supplementation in Pediatric Gastrointestinal Diseases. *Nutrients*, *15*(19), 4093. DOI: 10.3390/nu15194093 PMID: 37836377

Chinnasamy, E., Arulmani, S., Deepa, K., Kumar, D. S., Madhavan, J., & Senthil, S. (2019). Growth, Spectral, Optical, Studies of A Zinc Picolinate Dihydrate NLO Single Crystal. *Materials Today: Proceedings*, *8*, 264–270. DOI: 10.1016/j.matpr.2019.02.110

Classen, H.-G., Gröber, U., Löw, D., Schmidt, J., & Stracke, H. (2011). Zinc deficiency. Symptoms, causes, diagnosis and therapy. *Medizinische Monatsschrift fur Pharmazeuten*, *34*(3), 87–95. PMID: 21736013

Cummings, J. E., & Kovacic, J. P. (2009). The ubiquitous role of zinc in health and disease. *Journal of Veterinary Emergency and Critical Care (San Antonio, Tex.)*, *19*(3), 215–240. DOI: 10.1111/j.1476-4431.2009.00418.x PMID: 19691507

Damianaki, K., Lourenco, J. M., Braconnier, P., Ghobril, J.-P., Devuyst, O., Burnier, M., Lenglet, S., Augsburger, M., Thomas, A., & Pruijm, M. (2020). Renal handling of zinc in chronic kidney disease patients and the role of circulating zinc levels in renal function decline. *Nephrology, Dialysis, Transplantation*, *35*(7), 1163–1170. DOI: 10.1093/ndt/gfz065 PMID: 31006015

Deshpande, J., Joshi, M., & Giri, P. (2013). Zinc: The trace element of major importance in human nutrition and health. *International Journal of Medical Science and Public Health*, *2*(1), 1. DOI: 10.5455/ijmsph.2013.2.1-6

Dhaliwal, S., Nguyen, M., Vaughn, A. R., Notay, M., Chambers, C. J., & Sivamani, R. K. (2020). Effects of Zinc Supplementation on Inflammatory Skin Diseases: A Systematic Review of the Clinical Evidence. *American Journal of Clinical Dermatology*, *21*(1), 21–39. DOI: 10.1007/s40257-019-00484-0 PMID: 31745908

Duan, M., Li, T., Liu, B., Yin, S., Zang, J., Lv, C., Zhao, G., & Zhang, T. (2023). Zinc nutrition and dietary zinc supplements. *Critical Reviews in Food Science and Nutrition*, *63*(9), 1277–1292. DOI: 10.1080/10408398.2021.1963664 PMID: 34382897

Dumrongwongsiri, O., Suthutvoravut, U., Chatvutinun, S., Phoonlabdacha, P., Sangcakul, A., Siripinyanond, A., Thiengmanee, U., & Chongviriyaphan, N. (2015). Maternal zinc status is associated with breast milk zinc concentration and zinc status in breastfed infants aged 4-6 months. *Asia Pacific Journal of Clinical Nutrition*, *24*(2), 273–280. PMID: 26078244

El Din, E. M. S., Rabah, T. M., Metwally, A. M., Nassar, M. S., Elabd, M. A., Shalaan, A., Kandeel, W., El Etreby, L. A., & Shaaban, S. Y. (2019). Potential Risk Factors of Developmental Cognitive Delay in the First Two Years of Life. *Open Access Macedonian Journal of Medical Sciences*, *7*(12), 2024–2030. DOI: 10.3889/oamjms.2019.566 PMID: 31406549

Erick, M. (2018). Breast milk is conditionally perfect. *Medical Hypotheses*, *111*, 82–89. DOI: 10.1016/j.mehy.2017.12.020 PMID: 29407004

Faber, M., Berti, C., & Smuts, M. (2014). Prevention and control of micronutrient deficiencies in developing countries: Current perspectives. *Nutrition and Dietary Supplements*, *41*, 41. Advance online publication. DOI: 10.2147/NDS.S43523

Fallah, A., Mohammad-Hasani, A., & Colagar, A. H. (2018). Zinc is an essential element for male fertility: A review of Zn roles in men's health, germination, sperm quality, and fertilization. *Journal of Reproduction & Infertility*, *19*(2), 69. PMID: 30009140

Farias, P. M., Marcelino, G., Santana, L. F., De Almeida, E. B., Guimarães, R. D. C. A., Pott, A., Hiane, P. A., & Freitas, K. D. C. (2020). Minerals in Pregnancy and Their Impact on Child Growth and Development. *Molecules (Basel, Switzerland)*, *25*(23), 5630. DOI: 10.3390/molecules25235630 PMID: 33265961

Finzi, E., & Harrington, A. (2021). Zinc treatment of outpatient COVID-19: A retrospective review of 28 consecutive patients. *Journal of Medical Virology*, *93*(5), 2588–2590. DOI: 10.1002/jmv.26812 PMID: 33475170

Foster, M., & Samman, S. (2010). Zinc and Redox Signaling: Perturbations Associated with Cardiovascular Disease and Diabetes Mellitus. *Antioxidants & Redox Signaling*, *13*(10), 1549–1573. DOI: 10.1089/ars.2010.3111 PMID: 20568953

Gaffney-Stomberg, E. (2019). The Impact of Trace Minerals on Bone Metabolism. *Biological Trace Element Research*, *188*(1), 26–34. DOI: 10.1007/s12011-018-1583-8 PMID: 30467628

Garcia-Casal, M. N., Estevez, D., & De-Regil, L. M. (2018). Multiple micronutrient supplements in pregnancy: Implementation considerations for integration as part of quality services in routine antenatal care. Objectives, results, and conclusions of the meeting. *Maternal and Child Nutrition*, *14*(S5), e12704. DOI: 10.1111/mcn.12704 PMID: 30585705

Garner, T. B., Hester, J. M., Carothers, A., & Diaz, F. J. (2021). Role of zinc in female reproduction. *Biology of Reproduction*, *104*(5), 976–994. DOI: 10.1093/biolre/ioab023 PMID: 33598687

Gembillo, G., Visconti, L., Giuffrida, A. E., Labbozzetta, V., Peritore, L., Lipari, A., Calabrese, V., Piccoli, G. B., Torreggiani, M., Siligato, R., & Santoro, D. (2022). Role of zinc in diabetic kidney disease. *Nutrients*, *14*(7), 1353. DOI: 10.3390/nu14071353 PMID: 35405968

Gibbs, M. (2010). *Manufactured complementary foods for infant and young child feeding in Asia: Micronutrient adequacy and improvement* [PhD Thesis, University of Otago]. https://ourarchive.otago.ac.nz/handle/10523/369

Gibson, R. S. (1994). Zinc nutrition in developing countries. *Nutrition Research Reviews*, *7*(1), 151–173. DOI: 10.1079/NRR19940010 PMID: 19094296

Gibson, R. S. (2006). Zinc: The missing link in combating micronutrient malnutrition in developing countries. *The Proceedings of the Nutrition Society*, *65*(1), 51–60. DOI: 10.1079/PNS2005474 PMID: 16441944

Gibson, R. S. (2012). A historical review of progress in the assessment of dietary zinc intake as an indicator of population zinc status. *Advances in Nutrition*, *3*(6), 772–782. DOI: 10.3945/an.112.002287 PMID: 23153731

Gibson, R. S. (2015). Dietary-induced Zinc Deficiency in low Income Countries: Challenges and Solutions The Avanelle Kirksey Lecture at Purdue University. *Nutrition Today*, *50*(1), 49–55. DOI: 10.1097/NT.0000000000000070

Gibson, R. S., & Ferguson, E. L. (1998). Nutrition intervention strategies to combat zinc deficiency in developing countries. *Nutrition Research Reviews*, *11*(1), 115–131. DOI: 10.1079/NRR19980008 PMID: 19087462

Gibson, R. S., Raboy, V., & King, J. C. (2018). Implications of phytate in plant-based foods for iron and zinc bioavailability, setting dietary requirements, and formulating programs and policies. *Nutrition Reviews*, *76*(11), 793–804. DOI: 10.1093/nutrit/nuy028 PMID: 30010865

Gombart, A. F., Pierre, A., & Maggini, S. (2020). A review of micronutrients and the immune system–working in harmony to reduce the risk of infection. *Nutrients*, *12*(1), 236. DOI: 10.3390/nu12010236 PMID: 31963293

Grabrucker, M, A., Rowan, M., & C Garner, C. (2011). Brain-delivery of zinc-ions as potential treatment for neurological diseases: Mini review. *Drug Delivery Letters*, *1*(1), 13–23. PMID: 22102982

Grzeszczak, K., Kwiatkowski, S., & Kosik-Bogacka, D. (2020). The role of Fe, Zn, and Cu in pregnancy. *Biomolecules*, *10*(8), 1176. DOI: 10.3390/biom10081176 PMID: 32806787

Gupta, D. N., Rajendran, K., Mondal, S. K., Ghosh, S., & Bhattacharya, S. K. (2007). Operational feasibility of implementing community-based zinc supplementation: Impact on childhood diarrheal morbidity. *The Pediatric Infectious Disease Journal*, *26*(4), 306–310. DOI: 10.1097/01.inf.0000258692.65485.d9 PMID: 17414392

Gupta, M., Mahajan, V. K., Mehta, K. S., & Chauhan, P. S. (2014). Zinc therapy in dermatology: A review. *Dermatology Research and Practice*, *2014*, 1–11. https://www.hindawi.com/journals/drp/2014/709152/abs/. DOI: 10.1155/2014/709152 PMID: 25120566

Gupta, R. K., Gangoliya, S. S., & Singh, N. K. (2015). Reduction of phytic acid and enhancement of bioavailable micronutrients in food grains. *Journal of Food Science and Technology*, *52*(2), 676–684. DOI: 10.1007/s13197-013-0978-y PMID: 25694676

Haase, H., & Rink, L. (2014). Zinc signals and immune function. *BioFactors (Oxford, England)*, *40*(1), 27–40. DOI: 10.1002/biof.1114 PMID: 23804522

Hambidge, K. M., & Krebs, N. F. (2007). Zinc Deficiency: A Special Challenge1. *The Journal of Nutrition*, *137*(4), 1101–1105. DOI: 10.1093/jn/137.4.1101 PMID: 17374687

Hambidge, K. M., Miller, L. V., Westcott, J. E., Sheng, X., & Krebs, N. F. (2010). Zinc bioavailability and homeostasis. *The American Journal of Clinical Nutrition*, *91*(5), 1478S–1483S. DOI: 10.3945/ajcn.2010.28674I PMID: 20200254

Hassan, A., Sada, K.-K., Ketheeswaran, S., Dubey, A. K., & Bhat, M. S. (2020). Role of Zinc in Mucosal Health and Disease: A Review of Physiological, Biochemical, and Molecular Processes. *Cureus*. Advance online publication. DOI: 10.7759/cureus.8197 PMID: 32572355

Hemilä, H. (2017). Zinc lozenges and the common cold: A meta-analysis comparing zinc acetate and zinc gluconate, and the role of zinc dosage. *JRSM Open*, *8*(5), 205427041769429. DOI: 10.1177/2054270417694291 PMID: 28515951

Hemilä, H., & Chalker, E. (2015). The effectiveness of high dose zinc acetate lozenges on various common cold symptoms: A meta-analysis. *BMC Family Practice*, *16*(1), 24. DOI: 10.1186/s12875-015-0237-6 PMID: 25888289

Henkin, R. I. (1984). Zinc in taste function: A critical review. *Biological Trace Element Research*, *6*(3), 263–280. DOI: 10.1007/BF02917511 PMID: 24264025

Heyland, D. K., Jones, N., Cvijanovich, N. Z., & Wong, H. (2008). Zinc Supplementation in Critically Ill Patients: A Key Pharmaconutrient? *JPEN. Journal of Parenteral and Enteral Nutrition*, *32*(5), 509–519. DOI: 10.1177/0148607108322402 PMID: 18669902

Himoto, T., & Masaki, T. (2018). Associations between zinc deficiency and metabolic abnormalities in patients with chronic liver disease. *Nutrients*, *10*(1), 88. DOI: 10.3390/nu10010088 PMID: 29342898

Hobbs, R. P., & Bernstein, P. S. (2014). Nutrient supplementation for age-related macular degeneration, cataract, and dry eye. *Journal of Ophthalmic & Vision Research*, *9*(4), 487. DOI: 10.4103/2008-322X.150829 PMID: 25709776

Hoffman, H. N.II, Phyliky, R. L., & Fleming, C. R. (1988). Zinc-induced copper deficiency. *Gastroenterology*, *94*(2), 508–512. DOI: 10.1016/0016-5085(88)90445-3 PMID: 3335323

Hotz, C., & Brown, K. H. (2004). *Assessment of the risk of zinc deficiency in populations and options for its control.* https://citeseerx.ist.psu.edu/document?repid=rep1&type=pdf&doi=4fffa0f903be10224b0651fed1d27bb144feb1ac

Jankowska, M., Rutkowski, B., & Dębska-Ślizień, A. (2017). Vitamins and microelement bioavailability in different stages of chronic kidney disease. *Nutrients*, *9*(3), 282. DOI: 10.3390/nu9030282 PMID: 28294976

Jones, P. W., & Williams, D. R. (2004). The use and role of zinc and its compounds in wound healing. *Metal Ions in Biological Systems*, *41*, 139–184. DOI: 10.1201/9780203913703.ch5 PMID: 15206116

Kapper, C., Oppelt, P., Ganhör, C., Gyunesh, A. A., Arbeithuber, B., Stelzl, P., & Rezk-Füreder, M. (2024). Minerals and the Menstrual Cycle: Impacts on Ovulation and Endometrial Health. *Nutrients*, *16*(7), 1008. DOI: 10.3390/nu16071008 PMID: 38613041

Kaur, K., Gupta, R., Saraf, S. A., & Saraf, S. K. (2014). Zinc: The Metal of Life. *Comprehensive Reviews in Food Science and Food Safety*, *13*(4), 358–376. DOI: 10.1111/1541-4337.12067 PMID: 33412710

Khadamy, J. (n.d.). *Nutrients for Eye Health and Disease Management.* Retrieved May 25, 2024, from https://www.researchgate.net/profile/Joobin-Khadamy/publication/376582120_Nutrients_for_Eye_Health_and_Disease_Management/links/657df780aff8b16813ad8fda/Nutrients-for-Eye-Health-and-Disease-Management.pdf

Khayat, S., Fanaei, H., & Ghanbarzehi, A. (2017). Minerals in pregnancy and lactation: A review article. *Journal of Clinical and Diagnostic Research : JCDR*, *11*(9), QE01. DOI: 10.7860/JCDR/2017/28485.10626 PMID: 29207789

Khoo, H. E., Ng, H. S., Yap, W.-S., Goh, H. J. H., & Yim, H. S. (2019). Nutrients for prevention of macular degeneration and eye-related diseases. *Antioxidants*, *8*(4), 85. DOI: 10.3390/antiox8040085 PMID: 30986936

King, J. C., Brown, K. H., Gibson, R. S., Krebs, N. F., Lowe, N. M., Siekmann, J. H., & Raiten, D. J. (2016). Biomarkers of Nutrition for Development (BOND)—Zinc Review12345. *The Journal of Nutrition*, *146*(4), 858S–885S. DOI: 10.3945/jn.115.220079 PMID: 26962190

Krebs, N. F. (2013). Update on Zinc Deficiency and Excess in Clinical Pediatric Practice. *Annals of Nutrition & Metabolism*, *62*(Suppl. 1), 19–29. DOI: 10.1159/000348261 PMID: 23689110

Kumari, D., Garg, S., & Bhawrani, P. (2022). Zinc homeostasis in immunity and its association with preterm births. *Scandinavian Journal of Immunology*, *95*(4), e13142. DOI: 10.1111/sji.13142 PMID: 35007353

Kvamme, J.-M., Grønli, O., Jacobsen, B. K., & Florholmen, J. (2015). Risk of malnutrition and zinc deficiency in community-living elderly men and women: The Tromsø Study. *Public Health Nutrition*, *18*(11), 1907–1913. DOI: 10.1017/S1368980014002420 PMID: 25373445

Ladipo, O. A. (2000). Nutrition in pregnancy: Mineral and vitamin supplements. *The American Journal of Clinical Nutrition*, *72*(1), 280S–290S. DOI: 10.1093/ajcn/72.1.280S PMID: 10871594

Lamberti, L. M., Fischer Walker, C. L., Chan, K. Y., Jian, W.-Y., & Black, R. E. (2013). Oral zinc supplementation for the treatment of acute diarrhea in children: A systematic review and meta-analysis. *Nutrients*, *5*(11), 4715–4740. DOI: 10.3390/nu5114715 PMID: 24284615

Larson, C. P., Koehlmoos, T. P., Sack, D. A., & Team, S. U. (2012). Scaling up zinc treatment of childhood diarrhoea in Bangladesh: Theoretical and practical considerations guiding the SUZY Project. *Health Policy and Planning*, *27*(2), 102–114. DOI: 10.1093/heapol/czr015 PMID: 21343236

Lee, J., Tucker, R. M., Tan, S. Y., Running, C. A., Jones, J. B., & Mattes, R. D. (2015). Nutritional Implications of Taste and Smell Dysfunction. In Doty, R. L. (Ed.), *Handbook of Olfaction and Gustation* (1st ed., pp. 829–864). Wiley., DOI: 10.1002/9781118971758.ch37

Lee, S. R. (2018). Critical Role of Zinc as Either an Antioxidant or a Prooxidant in Cellular Systems. *Oxidative Medicine and Cellular Longevity*, *2018*(1), 1–11. DOI: 10.1155/2018/9156285 PMID: 29743987

Li, J., Cao, D., Huang, Y., Chen, B., Chen, Z., Wang, R., Dong, Q., Wei, Q., & Liu, L. (2022). Zinc intakes and health outcomes: An umbrella review. *Frontiers in Nutrition*, *9*, 798078. DOI: 10.3389/fnut.2022.798078 PMID: 35211497

Lin, P.-H., Sermersheim, M., Li, H., Lee, P., Steinberg, S., & Ma, J. (2017). Zinc in Wound Healing Modulation. *Nutrients*, *10*(1), 16. DOI: 10.3390/nu10010016 PMID: 29295546

Liu, H. Y., Gale, J. R., Reynolds, I. J., Weiss, J. H., & Aizenman, E. (2021). The multifaceted roles of zinc in neuronal mitochondrial dysfunction. *Biomedicines*, *9*(5), 489. DOI: 10.3390/biomedicines9050489 PMID: 33946782

Livingstone, C. (2015). Zinc: Physiology, Deficiency, and Parenteral Nutrition. *Nutrition in Clinical Practice*, *30*(3), 371–382. DOI: 10.1177/0884533615570376 PMID: 25681484

Lovat, L. B. (1996). Age related changes in gut physiology and nutritional status. *Gut*, *38*(3), 306–309. DOI: 10.1136/gut.38.3.306 PMID: 8675079

Maggini, S., Pierre, A., & Calder, P. (2018). Immune Function and Micronutrient Requirements Change over the Life Course. *Nutrients*, *10*(10), 1531. DOI: 10.3390/nu10101531 PMID: 30336639

McCusker, M. M., Durrani, K., Payette, M. J., & Suchecki, J. (2016). An eye on nutrition: The role of vitamins, essential fatty acids, and antioxidants in age-related macular degeneration, dry eye syndrome, and cataract. *Clinics in Dermatology*, *34*(2), 276–285. DOI: 10.1016/j.clindermatol.2015.11.009 PMID: 26903189

Mezzaroba, L., Alfieri, D. F., Simão, A. N. C., & Reiche, E. M. V. (2019). The role of zinc, copper, manganese and iron in neurodegenerative diseases. *Neurotoxicology*, *74*, 230–241. DOI: 10.1016/j.neuro.2019.07.007 PMID: 31377220

Mirnamniha, M., Faroughi, F., Tahmasbpour, E., Ebrahimi, P., & Beigi Harchegani, A. (2019). An overview on role of some trace elements in human reproductive health, sperm function and fertilization process. *Reviews on Environmental Health*, *34*(4), 339–348. DOI: 10.1515/reveh-2019-0008 PMID: 31203261

Mocchegiani, E., Romeo, J., Malavolta, M., Costarelli, L., Giacconi, R., Diaz, L.-E., & Marcos, A. (2013). Zinc: Dietary intake and impact of supplementation on immune function in elderly. *Age (Dordrecht, Netherlands)*, *35*(3), 839–860. DOI: 10.1007/s11357-011-9377-3 PMID: 22222917

Mohn, E., Kern, H., Saltzman, E., Mitmesser, S., & McKay, D. (2018). Evidence of Drug–Nutrient Interactions with Chronic Use of Commonly Prescribed Medications: An Update. *Pharmaceutics*, *10*(1), 36. DOI: 10.3390/pharmaceutics10010036 PMID: 29558445

Molenda, M., & Kolmas, J. (2023). The Role of Zinc in Bone Tissue Health and Regeneration—A Review. *Biological Trace Element Research*, *201*(12), 5640–5651. DOI: 10.1007/s12011-023-03631-1 PMID: 37002364

Montoro-Huguet, M. A., Belloc, B., & Domínguez-Cajal, M. (2021). Small and Large Intestine (I): Malabsorption of Nutrients. *Nutrients*, *13*(4), 1254. DOI: 10.3390/nu13041254 PMID: 33920345

Moser-Veillon, P. B. (1990). Zinc: Consumption patterns and dietary recommendations. *Journal of the American Dietetic Association*, *90*(8), 1089–1094. DOI: 10.1016/S0002-8223(21)01706-5 PMID: 2166098

Mossad, S. B., Macknin, M. L., Mendendorp, S. V., & Mason, P. (1996). Zinc Gluconate Lozenges for Treating the Common Cold: A Randomized, Double-Blind, Placebo-Controlled Study. *Annals of Internal Medicine*, *125*(2), 81–88. DOI: 10.7326/0003-4819-125-2-199607150-00001 PMID: 8678384

Mozaffar, B., Ardavani, A., Muzafar, H., & Idris, I. (2023). The Effectiveness of Zinc Supplementation in Taste Disorder Treatment: A Systematic Review and Meta-Analysis of Randomized Controlled Trials. *Journal of Nutrition and Metabolism, 2023*, 1–13. DOI: 10.1155/2023/6711071 PMID: 36937245

Naem, N. E., El-Sayed, N. M., Nossier, S. A., & Zeid, A. A. A. (2014). Zinc status and dietary intake of pregnant women, Alexandria, Egypt. *The Journal of the Egyptian Public Health Association*, *89*(1), 35–41. DOI: 10.1097/01.EPX.0000443987.44261.9b PMID: 24717399

Neufingerl, N., & Eilander, A. (2021). Nutrient intake and status in adults consuming plant-based diets compared to meat-eaters: A systematic review. *Nutrients*, *14*(1), 29. DOI: 10.3390/nu14010029 PMID: 35010904

Nriagu, J. (2007). Zinc toxicity in humans. *School of Public Health, University of Michigan*, 1–7.

Ogawa, Y., Kinoshita, M., Shimada, S., & Kawamura, T. (2018). Zinc and Skin Disorders. *Nutrients*, *10*(2), 199. DOI: 10.3390/nu10020199 PMID: 29439479

Oh, C., Keats, E. C., & Bhutta, Z. A. (2020). Vitamin and mineral supplementation during pregnancy on maternal, birth, child health and development outcomes in low- and middle-income countries: A systematic review and meta-analysis. *Nutrients*, *12*(2), 491. DOI: 10.3390/nu12020491 PMID: 32075071

Osredkar, J., & Sustar, N. (2011). Copper and zinc, biological role and significance of copper/zinc imbalance. *J Clinic Toxicol s, 3*(2161), 0495.

Patil, R., Sontakke, T., Biradar, A., & Nalage, D. (2023). Zinc: An essential trace element for human health and beyond. *Food and Health*, *5*(3), 13. DOI: 10.53388/FH2023013

Penny, M. E. (2013). Zinc Supplementation in Public Health. *Annals of Nutrition & Metabolism*, *62*(Suppl. 1), 31–42. DOI: 10.1159/000348263 PMID: 23689111

Petrilli, M. A., Kranz, T. M., Kleinhaus, K., Joe, P., Getz, M., Johnson, P., Chao, M. V., & Malaspina, D. (2017). The emerging role for zinc in depression and psychosis. *Frontiers in Pharmacology*, *8*, 414. DOI: 10.3389/fphar.2017.00414 PMID: 28713269

Plum, L. M., Rink, L., & Haase, H. (2010). The essential toxin: Impact of zinc on human health. *International Journal of Environmental Research and Public Health*, *7*(4), 1342–1365. DOI: 10.3390/ijerph7041342 PMID: 20617034

Prakash, A., Bharti, K., & Majeed, A. B. A. (2015). Zinc: Indications in brain disorders. *Fundamental & Clinical Pharmacology*, *29*(2), 131–149. DOI: 10.1111/fcp.12110 PMID: 25659970

Prasad, A. S. (1988). Zinc in growth and development and spectrum of human zinc deficiency. *Journal of the American College of Nutrition*, *7*(5), 377–384. DOI: 10.1080/07315724.1988.10720255 PMID: 3053862

Prasad, A. S. (1996). Zinc deficiency in women, infants and children. *Journal of the American College of Nutrition*, *15*(2), 113–120. DOI: 10.1080/07315724.1996.10718575 PMID: 8778139

Prasad, A. S. (2004). Zinc deficiency: Its characterization and treatment. *Metal Ions in Biological Systems*, *41*, 103–138. PMID: 15206115

Prasad, A. S. (2013). Discovery of human zinc deficiency: Its impact on human health and disease. *Advances in Nutrition*, *4*(2), 176–190. DOI: 10.3945/an.112.003210 PMID: 23493534

Qi, S., He, J., Zheng, H., Chen, C., Jiang, H., & Lan, S. (2020). Zinc Supplementation Increased Bone Mineral Density, Improves Bone Histomorphology, and Prevents Bone Loss in Diabetic Rat. *Biological Trace Element Research*, *194*(2), 493–501. DOI: 10.1007/s12011-019-01810-7 PMID: 31363990

Rajput, R. (2018). A scientific hypothesis on the role of nutritional supplements for effective management of hair loss and promoting hair regrowth. *Journal of Nutritional Health & Food Science*, *6*(3), 1–11. DOI: 10.15226/jnhfs.2018.001132

Read, S. A., Obeid, S., Ahlenstiel, C., & Ahlenstiel, G. (2019). The Role of Zinc in Antiviral Immunity. *Advances in Nutrition*, *10*(4), 696–710. DOI: 10.1093/advances/nmz013 PMID: 31305906

Reynolds, D. (2018). *Skin Conditions: From Acne to Eczema*. Greenhaven Publishing LLC.

Roohani, N., Hurrell, R., Kelishadi, R., & Schulin, R. (2013). Zinc and its importance for human health: An integrative review. *Journal of Research in Medical Sciences : the Official Journal of Isfahan University of Medical Sciences*, *18*(2), 144. PMID: 23914218

Ruiz-Tagle, S. A., Figueira, M. M., Vial, V., Espinoza-Benavides, L., & Miteva, M. (2018). Micronutrients in hair loss. *Our Dermatology Online. Nasza Dermatologia Online*, *9*(3), 320–328. https://www.odermatol.com/odermatology/20183/25.Micronutrients-Ruiz-TagleSA.pdf. DOI: 10.7241/ourd.20183.25

Rushton, D. H. (2002). Nutritional factors and hair loss. *Clinical and Experimental Dermatology, 27*(5), 396–404. DOI: 10.1046/j.1365-2230.2002.01076.x PMID: 12190640

Salgueiro, M. J., Zubillaga, M. B., Lysionek, A. E., Caro, R. A., Weill, R., & Boccio, J. R. (2002). The role of zinc in the growth and development of children. *Nutrition (Burbank, Los Angeles County, Calif.), 18*(6), 510–519. DOI: 10.1016/S0899-9007(01)00812-7 PMID: 12044825

Samtiya, M., Aluko, R. E., & Dhewa, T. (2020). Plant food anti-nutritional factors and their reduction strategies: An overview. *Food Production, Processing and Nutrition, 2*(1), 6. DOI: 10.1186/s43014-020-0020-5

Sandstead, H. H., & Freeland-Graves, J. H. (2014). Dietary phytate, zinc and hidden zinc deficiency. *Journal of Trace Elements in Medicine and Biology, 28*(4), 414–417. DOI: 10.1016/j.jtemb.2014.08.011 PMID: 25439135

Sangeetha, V. J., Dutta, S., Moses, J. A., & Anandharamakrishnan, C. (2022). Zinc nutrition and human health: Overview and implications. *eFood, 3*(5), e17. DOI: 10.1002/efd2.17

Saper, R. B., & Rash, R. (2009). Zinc: An essential micronutrient. *American Family Physician, 79*(9), 768. PMID: 20141096

Scarpellini, E., Balsiger, L. M., Maurizi, V., Rinninella, E., Gasbarrini, A., Giostra, N., Santori, P., Abenavoli, L., & Rasetti, C. (2022). Zinc and gut microbiota in health and gastrointestinal disease under the COVID-19 suggestion. *BioFactors (Oxford, England), 48*(2), 294–306. DOI: 10.1002/biof.1829 PMID: 35218585

Schaefer, E., & Nock, D. (2019). The Impact of Preconceptional Multiple-Micronutrient Supplementation on Female Fertility. *Clinical Medicine Insights: Women's Health, 12*, 1179562X1984386. DOI: 10.1177/1179562X19843868

Schwartz, J. R., Marsh, R. G., & Draelos, Z. D. (2005). Zinc and Skin Health: Overview of Physiology and Pharmacology. *Dermatologic Surgery, 31*(s1), 837–847. DOI: 10.1111/j.1524-4725.2005.31729 PMID: 16029676

Scrimgeour, A. G., Condlin, M. L., Otieno, L., & Bovill, M. E. (2011). Zinc Intervention Strategies: Costs and Health Benefits. In Gerald, J. K., Watson, R. R., & Preedy, V. R. (Eds.), *Nutrients, Dietary Supplements, and Nutriceuticals* (pp. 189–214). Humana Press., DOI: 10.1007/978-1-60761-308-4_13

Serhan, H., Alma'aitah, H., Irshaidat, S., Ameer, M., Asghar, M., & Tahir, M. (2022). Ophthalmic manifestations of nutritional deficiencies: A mini review. *Journal of Family Medicine and Primary Care, 11*(10), 5899–5901. DOI: 10.4103/jfmpc.jfmpc_790_22 PMID: 36618247

Severe, M. (n.d.). *Zinc: Everything you need to know about this vital mineral.* Retrieved May 25, 2024, from https://blog.cytoplan.co.uk/zinc-all-about-this-vital-mineral/

Sevryugin, O., Kasvis, P., Vigano, M., & Vigano, A. (2021). Taste and smell disturbances in cancer patients: A scoping review of available treatments. *Supportive Care in Cancer, 29*(1), 49–66. DOI: 10.1007/s00520-020-05609-4 PMID: 32734392

Shayganfard, M. (2022). Are Essential Trace Elements Effective in Modulation of Mental Disorders? Update and Perspectives. *Biological Trace Element Research, 200*(3), 1032–1059. DOI: 10.1007/s12011-021-02733-y PMID: 33904124

Shikora, S. A., Kim, J. J., & Tarnoff, M. E. (2007). Nutrition and Gastrointestinal Complications of Bariatric Surgery. *Nutrition in Clinical Practice, 22*(1), 29–40. DOI: 10.1177/011542650702200129 PMID: 17242452

Singh, P., & Prasad, S. (2023). A review on iron, zinc and calcium biological significance and factors affecting their absorption and bioavailability. *Journal of Food Composition and Analysis, 123*, 105529. DOI: 10.1016/j.jfca.2023.105529

Skalny, A. V., Aschner, M., Lei, X. G., Gritsenko, V. A., Santamaria, A., Alekseenko, S. I., Prakash, N. T., Chang, J.-S., Sizova, E. A., Chao, J. C., Aaseth, J., & Tinkov, A. A. (2021). Gut microbiota as a mediator of essential and toxic effects of zinc in the intestines and other tissues. *International Journal of Molecular Sciences, 22*(23), 13074. DOI: 10.3390/ijms222313074 PMID: 34884881

Squitti, R., Pal, A., Picozza, M., Avan, A., Ventriglia, M., Rongioletti, M. C., & Hoogenraad, T. (2020). Zinc Therapy in early Alzheimer's disease: Safety and potential therapeutic efficacy. *Biomolecules, 10*(8), 1164. DOI: 10.3390/biom10081164 PMID: 32784855

Stefanidou, M., Maravelias, C., Dona, A., & Spiliopoulou, C. (2006). Zinc: A multipurpose trace element. *Archives of Toxicology, 80*(1), 1–9. DOI: 10.1007/s00204-005-0009-5 PMID: 16187101

Swardfager, W., Herrmann, N., McIntyre, R. S., Mazereeuw, G., Goldberger, K., Cha, D. S., Schwartz, Y., & Lanctôt, K. L. (2013). Potential roles of zinc in the pathophysiology and treatment of major depressive disorder. *Neuroscience and Biobehavioral Reviews, 37*(5), 911–929. DOI: 10.1016/j.neubiorev.2013.03.018 PMID: 23567517

Szewczyk, B. (2013). Zinc homeostasis and neurodegenerative disorders. *Frontiers in Aging Neuroscience*, *5*. Advance online publication. DOI: 10.3389/fnagi.2013.00033 PMID: 23882214

Takeda, T., Miyazaki, S., Kobayashi, M., Nishino, K., Goto, T., Matsunaga, M., Ooi, M., Shirakawa, H., Tani, F., Kawamura, T., Komai, M., & Kambe, T. (2018). Zinc deficiency causes delayed ATP clearance and adenosine generation in rats and cell culture models. *Communications Biology*, *1*(1), 113. DOI: 10.1038/s42003-018-0118-3 PMID: 30271993

Ugarte, M., & Osborne, N. N. (2001). Zinc in the retina. *Progress in Neurobiology*, *64*(3), 219–249. DOI: 10.1016/S0301-0082(00)00057-5 PMID: 11240307

Upadhaya, S. D., & Kim, I. H. (2020). Importance of micronutrients in bone health of monogastric animals and techniques to improve the bioavailability of micronutrient supplements—A review. *Asian-Australasian Journal of Animal Sciences*, *33*(12), 1885–1895. DOI: 10.5713/ajas.19.0945 PMID: 32164057

Uriu-Adams, J. Y., & Keen, C. L. (2010). Zinc and reproduction: Effects of zinc deficiency on prenatal and early postnatal development. *Birth Defects Research. Part B, Developmental and Reproductive Toxicology*, *89*(4), 313–325. DOI: 10.1002/bdrb.20264 PMID: 20803691

Vickram, S., Rohini, K., Srinivasan, S., Nancy Veenakumari, D., Archana, K., Anbarasu, K., Jeyanthi, P., Thanigaivel, S., Gulothungan, G., Rajendiran, N., & Srikumar, P. S. (2021). Role of Zinc (Zn) in Human Reproduction: A Journey from Initial Spermatogenesis to Childbirth. *International Journal of Molecular Sciences*, *22*(4), 2188. DOI: 10.3390/ijms22042188 PMID: 33671837

Walke, G., Gaurkar, S. S., Prasad, R., Lohakare, T., & Wanjari, M. (2023). The impact of oxidative stress on male reproductive function: Exploring the role of antioxidant supplementation. *Cureus*, *15*(7). Advance online publication. https://www.cureus.com/articles/169642-the-impact-of-oxidative-stress-on-male-reproductive-function-exploring-the-role-of-antioxidant-supplementation.pdf. DOI: 10.7759/cureus.42583 PMID: 37641770

Wan, Y., & Zhang, B. (2022). The impact of zinc and zinc homeostasis on the intestinal mucosal barrier and intestinal diseases. *Biomolecules*, *12*(7), 900. DOI: 10.3390/biom12070900 PMID: 35883455

Wang, B., Fang, T., & Chen, H. (2023). Zinc and central nervous system disorders. *Nutrients*, *15*(9), 2140. DOI: 10.3390/nu15092140 PMID: 37432243

Wang, X., Valenzano, M. C., Mercado, J. M., Zurbach, E. P., & Mullin, J. M. (2013). Zinc Supplementation Modifies Tight Junctions and Alters Barrier Function of CACO-2 Human Intestinal Epithelial Layers. *Digestive Diseases and Sciences*, *58*(1), 77–87. DOI: 10.1007/s10620-012-2328-8 PMID: 22903217

Wang, X., Wu, W., Zheng, W., Fang, X., Chen, L., Rink, L., Min, J., & Wang, F. (2019). Zinc supplementation improves glycemic control for diabetes prevention and management: A systematic review and meta-analysis of randomized controlled trials. *The American Journal of Clinical Nutrition*, *110*(1), 76–90. DOI: 10.1093/ajcn/nqz041 PMID: 31161192

Wapnir, R. A. (2000). Zinc deficiency, malnutrition and the gastrointestinal tract. *The Journal of Nutrition*, *130*(5), 1388S–1392S. DOI: 10.1093/jn/130.5.1388S PMID: 10801949

Wegmüller, R., Tay, F., Zeder, C., Brnić, M., & Hurrell, R. F. (2014). Zinc absorption by young adults from supplemental zinc citrate is comparable with that from zinc gluconate and higher than from zinc oxide. *The Journal of Nutrition*, *144*(2), 132–136. DOI: 10.3945/jn.113.181487 PMID: 24259556

Wessells, K. R., & Brown, K. H. (2012). Estimating the global prevalence of zinc deficiency: Results based on zinc availability in national food supplies and the prevalence of stunting. *PLoS One*, *7*(11), e50568. DOI: 10.1371/journal.pone.0050568 PMID: 23209782

Wierdsma, N. J., Van Bokhorst-de van der Schueren, M., Berkenpas, M., Mulder, C., & Van Bodegraven, A. (2013). Vitamin and mineral deficiencies are highly prevalent in newly diagnosed celiac disease patients. *Nutrients*, *5*(10), 3975–3992. DOI: 10.3390/nu5103975 PMID: 24084055

Yamaguchi, M. (1998). Role of zinc in bone formation and bone resorption. *The Journal of Trace Elements in Experimental Medicine*, *11*(2–3), 119–135. DOI: 10.1002/(SICI)1520-670X(1998)11:2/3<119::AID-JTRA5>3.0.CO;2-3

Yamaguchi, M. (2007). Role of zinc in bone metabolism and preventive effect on bone disorder. *Biomedical Research on Trace Elements*, *18*(4), 346–366.

Yamaguchi, M., & Weitzmann, M. N. (2011). Zinc stimulates osteoblastogenesis and suppresses osteoclastogenesis by antagonizing NF-κB activation. *Molecular and Cellular Biochemistry*, *355*(1–2), 179–186. DOI: 10.1007/s11010-011-0852-z PMID: 21533765

Zand, N., Christides, T., & Loughrill, E. (2015). Dietary intake of minerals. In De La Guardia, M., & Garrigues, S. (Eds.), *Handbook of Mineral Elements in Food* (1st ed., pp. 23–39). Wiley., DOI: 10.1002/9781118654316.ch2

Chapter 7
Zinc Supplementation as a Preventive Measure for Zinc Deficiency

Paran Jyoti Borpatra
Banaras Hindu University, India

B. Shriya Saikia
Gauhati University, India

ABSTRACT

Zinc is an essential micronutrient crucial for various physiological functions within the human body, spanning from immune support to wound healing and DNA synthesis. Despite its importance, zinc deficiency remains a widespread health issue, affecting diverse populations across regions and age groups. Recognizing zinc's critical role in health, extensive research has been conducted to explore the potential benefits of zinc supplementation to prevent deficiency. By addressing the body's zinc requirements, it digs into various methods of zinc supplementation, including dietary modifications, fortifications, and oral supplements. Effective implementation strategies must consider dosage, duration, and target population characteristics, are crucial for maximizing efficacy while minimizing potential risks. This chapter will explore the impacts of zinc deficiency, the effectiveness and safety of supplementation, underscoring the significance of addressing zinc deficiency through public health initiatives. Additionally, it will outline future avenues for research in this crucial field.

DOI: 10.4018/979-8-3693-5355-4.ch007

1. INTRODUCTION

Zinc, a vital micronutrient, plays a crucial role in facilitating various enzymatic reactions, bolstering immune functions and regulating cellular activities in the human body. Despite its significance, the widespread issue of zinc deficiency persists worldwide, particularly in regions where diets are deficient in zinc-rich foods or where there are high rates of malnutrition. This deficiency impacts individuals of all ages and carries substantial implications for their overall health and welfare.

Zinc serves as a cofactor for over 300 enzymes involved in various biochemical reactions, encompassing protein synthesis, cell division and DNA synthesis (Gibson, 2006). Additionally, it holds pivotal significance in immune function, wound healing and maintaining the integrity of skin and mucosal membranes. Considering its multifaceted roles, ensuring sufficient zinc consumption is imperative for normal growth and development, particularly during critical periods such as infancy, childhood and pregnancy.

Despite its importance, zinc deficiency is widespread, affecting an estimated 17.3% of the global population, with the highest prevalence observed in low- and middle-income countries (Kumssa, 2015; Wessells & Brown, 2012). The ramifications of insufficient zinc levels can be severe and extensive. In children, it can lead to stunted growth, impaired cognitive development and increased susceptibility to infections. Pregnant women with zinc deficiency are at higher risk of complications such as preterm delivery, low birth weight and foetal malformations. Moreover, inadequate zinc levels compromise immune function, rendering individuals more susceptible to infectious diseases, notably respiratory illnesses and diarrhoea, which are leading causes of illness and death worldwide (Kay, 1975; Walsh et al., 1994). (Figure 1)

Figure 1. Effects of zinc deficiency in different stages of life

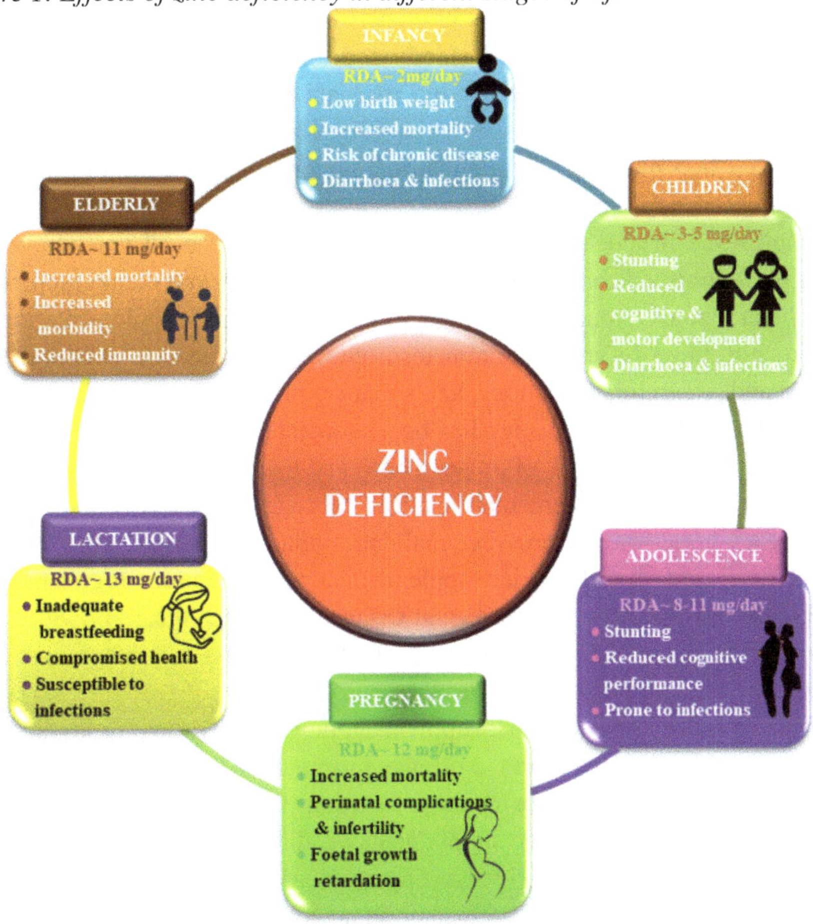
INFANCY
RDA~ 2mg/day
Low birth weight
Increased mortality
Risk of chronic disease
Diarrhoea & infections
CHILDREN
RDA~ 3-5 mg/day
Stunting
Reduced cognitive & motor development
Diarrhoea & infections
ADOLESCENCE
RDA~ 8-11 mg/day
Stunting
Reduced cognitive performance
Prone to infections
PREGNANCY
RDA~ 12 mg/day
Increased mortality
Perinatal complications & infertility
Foetal growth retardation
LACTATION
RDA~ 13 mg/day
Inadequate breastfeeding
Compromised health
Susceptible to infections
ELDERLY
RDA~ 11 mg/day
Increased mortality
Increased morbidity
Reduced immunity
ZINC DEFICIENCY

Recognizing the severity of zinc deficiency and its adverse effects on human health, researchers and public health experts have explored various strategies to address this issue. Zinc supplementation stands out as a promising preventive measure to combat zinc deficiency and its associated health consequences.

Zinc supplementation involves the administration of zinc-containing supplements, either in the form of tablets, capsules, syrups or fortified foods, with the aim of increasing zinc intake to meet recommended daily requirements. This intervention has been widely studied in both clinical and community settings, yielding valuable insights into its efficacy and potential benefits (Maret & Sandstead, 2006; Shankar et al., 2000).

One of the primary objectives of zinc supplementation is to ensure adequate zinc intake among populations at risk of deficiency, including infants, young children, pregnant and lactating women, the elderly and individuals with certain medical conditions that predispose them to zinc inadequacy. Through the provision of supplemental zinc, either independently or alongside other nutrients like vitamins or minerals, it becomes feasible to enhance zinc levels and alleviate the negative impacts of deficiency (Penny, 2013).

Multiple research endeavours have demonstrated the efficacy of zinc supplementation in preventing and correcting zinc deficiency across various demographics and geographical regions (Roohani et al., 2013). In children, zinc supplementation has been shown to improve growth parameters, reduce the incidence and severity of diarrhoea and respiratory infections, and enhance immune function. Additionally, supplementation during pregnancy has been associated with improved birth outcomes, including reduced risk of preterm birth and low birth weight.

The success of zinc supplementation initiatives relies not solely on the intervention's efficacy but also on addressing challenges related to access, adherence and sustainability. Efforts to scale up zinc supplementation programs require collaboration between governments, non-governmental organizations, healthcare providers and communities to ensure equitable access, promote awareness and integrate supplementation with existing healthcare services.

Despite its proven benefits, zinc supplementation is not without limitations and considerations. Challenges related to dosage, formulation, adherence and potential interactions with other nutrients or medications require thorough assessment to ensure the safe and effective use of zinc supplements. Additionally, on-going research is needed to further elucidate the optimal dosing regimens, duration of supplementation and long-term effects of zinc supplementation on health outcomes across different populations and settings.

In conclusion, zinc supplementation represents a valuable preventive measure for addressing zinc deficiency and mitigating its adverse health consequences. Through enhancing immune responses, aiding in growth and development, and enhancing outcomes in maternal and child health, zinc supplementation emerges as a cost-efficient intervention with extensive public health advantages. Sustained efforts in research, program execution and policy formulation are crucial to optimizing the effectiveness of zinc supplementation and attaining lasting enhancements in public health.

2. PHYSIOLOGY OF ZINC

The physiology of zinc delves into the intricate mechanisms through which this essential micronutrient operates within the human body, influencing a myriad of biological functions crucial for health and well-being (Kambe et al., 2015). It is an essential micronutrient which acts as a cofactor for numerous enzymes, facilitating their function in biochemical reactions. Here is a detailed explanation of the physiology of zinc:

2.1 Biological Functions of Zinc

Zinc is present in cells across the body, crucial for the immune system's effectiveness. It aids in cell division, growth, wound healing and carbohydrate breakdown. Zinc is also essential for the senses of smell and taste. Its necessity is heightened during pregnancy, infancy and childhood for proper growth and development. Some of the significant biological functions of zinc are:

- **Enzyme Function:** Zinc plays a vital role in more than 300 enzymes crucial for various biochemical pathways necessary for cellular metabolism. These enzymes participate in processes such as DNA synthesis, protein metabolism, cell division and wound healing. Without adequate zinc, these enzymatic reactions would be impaired, affecting overall cellular function.
- **Gene Expression:** Zinc is crucial for controlling gene expression through its influence on the activity of transcription factors. This regulation influences the production of various proteins essential for cellular function and development.
- **Immune System:** Zinc is essential for the immune system's optimal performance, supporting the growth and function of immune cells such as T cells, B cells, and macrophages. Zinc deficiency can weaken immune responses, making individuals more susceptible to infections and impairing wound healing.
- **Growth and Development:** Zinc is vital for proper growth and development, especially during phases of rapid growth like infancy, childhood, and adolescence. It is necessary for cell division, protein synthesis and tissue repair. Zinc deficiency in children can result in stunted growth, delayed sexual development, and hindered cognitive progress.
- **Skin Health:** Zinc is important for maintaining the integrity of the skin and mucous membranes. It is involved in processes such as wound healing, skin regeneration, and the formation of the skin barrier. Zinc deficiency can result in skin conditions such as dermatitis and impaired wound healing.

- **Reproductive Health:** Zinc plays a role in reproductive health and fertility. It is involved in sperm production, ovulation and fetal development during pregnancy. Zinc deficiency in pregnant women can lead to complications such as preterm birth, low birth weight and congenital abnormalities in the fetus.
- **Neurological Function:** Zinc is implicated in neurological function and cognitive processes. It contributes to neurotransmitter release, synaptic transmission and neuronal signaling. Zinc deficiency has been linked to cognitive impairments, mood disorders and neurodegenerative diseases such as Alzheimer's disease.
- **Antioxidant Defense:** Zinc functions as an antioxidant, protecting cells against the oxidative damage inflicted by free radicals. It scavenges free radicals and helps maintain the balance of antioxidant systems in the body, reducing the risk of oxidative stress-related damage.

2.2 Dietary Sources of Zinc

Dietary sources of zinc include both animal and plant-based foods. However, animal sources tend to have higher bioavailability of zinc compared to plant sources. Some of the good dietary sources of zinc include:

- **Vegetarian Sources:**

  a) Legumes & pulses
  b) Nuts & seeds
  c) Whole grains
  d) Dairy products
  e) Fruits & vegetables
  f) Dark chocolate

- **Non-Vegetarian Sources:**

  a) Shellfish
  b) Meat
  c) Eggs
  d) Organ meats

2.3 Absorption and Metabolism of Zinc

Zinc absorption occurs primarily in the small intestine, particularly the jejunum and duodenum (Lee et al., 1989). Various factors influence zinc absorption, including dietary zinc intake, the presence of other nutrients (such as protein) and the zinc status of the individual. Zinc absorption is regulated by proteins such as metallothionein and zinc transporters.

Once absorbed, zinc is transported in the bloodstream bound to carrier proteins and distributed to various tissues and organs throughout the body. Zinc is stored primarily in the liver, pancreas, kidneys, bones, muscles and skin. Excess zinc is excreted primarily through feces, with smaller amounts excreted in urine and sweat.

In conclusion, the physiology of zinc underscores its indispensable role in maintaining optimal health and functioning of the human body. From enzymatic reactions to immune response and beyond, zinc is an essential micronutrient with far-reaching implications for overall well-being. It is found in a variety of foods and is absorbed and metabolized primarily in the small intestine. Maintaining adequate zinc levels is essential for overall health and well-being, as deficiency can have widespread implications for physiological processes and disease susceptibility.

3. ZINC DEFICIENCY: CAUSES AND CONSEQUENCES

Zinc, a most important trace element, functions as a cornerstone of numerous physiological processes vital for human health. Despite its importance, however, zinc deficiency remains a pervasive nutritional challenge worldwide, affecting individuals across all age groups and socioeconomic strata. Understanding the intricate interplay of factors contributing to zinc deficiency and its far-reaching consequences is paramount for addressing this public health concern effectively. In this discourse, we delve into the causes and consequences of zinc deficiency, shedding light on the mechanisms underlying its onset and the multifaceted impacts it exerts on human health.

3.1 Causes of Zinc Deficiency

Zinc deficiency generally arises from several factors, including insufficient intake, increased losses, heightened requirements, malabsorption and inadequate utilization (King et al., 2016). The most common cause is diet lacking in absorbable zinc, which can occur due to low zinc intake in the diet or a dependence on foods with minimal or inadequate zinc absorption. Many regions around the world experience prevalent inadequate dietary zinc intake, a problem often worsened by physiological conditions that elevate zinc requirements (King et al., 2016; Lönnerdal, 2000).

Zinc malabsorption may occur in various disorders, such as acrodermatitis enteropathica (Van Wouwe, 1989). Secondary zinc deficiency may result the malabsorption syndromes and inflammatory bowel diseases, which cause poor zinc absorption and loss of zinc, especially when dietary intake is marginal (King et al., 2016).

Intestinal integrity impairs zinc absorption and leads to enhanced endogenous zinc losses. Acute diarrhoea exacerbates this issue by raising fecal zinc excretion, though it is unclear how much of this zinc is unabsorbed versus of endogenous origin (Brown et al., 1998). In many underdeveloped countries, diarrhoeal diseases are common. Zinc deficiency heightens susceptibility to diarrhoea in children, and the increased endogenous zinc losses during diarrhoea further deplete the body's zinc levels (Maret, 2001; Nazanin et al., 2013).

3.2 Consequences of Zinc Deficiency

Zinc plays a crucial role in various biochemical functions within human cells, leading to a wide array of physiological symptoms when zinc deficiency occurs. The severity of these symptoms can vary. Zinc deficiency is known to impact various organ systems, including the gastrointestinal tract, skin, central nervous system, skeletal structure, immune and reproductive system (Hambidge & Walravenf, 1982).

Severe zinc deficiency, seen in industrialized nations and in those with acrodermatitis enteropathica (an inherited disorder affecting zinc absorption), can also occur due to other causes like prolonged parenteral nutrition lacking zinc (Van Wouwe, 1989). While severe cases show striking symptoms, milder zinc deficiencies are more common and can exhibit similar but less severe clinical signs. Community-based studies often identify functional impairments associated with mild to moderate zinc deficiency, resembling those seen in acrodermatitis enteropathica (Hambidge, 2000). Some of these impairments include:

- **Growth and Development:** One of the extensively well-researched clinical aspects associated with zinc deficiency is the physical development and growth impediment (Brown et al., 2002). Nonetheless, the underlying mechanisms remain incompletely understood. This impact is particularly significant during ages of rapid growth, such as pregnancy, infancy and puberty, when zinc demands are at their peak (Nazanin et al., 2013).
- **Risk of Infections:**

  Diarrhoea often presents as a distinct feature of acrodermatitis enteropathica, though not invariably (Hambidge, 1992). Plausible reasons for the connection between diarrhoea and zinc deficiency involve the compromised immune system and dysfunction of intestinal mucosal cell transport (Ghishan, 1984). The favourable effects of zinc supplements and the simultaneous increase in growth velocity suggest a causal connection between diarrhoea and zinc deficiency (Brown et al., 1998).

The extent to which oral zinc supplementation can decrease malaria episodes in endemic regions remains uncertain. Some studies suggest a reduction in malaria incidence with zinc supplementation, while others show no significant effect (Shankar et al., 2000; Veenemans et al., 2011).

Community-based zinc supplementation research involving infants in underdeveloped nations have shown a considerable and statistically significant decrease in pneumonia occurrence (Bhutta et al., 1999).

3.3 The Correlation between Zinc Deficiency and Age

Age-related degenerative changes, such as diminished immunocompetence, delayed wound healing, specific neurological and psychological alterations, may be partially attributed to zinc deficiency (Whittaker, 1998).

In general, across different age groups, the clinical indicators of zinc deficiency exhibit variation. Diarrhoea often stands out as an observable symptom in the early stages of infancy. Zinc deficiency can also result in impaired cognitive function, memory problems, behavioral issues, learning disabilities and neuronal atrophy (Brown et al., 2004; Nazanin et al., 2013). As children mature, skin problems become more prevalent, with alopecia, recurrent infections and growth retardation being common during school-age children. Among the elderly, chronic non-healing skin ulcers and repeated infections are frequent. Randomized clinical trials have demonstrated beneficial impacts to supplemental zinc in alleviating these effects (Nazanin et al. 2013). Globally, malnutrition and infectious diseases are the primary causes of mortality and morbidity among young kids.

Ensuring sufficient zinc intake could serve as an effective preventive measure to reduce morbidity and mortality rates in children in developing regions, particularly when vitamin A or iron deficiencies are not present. The prevalence of childhood obesity and its associated conditions, including metabolic syndrome and insulin resistance, is escalating, posing significant health challenges. Zinc supplementation might prove beneficial in managing certain metabolic aspects of these conditions. Furthermore, lower serum zinc levels have been observed in children of parents with premature atherosclerosis, suggesting a potential protective role of zinc in inflammation and the improvement of atherosclerosis (Kelishadi et al., 2002).

Addressing zinc deficiency requires a multifaceted approach, including promoting dietary diversity, fortifying foods with zinc in at-risk populations, supplementation when necessary, and addressing underlying health conditions contributing to malabsorption. By understanding the causes and consequences of zinc deficiency, healthcare providers and policymakers can implement targeted intermediations to improve public health outcomes and mitigate the problem of this preventable nutritional disorder.

4. RATIONALE FOR ZINC SUPPLEMENTATION

Zinc is vital for the activity of over 300 enzymes associated with numerous metabolic pathways, thus playing a crucial role in various immunological, biochemical and clinical functions (Gibson, 2006). Consequently, zinc deficiency affects multiple bodily functions, including immune response, reproductive function, physical growth and neuro-behavioral development. The health implications of zinc deficiency vary across different age groups. Infants commonly experience diarrhea, low weight gain, anorexia and neuro-behavioral abnormalities, while toddlers and school-age children may exhibit blepharo-conjunctivitis, skin changes and impaired linear growth (Hambidge, 1989). Among the elderly, manifestations can include hypogeusia (reduced taste sensitivity), chronic non-healing leg ulcers and persistent infections (Kohn et al., 2000).

The first Randomized Controlled Trial (RCT) on zinc and growth was conducted in 1976 among US infants, revealing positive effects on growth from zinc supplementation (Walravens et al., 1976). Since then, about 100 RCTs and various meta-analyses have investigated zinc's impact on children's growth. According to the thirty-three RCTs, zinc supplementation significantly improved linear growth and weight loss, especially in stunted or underweight children. The benefits were more pronounced in males than females.

In the past decade, RCTs targeting high-risk populations including infants, young children and expectant mothers have demonstrated zinc's preventive health benefits (Bhutta et al., 1999). A comprehensive analysis of studies conducted in underdeveloped nations revealed that zinc supplementation decreased frequency of diarrhoeal infections and acute lower respiratory infections in young children by 18% and 41%, respectively. Zinc also appeared to reduce the severity of malaria caused by Plasmodium falciparum (Shankar et al., 2000). Though fewer studies have explored zinc's impact on mortality, significant reductions were observed in small-for-gestational-age infants in North India and older children in Burkina Faso, with mortality reductions of 67% and 50%, respectively (Sazawal et al. 2001; Muller et al. 2001).

RCT results on pregnancy and maternal health outcomes have been inconsistent, possibly due to variations in assessed outcomes, study location, design and other factors. Few studies, especially in underdeveloped countries, have explored the impact of zinc supplementation on maternal health during pregnancy (Gibson, 2006). While some studies have reported positive responses in baby weight and gestational age with zinc supplementation, others have not observed such effects. For instance, RCTs in Latin America and Asia found no positive impact on baby weight or pregnancy duration with zinc supplementation. However, supplementation with zinc, iron and folate in Peruvian mothers has shown benefits in fetal neuro-behavioral development compared to iron and folate alone. Additionally, low birth weight infants whose mothers received zinc supplements throughout pregnancy have shown decreased rates of diarrhoea, dysentery, and impetigo. Recent zinc supplementation trials have focused on neuro-behavioral function in infants and early childhood, with mixed results indicating potential improvements in activity levels, developmental scores and neuropsychological test performance (Gibson, 2006).

5. METHODS OF ZINC SUPPLEMENTATION

Various strategies have proven effective in addressing zinc deficiency. These include supplementation programs, fortification initiatives, bio-fortification approaches and dietary diversification. Selecting an intervention relies on the particular reason for the deficiency and the availability of resources, technologies and infrastructure (Brown et al., 2004).

5.1 Supplementation

Supplementation is an effective immediate measure to replenish zinc levels in at-risk cohorts. It provides a feasible approach for reaching the target groups unable to access zinc-rich foods when fortification or dietary interventions are inadequate. Zinc supplementation helps prevent diarrhoea, pneumonia, lung-related infections, infantile mortality, and unfavourable pregnancy outcomes in women, particularly in low- to middle-income countries.

Selecting a chemical form of zinc for supplementation is crucial, considering its bioavailability, safety and cost-effectiveness. Options like zinc chloride, citrate, acetate, oxide, lactate, gluconate, sulfate, stearate and methionine are available. Zinc acetate, sulfate and gluconate are more soluble in water than other forms, making them preferable. Notably, zinc oxide absorption is slightly lower when ingested without food (Brown et al., 2004). WHO recommends dispersible tablets or syrups of zinc acetate (30% Zn), zinc sulfate (23% Zn), or zinc gluconate (14% Zn) for diarrhoea management (WHO, 2006). Studies comparing zinc absorption found zinc citrate effective, with zinc gluconate being a good alternative.

Several studies demonstrate the benefits of zinc supplementation. In Iran, supplementation with 5 mg of elemental zinc per day for six months prevented growth retardation in children aged 6–24 months (Abdollahi et al., 2019). Similarly, a meta-analysis showed increased height, weight and serum zinc levels in prepubescent children receiving zinc supplementation. Enteral zinc supplementation in infants accelerated weight loss and linear growth (Alshaikh et al., 2022). According to a meta-analysis, the growth was significantly increased in children under the age of five who received a dosage of 10 mg zinc per day for 24 weeks. Nevertheless, a daily dose of 7 mg of zinc per day was inadequate to improve cytokine or T-cell levels in rural Laotian children between 6-23 months old (Kewcharoenwong et al., 2020).

In accordance with UNICEF and WHO recommendations, zinc supplementation is implemented in several Asian and African nations, as well as parts of South America, to address diarrhoea in children under 5 years old. Guidelines suggest administering children under 3 years old 10 mg of zinc per day and older children (3–5 years) 20 mg of zinc per day over a period of 10–14 days. However, this strategy alone may not adequately prevent zinc deficiency in children, as supplementation occurs only during diarrhoeal episodes. Despite the fact of its beneficial effects on child growth is established, further scientific research is necessary to ascertain the benefits of zinc supplementation for adults, especially expectant mothers (Sangeetha et al., 2022).

Supplementation programs face challenges like cost, donor dependency and compliance. In Mexico, zinc supplementation reduced deficiency among pre-schoolers by 58.6 percentage points and decreased diarrhoea duration and incidence in children under 5. Despite these successes, issues like distribution, regulation and non-patented supplements hinder progress. A reliable system for continuous supply, distribution and monitoring is essential (Sangeetha et al., 2022). To address multiple micronutrient deficiencies, integrating zinc into existing interventions is crucial, requiring collaboration among public health experts, governments, and funding agencies.

Multiple Micronutrient Powders (MNPs) containing zinc have shown promise in reducing diarrhoea but lack strong evidence for improving zinc status compared to single micronutrient supplements (Lamberti et al., 2016). Potential risks of MNPs, such as intestinal inflammation and altered gut microbiota, have raised concerns. Zinc absorption is most effective with meals and without other micronutrients. More research is needed to evaluate MNP effectiveness and risks, especially with phytate-containing foods. In particularly for children, exploring personalized foods including gels, texturized products, and 3D-printed foods could help fulfill the Recommended Daily Allowance (RDA) of zinc (Sangeetha et al., 2022).

5.2 Fortification

Food fortification offers an affordable and sustainable solution for addressing micronutrient deficiency compared to supplementation. For communities where deficiency is widespread and dietary modification is challenging, fortifying commonly processed foods presents a viable solution. Mexico exemplifies a country with a national zinc fortification initiative, enriching corn flours and wheat utilized in essential foods such as bread and tortillas with micronutrients. When implementing multiple interventions, it's essential to consider both antagonistic and synergistic interactions amongst micronutrients when developing appropriate formulations (Sangeetha et al., 2022; Nazanin et al., 2013).

Fortification programs can help high-risk groups, like infants and young children, by adding zinc and other micronutrients to their foods. Many infant formulae and complementary foods are already fortified with zinc at about 1 mg/L. The chosen food for fortification should be widely and consistently consumed. Zinc sulfate and zinc oxide are commonly used due to their cost-effectiveness, with recommended fortification levels for flour between 30 and 70 mg/kg. Although zinc sulfate is theoretically more absorbable because of its higher solubility, human studies have not consistently demonstrated significant differences in absorption between zinc oxide and zinc sulfate (Sangeetha et al., 2022; Nazanin et al., 2013).

5.3 Bio-Fortification

Plant breeding and genetic engineering strategies are being explored to boost the bioavailability of zinc in vegetable foods. These methods aim to increase zinc levels, reduce inhibitors like phytate and enhance compounds that aid zinc absorption, such as amino acids. Bio-fortification, unlike ordinary fortification, enriches plant parts with micronutrients during growth, providing nutrients directly in the food source without the need for external processing. This approach is especially beneficial for rural communities where access to commercially fortified foods is limited (Lönnerdal, 2003). Bio-fortification is considered a promising strategy for addressing micronutrient deficiencies in the underdeveloped countries, offering greater advantages like increased crop production and vitality of zinc-enriched seedlings (Sangeetha et al., 2022).

5.4 Bio-Fortification Methods

Bio-fortification is an agricultural approach aiming to boost the levels of essential micronutrients, such as zinc, in staple crops like wheat, maize, rice, and pearl millet. Strategies involve using zinc fertilizers and developing crop varieties that absorb and accumulate more zinc from the soil into edible parts. By capitalizing on the daily intake of staple foods by all family, especially women and children who are more susceptible to malnutrition, bio-fortification effectively focuses on low-income households (Sangeetha et al., 2022).

Increasing dietary zinc intake can be achieved through various interventions, including agronomic and genetic techniques (Stein, 2010; Sangeetha et al., 2022). Agronomic bio-fortification involves enhancing the availability of zinc in the soil or applying zinc fertilizers, requiring suitable infrastructure but proving successful where mineral fertilizers are used. Genetic bio-fortification aims to enhance zinc uptake from the soil and its concentration in edible plant parts, making use of the existing zinc content in agricultural soils. Economic analyses often favour genetic bio-fortification as a practical, long-lasting and cost-effective approach compared to other strategies like supplementation, food fortification or dietary diversification for vulnerable populations (Nazanin et al., 2013; Sangeetha et al., 2022).

Applying zinc to the soil via fertilizers or as foliar sprays is an effective method for increasing zinc level, known as agronomic bio-fortification. The HarvestPlus program evaluates this approach for cereals like wheat, rice and maize in various countries. This method complements breeding programs for high-zinc grain genotypes. Research shows that soil and foliar zinc applications significantly boost grain zinc levels, with $ZnSO_4$ being a popular choice due to its affordability and solubility. $ZnSO_4$ applications have doubled wheat grain zinc concentrations in Central Anatolia, with foliar applications showing even greater increases. The most effective method to maximize zinc accumulation, improve plant growth, and increase grain yield is to use both soil and foliar applications (Sangeetha et al., 2022).

5.5 Dietary Diversification

Dietary diversification is a sustainable method for boosting the intake of multiple nutrients, including zinc (Gibson & Anderson, 2009). Approaches at the community level can enhance the availability of bioavailable zinc, such as:

- Agricultural interventions
- Promoting animal-source foods through aquaculture or animal husbandry
- Methods of processing to improve the absorption of zinc from plant-based diets

While plant-focused agricultural interventions may have limited impact on bio-available zinc intake, combining them with processing methods to reduce inhibitors like phytate can help. Efforts in animal husbandry that boost the consumption of milk, cheese, liver, and red meat can enhance zinc intake since these foods generally provide zinc in a form that is easily absorbed. Educating people about nutrition and encouraging a varied diet can result in increased consumption of animal-based foods and zinc that is easily absorbed by the body. However, caution is necessary to avoid potential adverse effects, such as aflatoxin contamination or loss of nutrients during food processing (Sangeetha et al., 2022). Despite being the most sustainable approach, dietary modification can be challenging due to entrenched dietary preferences and the high cost of foods rich in bioavailable zinc, like red meat.

6. FACTORS INFLUENCING EFFICACY AND SAFETY OF ZINC SUPPLEMENTATION

Supplementing with zinc has become a promising strategy to address zinc deficiency and mitigate its negative health impacts. However, the safety and efficacy of zinc supplementation are influenced by a multitude of factors, ranging from dosage and formulation to individual characteristics and concurrent health conditions. Comprehending these factors is vital in order to optimize the benefits of zinc supplementation while minimizing potential risks. In this discussion, we explore the various factors that affect the efficiency and safety of zinc supplementation, providing insights into how healthcare providers and policymakers can tailor supplementation strategies to maximize effectiveness and promote overall well-being.

6.1 General Issues of Supplementation Programs

Supplementation involves providing additional nutrients in chemical form rather than through food. It's a valuable short-term approach for enhancing the nutritional status of vulnerable populations, such as those without access to fortified foods or pregnant women needing iron and folate. In wealthier nations, certain populations still rely on supplementation. While it may be necessary until the benefits of fortification and dietary diversification are realized, some groups might need long-term supplementation.

For supplementation programs to succeed, they need a reliable supply, effective distribution, and proper delivery of supplements, along with efforts to encourage their use. Many programs fail due to lack of commitment, inconsistent supply, poor coverage, ineffective communication and low compliance. Overburdened healthcare systems also play a role. Compliance issues, particularly with iron supplements, often stem from side effects and behavioral barriers. Successful programs typically employ social marketing, effective targeting, extended outreach and improved service quality. Developing successful supplemental programs require careful consideration of the following factors:

- Selecting the appropriate zinc forms, physical and chemical
- Determining the appropriate dosage level and frequency of administration
- Deciding whether to include other micronutrients in the supplement
- Administering supplements with or without food
- Establishing an efficient packaging and distribution system
- Assessing any potential risks of toxicity

6.2 Selecting a Supplement Type, Dosage and Administration Method

- **Chemical form of the Supplement:** Choosing the appropriate chemical form of zinc for supplements depends on solubility, cost, taste, side effects and safety. Water-soluble substances like zinc acetate, gluconate and sulfate are generally preferred for their efficient absorption. Research on various forms, including zinc acetate, ascorbate, aminoate, citrate, gluconate, oxide, histidine, methionine, picolinate and sulfate, shows variable and sometimes conflicting absorption rates (Barrie et al., 1987). Zinc oxide, for example, is less absorbable due to its low solubility at neutral pH, which can be problematic in cases of reduced gastric acidity, such as in malnourished children. Research demonstrates that zinc sulfate is more efficient than zinc oxide in increasing plasma levels of zinc. Zinc histidine and methionine, despite potentially better absorption due to amino acid ligands, may not be cost-effective (Scholmerich et al., 1987).
- **Physical form of the Supplement:** Zinc supplements for infants and young children are frequently used as flavored syrups or chewable tablets. For school-age children, tablets can be either chewable or dispersible in fluids. Recently, zinc has been added to high-fat spreads, single-dose sachets (sprinkles) and crushable tablets added to food at serving. The ideal form is contingent upon the age range, cultural inclinations and the need for additional nutrients. Liquid or easily mixable supplements are best for young children, while dry forms (capsules, powders, tablets) are cheaper, more stable and can include a wider variety of nutrients. High-fat, micronutrient-fortified spreads offer another option, but further research are needed to evaluate their acceptability, effectiveness and influence on standard diets (Cavan et al., 1993).
- **Considerations for Administering Zinc Supplements alongside other Nutrients or Meals:** Zinc can be taken on its own or as part of multi-nutrient supplements, such as those containing iron and folate for prenatal use, and it can be consumed with meals or between meals. Absorption is higher on an empty stomach since dietary phytates inhibit it. To minimize interactions with minerals like calcium, iron and copper, easily absorbed zinc salts are

preferred in multi-nutrient supplements. Although food ligands can lessen the inhibitory impact of non-heme iron on zinc absorption, zinc is generally absorbed more efficiently when taken without food (Valberg et al., 1984; Sandstrom et al., 1985). Adding ligands like histidine to zinc supplements can enhance absorption, though many trials do not specify if supplements were taken with food, complicating the assessment of nutrient interactions.

- **Frequency of Administration:** Frequent administration of zinc supplements might be necessary because the majority of zinc in the body is stored in stable, non-labile pools that are not readily released during periods of deficiency. However, some studies suggest less frequent dosing could still be effective. A trial with Vietnamese infants found that administering daily (5 mg) and weekly (17 mg) supplements of zinc enhanced both linear growth and serum zinc levels in children suffering from stunted growth (Thu et al., 1999). The finding suggested that the benefits of zinc supplementation might extend beyond the immediate increase in zinc levels. Nonetheless, a rat study indicated that daily zinc was necessary for optimal growth response. Due to limited comparative studies, daily zinc supplementation (5-7 days a week) is currently suggested.
- **Guideline Daily Dosage Levels:** The ideal zinc dosage to avoid deficiency across age groups and clinical conditions lacks systematic study. Tentative recommendations, based on RDAs and clinical trial dosages, aim to avoid chronic over-dosage. It is recommended that children aged 7 months to 3 years receive 5 mg of zinc per day, while those older than 3 years should receive 10 mg per day. A meta-analysis of studies involving children aged 6 months to 10 years showed that zinc dosages between 1 and 20 mg per day led to positive growth responses. The lack of a clear dose-response relationship suggests that even lower doses might be effective in preventing growth retardation caused by zinc deficiency (Brown et al., 2002). For young children recuperating from severe malnutrition (weight-for-height Z-score < –3), 10 mg/day is recommended to meet increased catch-up growth needs, as their physiological zinc requirements are roughly doubled. Pregnant women are generally advised to take 15–30 mg of elemental zinc daily, usually most commonly in the form of sulfate.

6.3 Expense of Incorporating Zinc in Ongoing Supplementation Regimens

Incorporating zinc into programs that provide daily or weekly nutrient supplements, such as those with iron, is both feasible and cost-effective. The additional expenses would primarily involve the cost of zinc, quality control during manufacturing, and impact measurement. With zinc sulfate priced at $25.7 per kg, the extra cost would be $0.05–0.19 per person annually. Iron supplementation programs currently cost $3.17–5.30 per person annually, indicating the minimal cost increase for adding zinc. For program monitoring, using a cost-model for wheat flour fortification as a reference, reaching 1,290,000 pre-school children with evaluation activities would incur an extra $6,000 annually for zinc status biochemical analysis. This translates to less than $0.01 per person per year for monitoring, making the overall additional cost of including zinc negligible (Fink & Heitner, 2014).

7. PUBLIC HEALTH IMPLICATIONS

Zinc supplementation is a vital resource in public health efforts, addressing the pervasive issue of zinc deficiency. Zinc, an indispensable micronutrient, serves diverse functions within the body, impacting immune responses, the progression of growth and development, wound repair and cognitive abilities. Consequently, its deficiency can lead to a spectrum of health complications, ranging from increased susceptibility to infections to impaired growth and neurodevelopment.

7.1 Role of Zinc Supplementation in Public Health Programs

Zinc is crucial for numerous essential bodily functions that are vital for human well-being. Yet, the problem of zinc deficiency persists as a major worldwide public health issue, especially among communities with restricted dietary options. To counter this challenge, zinc supplementation has become a cornerstone in public health strategies, aiming to combat deficiencies and promote better health outcomes. Integrating zinc supplementation into existing health initiatives, such as maternal and child health programs, nutrition interventions and infectious disease prevention efforts, has the potential to improve immune function, support growth and development, and mitigate the adverse effects of deficiency on maternal and child health (Roohani et al., 2013).

7.2 Challenges and Opportunities in Zinc Supplementation: Toward Smarter, Scalable Solutions

While zinc supplementation offers promise in addressing nutritional deficiencies, several challenges need addressing to optimize its efficacy in public health initiatives.

- **Challenges of Zinc Supplementation:**

Bioavailability and Nutrient Interactions: One of the most pressing challenges in zinc supplementation lies in achieving optimal bioavailability. Zinc uptake is significantly hindered by phytates—antinutritional factors prevalent in cereals and legumes—which form insoluble complexes with zinc. Additionally, zinc competes with minerals like iron, calcium, and copper for absorption, posing a challenge in multi-micronutrient formulations. To address these constraints, future research and formulation strategies should prioritize on enhancing zinc bioavailability through innovative delivery systems such as chelated forms, enzymatic phytate degradation, and optimized meal timing to minimize antagonistic interactions.

Adherence and Acceptability: Adherence to zinc supplementation programs remains a significant challenge, largely due to the unfavourable organoleptic characteristics of zinc salts, which are known to cause nausea, metallic taste, and gastrointestinal discomfort—symptoms that are particularly detrimental in paediatric populations. In addition, sociocultural resistance, misinformation, and limited public awareness further impede compliance. To improve adherence and maximize program efficacy, it is imperative to improve the palatability of zinc supplements, develop age-appropriate formulations such as flavoured dispersible tablets or powders, and implement comprehensive, community-based educational campaigns.

Programmatic and Logistical Barriers: Zinc supplementation programs in many low- and middle-income countries are hindered by fragmented supply chains, limited financial resources, and underdeveloped distribution infrastructures, leading to irregular access to zinc supplements at both healthcare and community levels. Strengthening supply chain resilience through localized production, strategic public-private collaborations, and decentralized delivery systems is critical to addressing these challenges. Furthermore, the integration of digital technologies can facilitate real-time inventory tracking, minimize product wastage, and enhance the efficiency and timeliness of distribution.

Equity and Targeting: Zinc supplementation initiatives may inadvertently exclude the most vulnerable populations, such as individuals in remote rural areas, conflict zones, or marginalized urban communities. These groups frequently face layered challenges to healthcare access, such as inadequate infrastructure, financial constraints, and social exclusion. To mitigate these disparities, health systems should employ geospatial analysis and demographic data to accurately pinpoint underserved populations. Customized outreach interventions—such as mobile health services and networks of community health workers—can play a pivotal role in promoting equitable access to supplementation efforts.

Monitoring and Evaluation: The monitoring and evaluation of zinc supplementation programs remain suboptimal, especially with respect to real-time assessment of zinc status, adherence, and associated health outcomes. Conventional evaluation methods are often resource-intensive and may lack the sensitivity required for timely and accurate insights. Integrating biomarkers for zinc status, mobile health technologies, and community-driven surveillance systems can enhance data collection efficiency and support dynamic program refinement. Establishing continuous learning mechanisms and feedback loops is crucial for adaptive program management and ensuring long-term sustainability.

However, despite these challenges, there exist substantial prospects to utilize zinc supplementation within comprehensive public health strategies to improve health outcomes and diminish the impact of preventable diseases (Gupta et al., 2020).

- **Opportunities in Zinc Supplementation:**

  Integration with Broader Health Systems: Zinc supplementation presents a valuable opportunity for integration into established maternal and child health services, immunization efforts, and school-based nutrition programs. Embedding zinc delivery within comprehensive public health platforms can enhance the efficiency of resource use and extend program reach.

  Innovation in Delivery Platforms: Recent advancements in pharmaceutical and food technologies offer promising avenues for the development of innovative zinc delivery systems. Nanoformulations, targeted delivery mechanisms, and lipid-based carriers can enhance zinc bioavailability and therapeutic effectiveness. Additionally, development of culturally acceptable and age-specific products, such as micronutrient-enriched snacks, oral gels, or 3D-printed personalized nutrition solutions, has the potential to transform supplementation strategies.

  Bio-fortification Synergies: Integrating zinc supplementation with the bio-fortification of staple crops presents a sustainable approach to addressing chronic zinc deficiency. Agronomic methods, such as the use of zinc-enriched fertilizers, and genetic bio-fortification, including the development of high-zinc varieties of wheat, rice, or maize, have demonstrated potential in enhancing the zinc content of diets. These strategies are especially beneficial in rural areas where access to commercial supplements may be restricted. Aligning bio-fortification initiatives with national nutrition policies can amplify their effectiveness and reach.

Cross-Sector Collaboration: The multifaceted nature of zinc deficiency necessitates collaboration across health, agriculture, education, and technology sectors. Joint initiatives can enhance nutrition literacy, dietary diversity, and supplement distribution. Cross-sector partnerships also enable resource pooling and foster innovation in delivery models.

Tailored Supplementation Based on Genomics and Biomarkers: Emerging research in nutrigenomics and personalized medicine highlights the potential of tailoring zinc supplementation to individual genetic profiles and physiological needs. Genetic polymorphisms influencing zinc absorption and metabolism may guide the development of individualized supplementation protocols. Furthermore, the application of non-invasive biomarkers and artificial intelligence–driven predictive models offers promising tools for identifying at-risk populations and monitoring treatment responses, thereby paving the way for precision public health.

A more thorough exploration of these issues would facilitate a shift from broad, generalized recommendations toward more context-sensitive, scalable, and innovative interventions—an essential progression for informing effective policymaking and public health program design.

7.3 Addressing Zinc Deficiency through Intervention Programs

Public health interventions addressing zinc deficiency employ diverse strategies to encourage sufficient zinc intake and supplementation. These interventions often target vulnerable populations, such as pregnant women, infants and young children, who are at increased risk of zinc deficiency and its associated health consequences. Integrating supplementation programs into routine healthcare services, such as antenatal care, child health visits and community outreach efforts, facilitates reaching underserved populations and achieving broad coverage. Additionally, efforts to improve dietary diversity and quality complement supplementation initiatives, addressing underlying nutritional deficiencies comprehensively and promoting long-term health outcomes (Chaudhary et al., 2022).

7.4 Importance of Awareness and Education

At the core of effective zinc supplementation initiatives lies the critical need for awareness and education among healthcare providers, policymakers, and communities. Increasing awareness of the health benefits of zinc, the consequences of deficiency and the availability of supplementation programs can encourage uptake and adherence among target populations. Health education endeavors, comprising counseling sessions, informative resources and community workshops, are pivotal in empowering individuals and communities to make knowledgeable health choices. Furthermore, integrating zinc education into school curricula and training programs for healthcare professionals can help ensure sustained support for supplementation efforts and foster a culture of preventive healthcare.

In conclusion, zinc supplementation holds significant promise as a preventive measure for addressing zinc deficiency and improving public health outcomes. By integrating supplementation into existing health programs, addressing logistical challenges and prioritizing awareness and education, public health efforts can maximize the influence of zinc supplementation in reducing the burden of preventable diseases and promoting health and well-being for individuals and communities worldwide.

8. RECOMMENDATIONS FOR STAKEHOLDERS

In light of the extensive evidence on the causes, consequences, and interventions for zinc deficiency, it is essential to tailor actionable strategies for key stakeholders—including healthcare providers, policymakers, and researchers—to optimize zinc supplementation efforts and reduce public health burdens. The specific recommendations for zinc supplementation are indicated in Table 1.

Table 1. Stakeholder-specific recommendations for zinc supplementation

Stakeholder	Key Recommendations
Healthcare Providers	• Integrate zinc screening in routine antenatal, paediatric, and geriatric visits. • Administer age- and condition-specific doses of zinc based on WHO and national guidelines. • Choose appropriate forms (e.g., zinc sulfate or gluconate) based on bioavailability and patient tolerance. • Promote consumption of bioavailable zinc sources (meat, dairy, legumes) and educate patients on food preparation methods that reduce inhibitors like phytates. • Incorporate zinc supplementation in existing maternal and child health programs. • Scale up national zinc supplementation programs targeting high-risk groups using WHO-recommended protocols.
Policymakers	• Mandate zinc fortification in staple foods (e.g., wheat flour, maize meal) especially in populations with poor dietary diversity. • Promote inter-sectoral collaboration with agriculture and education sectors. • Establish national surveillance systems for tracking zinc deficiency prevalence and supplementation program outcomes. • Conduct comparative studies to determine the most effective formulations, dosing regimens, and administration methods for diverse populations. • Focus on vulnerable groups such as pregnant women, infants, and the elderly to generate population-specific recommendations and improve intervention targeting.
Researchers	• Research adherence barriers and design behavioural interventions. • Initiate long-term studies assessing the sustained impact of zinc supplementation on immunity, growth, cognitive development, and chronic disease prevention. • Analyse socio-economic and geographic disparities in access to zinc-rich diets and supplements, and develop solutions accordingly.

By implementing these tailored recommendations, stakeholders can significantly contribute in mitigating zinc deficiency, advancing health outcomes, and improving the overall well-being of vulnerable populations worldwide.

9. ADVANCING ZINC SUPPLEMENTATION: INNOVATIONS, RESEARCH SIGNIFICANCES AND STRATEGIC INTEGRATION

As our comprehension of zinc's role in human health progresses, we uncover numerous avenues for additional research and observe emerging trends in zinc supplementation. These paths not only involve enhancing current strategies but also delve into novel approaches to maximize the benefits of zinc supplementation (Pérez-Escamilla & Engmann, 2019).

9.1 Emerging Trends in Zinc Supplementation Research

Zinc supplementation research has undergone significant evolution, spurred by advancements in understanding the critical role of zinc in human health. As our knowledge expands, emerging trends in zinc supplementation research have begun to shape the landscape of preventive healthcare. This briefing outlines an overview of these emerging trends, which encompass novel approaches, cutting-edge technologies and interdisciplinary collaborations aimed at optimizing the effectiveness of zinc supplementation interventions.

- **Nanoformulations:** Investigating the use of nanoformulations to enhance the bioavailability and efficacy of zinc supplementation.
- **Genetic Factors:** Exploring genetic variations that influence zinc metabolism and responsiveness to supplementation, leading to personalized approaches.
- **Combined Supplementation:** Studying the synergistic effects of combining zinc with other micronutrients or bioactive compounds to amplify health benefits.
- **Targeted Delivery Systems:** Developing targeted delivery systems to deliver zinc specifically to tissues or organs where it is most needed.
- **Gut Microbiota:** Investigating the interplay between zinc supplementation and the gut microbiota, and how microbial composition influences zinc absorption and utilization.

9.2 Priority Areas for Future Research on Zinc Supplementation

Although zinc supplementation has demonstrated potential as a preventative method for managing zinc deficiency, numerous unaddressed aspects necessitate additional exploration. This overview examines the primary domains necessitating further research and inquiry into zinc supplementation to prevent zinc deficiency. Through an exploration of these domains, our objective is to expand our comprehension, enhance current methodologies and devise more impactful interventions to address this prevalent nutritional issue.

- **Optimizing Dosage and Formulation:** Research should focus on determining the optimal dosage and formulation of zinc supplements for different age groups, populations and health conditions. This includes investigating the bioavailability of various zinc compounds and delivery methods to ensure maximum absorption and effectiveness.
- **Identifying At-Risk Populations:** Further research is needed to identify and characterize populations most at risk of zinc deficiency, including pregnant women, infants, young children, the elderly and individuals with specific medical conditions or dietary restrictions. Understanding the factors contributing to zinc deficiency in these groups can inform targeted intervention strategies.

- **Integration with Healthcare Services:** Future studies should explore strategies for integrating zinc supplementation into routine healthcare services, including antenatal care, pediatric visits and primary care settings. This could involve training healthcare providers on the importance of zinc supplementation, developing guidelines for screening and monitoring zinc status, and incorporating zinc supplementation into standard clinical protocols.
- **Long-Term Health Outcomes:** Research should investigate the long-term health outcomes associated with zinc supplementation, including its effects on immune function, growth and development, cognitive function and the prevention of chronic diseases. Longitudinal studies are needed to assess the effect of zinc supplementation over extended periods and across different stages of the life course.
- **Nutritional Education and Behavioral Interventions:** There is a need for research on effective strategies to promote zinc-rich diets and improve dietary diversity among at-risk populations. Nutritional education programs, behavioral interventions and community-based initiatives can play a crucial role in increasing awareness of zinc-rich foods and promoting healthy eating habits.
- **Addressing Equity and Access:** Efforts should be made to address barriers to equitable access to zinc supplementation, particularly in low-income and marginalized communities. This includes exploring innovative delivery models, reducing cost barriers and ensuring availability of zinc supplements in remote or underserved areas.

To concisely present the key priority areas for future research, a summary has been organized in tabular format, as shown in Table 2.

Table 2. Priority research areas in zinc supplementation

Research Area	Key Gaps	Recommended Research
Optimal Dosing and Formulations	Lack of consensus on age-, sex-, and condition-specific dosing and duration	• Dose-response trials by age and condition • Compare absorption across zinc salts (e.g., gluconate vs. citrate) • Formulation trials comparing tablets, syrups, micronutrient powders (MNPs), and novel delivery systems (e.g., nano-encapsulation)
Zinc in Comorbid Conditions	Limited data on effects in chronic and inflammatory diseases	• Efficacy and safety of zinc in managing comorbidities such as diabetes, cardiovascular disease, and obesity • Studies on zinc's interaction with iron, calcium, and other micronutrients in poly-supplementation contexts
Maternal and Neonatal Outcomes	Inconclusive evidence on benefits of zinc during pregnancy and its effect on neonates	• Large RCTs assessing outcomes like low birth weight, preterm birth • Follow-up studies on child development
Cognitive and Neurobehavioral Impacts	Sparse evidence linking zinc to cognition	• Neurodevelopmental studies in children • Zinc's potential in managing attention-deficit/hyperactivity disorder (ADHD), autism spectrum disorder (ASD), depression
Personalized Supplementation	One-size-fits-all approaches overlook individual variability	• Genetic studies on zinc transporter variants • Microbiome- and diet-based personalization
Zinc–Gut Microbiota Interactions	Insufficient understanding of zinc's influence on gut microbiota composition and vice versa	• Metagenomic studies assessing how zinc alters microbial diversity and function • Research in malnourished/ immunocompromised groups
Implementation and Equity	Coverage, adherence, and equity remain operational challenges	• Studies on cost-effective, culturally appropriate delivery models • Equity-focused access analyses
Agricultural Biofortification Effects	Long-term ecological and nutritional outcomes not well studied	• Trials on environmental impact of zinc-fertilized crops • Consumer acceptability and nutrient yield in biofortified foods

By delving into these areas of research, we can not only expand our knowledge of zinc supplementation but also tailor interventions more effectively to improve health outcomes and address nutritional deficiencies on a global scale. Furthermore, embracing emerging trends in zinc supplementation research allows us to stay at the forefront of innovation and contribute to the advancement of public health strategies aimed at promoting well-being and reducing the burden of preventable diseases.

10. CONCLUSION

In conclusion, zinc supplementation remains a highly effective intervention for preventing zinc deficiency, offering a focused and evidence-based means of ensuring adequate intake of this essential micronutrient. It is especially beneficial for high-risk groups such as young children and pregnant women, given its crucial role in immune function, growth, and overall development. To maximize its public health impact, implementation must be tailored to local contexts, addressing key barriers such as limited bioavailability, poor adherence, health inequities, and the need for integration within existing healthcare infrastructures. Advancing this agenda will require sustained research, robust policy backing, and active community involvement. Additionally, strengthening program monitoring, fostering innovation, and enhancing health education efforts are critical for improving outcomes. A collaborative and data-driven approach can firmly position zinc supplementation at the heart of global strategies to reduce nutritional deficiencies and promote health equity.

REFERENCES

Abdollahi, M., Ajami, M., Abdollahi, Z., Kalantari, N., Houshiarrad, A., Fozouni, F., Fallahrokni, A., & Mazandarani, F. S. (2019). Zinc supplementation is an effective and feasible strategy to prevent growth retardation in 6 to 24 month children: A pragmatic double blind, randomized trial. *Heliyon*, *5*(11), e02581. DOI: 10.1016/j.heliyon.2019.e02581 PMID: 31720482

Alshaikh, B., Abo Zeed, M., Yusuf, K., Guin, M., & Fenton, T. (2022). Effect of enteral zinc supplementation on growth and neurodevelopment of preterm infants: A systematic review and meta- analysis. *Journal of Perinatology*, *42*(4), 430–439. DOI: 10.1038/s41372-021-01094-7 PMID: 34006967

Barrie, S. A., Wright, J. V., Pizzorno, J. E., Kutter, E., & Barron, P. C. (1987). Comparative absorption of zinc picolinate, zinc citrate and zinc gluconate in humans. *Agents and Actions*, *21*(1-2), 223–228. DOI: 10.1007/BF01974946 PMID: 3630857

Bhutta, Z. A., Black, R. E., Brown, K. H., Gardner, J. M., Gore, S., Hidayat, A., Khatun, F., Martorell, R., Ninh, N. X., Penny, M. E., Rosado, J. L., Roy, S. K., Ruel, M., Sazawal, S., & Shankar, A. (1999). Prevention of diarrhea and pneumonia by zinc supplementation in children in developing countries: Pooled analysis of randomized controlled trials. Zinc Investigators' Collaborative Group. *The Journal of Pediatrics*, *135*(6), 689–697. DOI: 10.1016/S0022-3476(99)70086-7 PMID: 10586170

Brown, K. H., Peerson, J. M., & Allen, L. H. (1998). Effect of zinc supplementation on children's growth: A meta-analysis of intervention trials. *Bibliotheca Nutritio et Dieta*, *54*, 76–83. PMID: 9597173

Brown, K. H., Peerson, J. M., Rivera, J., & Allen, L. H. (2002). Effect of supplemental zinc on the growth and serum zinc concentrations of prepubertal children: A meta-analysis of randomized controlled trials. *The American Journal of Clinical Nutrition*, *75*(6), 1062–1071. DOI: 10.1093/ajcn/75.6.1062 PMID: 12036814

Brown, K. H., Rivera, J. A., Bhutta, Z., Gibson, R. S., King, J. C., Lönnerdal, B., Ruel, M. T., Sandtröm, B., Wasantwisut, E., & Hotz, C. (2004). International Zinc Nutrition Consultative Group (IZiNCG) technical document #1. Assessment of the risk of zinc deficiency in populations and options for its control. *Food and Nutrition Bulletin*, *25*, S99–S203. PMID: 18046856

Cavan, K. R., Gibson, R. S., Grazioso, C. F., Isalgue, A. M., Ruz, M., & Solomons, N. W. (1993). Growth and body composition of periurban Guatemalan children in relation to zinc status: A longitudinal zinc intervention trial. *The American Journal of Clinical Nutrition*, *57*(3), 344–352. DOI: 10.1093/ajcn/57.3.344 PMID: 8438768

Chaudhary, V., Saraswathy, K. N., & Sarwal, R. (2022). Dietary diversity as a sustainable approach towards micronutrient deficiencies in India. *The Indian Journal of Medical Research, 156*(1), 31–45. DOI: 10.4103/ijmr.ijmr_3314_21 PMID: 36510896

Fink, G., & Heitner, J. (2014). Evaluating the cost-effectiveness of preventive zinc supplementation. *BMC Public Health, 14*(1), 852. DOI: 10.1186/1471-2458-14-852 PMID: 25128210

Ghishan, F. K. (1984). Transport of electrolytes, water, and glucose in zinc deficiency. *Journal of Pediatric Gastroenterology and Nutrition, 3*, 608–612. PMID: 6090631

Gibson, R. S. (2006). Zinc: The missing link in combating micronutrient malnutrition in developing countries. *The Proceedings of the Nutrition Society, 65*(1), 51–60. DOI: 10.1079/PNS2005474 PMID: 16441944

Gibson, R. S., & Anderson, V. P. (2009). A review of interventions based on dietary diversification or modification strategies with the potential to enhance intakes of total and absorbable zinc. *Food and Nutrition Bulletin, 30*(1_suppl1), S108–S143. DOI: 10.1177/15648265090301S107 PMID: 19472604

Gupta, S., Brazier, A. K. M., & Lowe, N. M. (2020). Zinc deficiency in low- and middle-income countries: Prevalence and approaches for mitigation. *Journal of Human Nutrition and Dietetics, 33*(5), 624–643. DOI: 10.1111/jhn.12791 PMID: 32627912

Hambidge, K. M. (1989). Mild zinc deficiency in children. In Mills, C. F. (Ed.), *Zinc in Human Biology* (pp. 285–295). Springer-Verlag. DOI: 10.1007/978-1-4471-3879-2_18

Hambidge, K. M. (1992). Zinc and diarrhea. *Acta Paediatrica (Oslo, Norway), 381*(s383), 82–86. DOI: 10.1111/j.1651-2227.1992.tb12377.x PMID: 1421947

Hambidge, K. M. (2000). Human zinc deficiency. *The Journal of Nutrition, 130*(5), S1344–S1349. DOI: 10.1093/jn/130.5.1344S PMID: 10801941

Hambidge, K. M., & Walravens, P. A. (1982). Disorders of mineral metabolism. *Clinics in Gastroenterology, 11*(1), 87–117. DOI: 10.1016/S0300-5089(21)00496-X PMID: 6277535

Kambe, T., Tsuji, T., Hashimoto, A., & Itsumura, N. (2015). The Physiological, Biochemical, and Molecular Roles of Zinc Transporters in Zinc Homeostasis and Metabolism. *Physiological Reviews, 95*(3), 749–784. DOI: 10.1152/physrev.00035.2014 PMID: 26084690

Kay, R. G. (1975). Tasman-Jones C. Acute zinc deficiency in man during intravenous alimentation. *ANZ Journal of Surgery*, *45*, 325–330. PMID: 813623

Kelishadi, R., Alikhassy, H., & Amiri, M. (2002). Zinc and copper status in children with high family risk of premature cardiovascular disease. *Annals of Saudi Medicine*, *22*(5-6), 291–294. DOI: 10.5144/0256-4947.2002.291 PMID: 17146244

Kewcharoenwong, C., Schuster, G. U., Wessells, K. R., Hinnouho, G.-M., Barffour, M. A., Kounnavong, S., Brown, K. H., Hess, S. Y., Samer, W., Tussakhon, I., Peerson, J. M., Lertmemongkolchai, G., & Stephensen, C. B. (2020). Daily preventive zinc supplementation decreases lymphocyte and eosinophil concentrations in rural Laotian children from communities with a high prevalence of zinc deficiency: Results of a randomized controlled trial. *The Journal of Nutrition*, *150*(8), 2204–2213. DOI: 10.1093/jn/nxaa037 PMID: 32119742

King, J. C., Brown, K. H., Gibson, R. S., Krebs, N. F., Lowe, N. M., Siekmann, J. H., & Raiten, D. J. (2016). Biomarkers of nutrition for development (BOND)-Zinc Review. *The Journal of Nutrition*, *146*(4), 858S–885S. DOI: 10.3945/jn.115.220079 PMID: 26962190

Kohn, S., Kohn, D., & Schiller, D. (2000). Effect of zinc supplementation on epidermal Langerhans'cells of elderly patients with decubital ulcers. *The Journal of Dermatology*, *27*(4), 2558–2563. DOI: 10.1111/j.1346-8138.2000.tb02161.x PMID: 10824490

Kumssa, D. B., Joy, E. J. M., Ander, E. L., Watts, M. J., Young, S. D., Walker, S., & Broadley, M. R. (2015). Dietary calcium and zinc deficiency risks are decreasing but remain prevalent. *Scientific Reports*, *5*(1), 10974. DOI: 10.1038/srep10974 PMID: 26098577

Lamberti, L. M., Walker, C. L. F., & Black, R. E. (2016). Zinc deficiency in childhood and pregnancy: Evidence for intervention effects and program responses, Hidden hunger. *Karger Publishers, 115*, 125–133.

Lee, H. H., Prasad, A. S., Brewer, G. J., & Owyang, C. (1989). Zinc absorption in human small intestine. *The American Journal of Physiology*, *256*, G87–G91. PMID: 2912154

Lönnerdal, B. (2000). Dietary factors influencing zinc absorption. *The Journal of Nutrition*, *130*(5), S1378–S1383. DOI: 10.1093/jn/130.5.1378S PMID: 10801947

Lönnerdal, B. (2003). Genetically modified plants for improved trace element nutrition. *The Journal of Nutrition*, *133*(5), 1490S–S1493. DOI: 10.1093/jn/133.5.1490S PMID: 12730450

Maret, W. (2001). Zinc biochemistry, physiology, and homeostasis: Recent insights and current trends. *Biometals*, *14*(3/4), 187–190. DOI: 10.1023/A:1012945110820

Maret, W., & Sandstead, H. H. (2006). Zinc requirements and the risks and benefits of zinc supplementation. *Journal of Trace Elements in Medicine and Biology*, *20*(1), 3–18. DOI: 10.1016/j.jtemb.2006.01.006 PMID: 16632171

Muller, O., Becher, H., van Zweeden, A. B., Ye, Y., Diallo, D. A., Konate, A. T., Gbangou, A., Kouyate, B., & Garenne, M. (2001). Effect of zinc supplementation on malaria and other causes of morbidity in west African children: Randomised double blind placebo-controlled trial. *British Medical Journal*, *322*(7302), 1567–1574. DOI: 10.1136/bmj.322.7302.1567 PMID: 11431296

Nazanin, R., Richard, H., Roya, K., & Rainer, S. (2013). Zinc and its importance for human health: An integrative review. *Journal of Research in Medical Sciences : the Official Journal of Isfahan University of Medical Sciences*, *18*, 144–157. PMID: 23914218

Penny, M. E. (2013). Zinc Supplementation in Public Health. *Annals of Nutrition & Metabolism*, *62*(Suppl. 1), 31–42. DOI: 10.1159/000348263 PMID: 23689111

Pérez-Escamilla, R., & Engmann, C. (2019). Integrating nutrition services into health care systems platforms: Where are we and where do we go from here. *Maternal and Child Nutrition*, *15*(S1), e12743. DOI: 10.1111/mcn.12743 PMID: 30748115

Roohani, N., Hurrell, R., Kelishadi, R., & Schulin, R. (2013). Zinc and its importance for human health: An integrative review. *Journal of Research in Medical Sciences : the Official Journal of Isfahan University of Medical Sciences*, *18*, 144–157. PMID: 23914218

Sandstrom, B., Davidsson, L., Cederblad, A., & Lönnerdal, B. (1985). Oral iron, dietary ligands and zinc absorption. *The Journal of Nutrition*, *115*(3), 411–414. DOI: 10.1093/jn/115.3.411 PMID: 3973750

Sangeetha, V. J., Dutta, S., Moses, J. A., & Anandharamakrishnan, C. (2022). Zinc nutrition and human health: Overview and implications. *eFood*, *3*(5), e17. DOI: 10.1002/efd2.17

Sazawal, S., Black, R. E., Menon, V. P., Dinghra, P., Caulfield, L. E., Dhingra, U., & Bagati, A. (2001). Zinc supplementation in infants born small for gestational age reduces mortality: A prospective, randomized, controlled trial. *Pediatrics*, *108*(6), 1280–1286. DOI: 10.1542/peds.108.6.1280 PMID: 11731649

Scholmerich, J., Freudemann, A., Kottgen, E., Wietholtz, H., Steiert, B., Lohle, E., Haussinger, D., & Gerok, W. (1987). Bioavailability of zinc from zinc-histidine complexes. I. Comparison with zinc sulfate in healthy men. *The American Journal of Clinical Nutrition, 45*(6), 1480–1486. DOI: 10.1093/ajcn/45.6.1480 PMID: 3591728

Shankar, A. H., Genton, B., Baisor, M., Paino, J., Tamja, S., Adiguma, T., Wu, L., Rare, L., Bannon, D., Tielsch, J. M., West, K. P., & Alpers, M. P. (2000). The influence of zinc supplementation on morbidity due to Plasmodium falciparum: Arandomized trial in preschool children in Papua New Guinea. *The American Journal of Tropical Medicine and Hygiene, 62*(6), 663–669. DOI: 10.4269/ajtmh.2000.62.663 PMID: 11304051

Stein, A. J. (2010). Global impacts of human mineral malnutrition. *Plant and Soil, 335*(1-2), 133–154. DOI: 10.1007/s11104-009-0228-2

Thu, B. D., Schultink, W., Dillon, D., Gross, R., Leswara, N. D., & Khoi, H. H. (1999). Effect of daily and weekly micronutrient supplementation on micronutrient deficiencies and growth in young Vietnamese children. *The American Journal of Clinical Nutrition, 69*(1), 80–86. DOI: 10.1093/ajcn/69.1.80 PMID: 9925127

Valberg, L. S., Flanagan, P. R., & Chamberlain, M. J. (1984). Effects of iron, tin, and copper on zinc absorption in humans. *The American Journal of Clinical Nutrition, 40*(3), 536–541. DOI: 10.1093/ajcn/40.3.536 PMID: 6475824

Van Wouwe, J. P. (1989). Clinical and laboratory diagnosis of acrodermatitis enteropathica. *European Journal of Pediatrics, 149*(1), 2–8. DOI: 10.1007/BF02024322 PMID: 2691254

Veenemans, J., Milligan, P., Prentice, A. M., Schouten, L. R. A., Inja, N., Heijden, A. C., de Boer, L. C. C., Jansen, E. J. S., Koopmans, A. E., Enthoven, W. T. M., Kraaijenhagen, R. J., Demir, A. Y., Uges, D. R. A., Mbugi, E. V., Savelkoul, H. F. J., & Verhoef, H. (2011). Effect of supplementation with zinc and other micronutrients on malaria in Tanzanian children: A randomised trial. *PLoS Medicine, 8*(11), e1001125. DOI: 10.1371/journal.pmed.1001125 PMID: 22131908

Walravens, P. A., & Hambidge, K. M. (1976). Growth of infants fed a zinc supplemented formula. *The American Journal of Clinical Nutrition, 29*(10), 1114–1121. DOI: 10.1093/ajcn/29.10.1114 PMID: 788494

Walsh, C. T., Sandstead, H. H., Prasad, A. S., Newberne, P. M., & Fraker, P. J. (1994). Zinc health effects and research priorities for the 1990's. *Environmental Health Perspectives, 102*, 5–46. PMID: 7925188

Wessells, K. R., & Brown, K. H. (2012). Estimating the global prevalence of zinc deficiency: Results based on zinc availability in national food supplies and the prevalence of stunting. *PLoS One*, *7*(11), e50568. DOI: 10.1371/journal.pone.0050568 PMID: 23209782

Whittaker, P. (1998). Iron and zinc interactions in humans. *The American Journal of Clinical Nutrition*, *68*(2), S442–S446. DOI: 10.1093/ajcn/68.2.442S PMID: 9701159

WHO (World Health Organization) (2006). Implementing the new recommendations on the clinical management of diarrhoea: Guidelines for policy makers and programme managers.

Chapter 8

The Role of Phytochemicals in Alleviating Zinc Deficiency in Humans

Smita Narwal
https://orcid.org/0009-0000-6506-9234
Global Research Institute of Pharmacy, India

Neha Yadav
https://orcid.org/0009-0008-2377-921X
Global Research Institute of Pharmacy, India

Ankit Ab
Global Research Institute of Pharmacy, India

Preeti Garg
Global Research Institute of Pharmacy, India

Gurvirender Singh
Kurukshetra University, India

Ashwani K. Dhingra
Global Research Institute of Pharmacy, India

Nisha Grewal
Global Research Institute of Pharmacy, India

Bhawna Chopra
https://orcid.org/0000-0003-2251-2034
Guru Gobind Singh College of Pharmacy, India

ABSTRACT

Zinc insufficiency in humans has been recognized as a significant global nutritional issue since from 1961 in Iranian males. It is more common in regions with a high diet of cereal and low consumption of animal food. While the dietary intake of zinc may not be inherently deficient, the bio-availability of zinc significantly influences its absorption. A severe zinc shortage can lead to several health issues. Therefore,

DOI: 10.4018/979-8-3693-5355-4.ch008

further research is frequently required to determine its prevalence and the issues it causes, such as growth retardation, diarrhea, infections, difficulties thinking clearly, and birth deformities. Phytochemicals, which are unique substances found in plant-based diets, improve how well our systems absorb zinc. The chapter provides an insight about the zinc deficiency, its prevalence on human health and various ways to overcome this issue.

1. INTRODUCTION

An essential element that may be found all around the world is zinc, the 23rd most prevalent metal in the crust. Its mass is 65.37 and its atomic number is 30. Shiny and bluish-white, pure zinc is a metal that can function as both a base and an acid, (Gondal et al., 2021). Most instruments are unable to detect it since it is colorless and lacks magnetic characteristics. It is essential for several processes in our bodies and promotes the growth of bacteria. Zinc is also necessary for animals and plants. Majority of it is present in our tissues and physiological fluids, namely in our muscles and bones. Zinc concentrations are higher in the prostate and eyes, (Fallah, Mohammad-Hasani, & Colagar, 2018). Adults typically have between 1.4 and 2.3 grams of zinc, (Hennigar et al., 2018) (Coleman, 1992). One third of the world's population may not get enough zinc, with children under the age of five being the most at danger due to their critical requirement for zinc for healthy growth and development, (Lassi et al., 2020). Worldwide, lack of nutrition is a major issue that impacts both developed and developing nations. In children specifically, it can lead to problems with behavior and mobility, poor development, weakened immune systems, difficulties learning and thinking effectively, and more, (Liu et al., 2018). Because zinc is essential to our bodies, it should be a significant component of our diets. It performs a variety of functions, including being a component of many proteins, supporting the normal function of enzymes, and being involved in several critical bodily processes. Zinc is a vital mineral that aids in the production of DNA, strengthens our immune system, and promotes wound healing, among many other processes, (Chasapis et al., 2020) (Skrajnowska & Bobrowska-Korczak, 2019). However, a lot of individuals lack access to healthy food, which prevents them from getting enough zinc, particularly in developing nations. A deficiency in zinc can lead to a number of health issues, including impaired growth, increased susceptibility to illness, and weakened immune system. Although zinc supplements are commonly used to address this, recent studies have shown that some compounds included in plant-based diets can also improve our body's absorption of zinc, (Singh et al., 2021). These substances, referred to as phytochemicals. Knowing how these plant compounds interact with zinc may lead to improved methods of living and eating.

2. GLOBAL PREVALENCE AND SIGNIFICANCE OF ZINC DEFICIENCY IN HUMAN

Zinc deficiency affects around 2 billion people, a significant issue in many poor nations. Their diets are rich in grain proteins that include phytate, which might prevent the absorption of zinc, which is one of the main causes of this, (Khan et al., 2022). Low zinc levels can also be brought on by several medical disorders, including liver illness and malabsorption syndrome, (Himoto & Masaki, 2018). A zinc shortage can lead to major health concerns such as immune system weakness, stunted development, and cognitive impairments. In 1960, the importance of Zn for animal growth focusing on multiple species was studied and documented, (Hussain et al., 2022). In 1961, zinc deficiency was observed for the first time, in the Iranian population and was found to be associated with dwarfism and delayed sexual development, (Gonoodi et al., 2018). In 1963, we were only aware of a small number of enzymes that required zinc for normal function; today, we know that zinc is necessary for approximately 300 enzymes and 1000 transcription factors, (Li et al., 2022). Nevertheless, in recent decades, there has been a focus on Zn research in various fields, particularly in using Zn supplements to combat health problems in humans. Zinc deficiency can result in human diseases that give rise to significant clinical complications. Furthermore, the elderly population commonly experiences a zinc deficiency due to a reduced intake of zinc in their diet, changes in their lifestyle, and the fact that 65% of the global population is suffering from general food scarcity and living below the poverty line, (Hussain et al., 2022). Approximately two billion people worldwide are at risk of developing clinical illness because of zinc deficiency. Recent estimates indicate that around 17.3% of the global population is exposed to the risk of consuming dietary commodities that are deficient in Zn, (Noulas, Tziouvalekas, & Karyotis, 2018). Adults who are deficient in zinc are more likely to have life-threatening medical conditions such as cancer, diabetes, and chronic and oxidative stressors. Insufficient zinc concentrations in human meals can also be observed through short-term memory issues, structural malformation of the brain, reduced cognitive activity, and behavioral problems in adulthood. Severe zinc deficiency results in excessive excretion of zinc in the urine (hyperzincuria), accelerated destruction of red blood cells (hemolysis) resulting to impaired growth, weakened immune system, inability to conceive (infertility), elevated levels of ammonia in the blood (hyperammonemia), reduced function of the reproductive glands in men (hypogonadism), and shrinkage of the thymus gland (thymic atrophy), (Hussain et al., 2022).

3. ZINC IMPACT ON HUMAN LIFE

Zinc plays a critical role in growth, reproduction, vision, and immune system function. For this reason, behind iron, it is the second most vital metal for fish also. In their diet, fish require 230–460 mol (15–30 mg) of zinc per kilogram of dry food, (Kumar, Krishnani, & Singh, 2018). Zinc is incredibly important for human health, and even a small shortage can cause big problems. Without enough zinc, people can lose their appetite, sense of taste and smell, and experience other symptoms like weakened immune systems, heart problems, and anemia, (Khalid et al., 2020). In fact, zinc is the only natural substance that stimulates certain immune cells. It is essential for making enzymes, DNA, and RNA in the body, (Coleman, 1992) (Frassinetti et al., 2006). Not getting enough zinc can lead to complications during pregnancy, slow growth in children, and birth defects in babies(19).Unfortunately, zinc deficiency causes a lot of fatalities every year.

Figure 1. Impact of zinc on human life

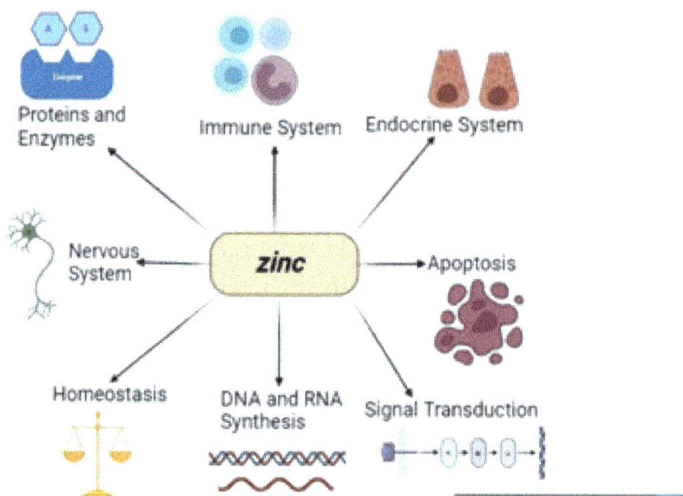

4. ZINC DEFICIENCY IN HUMANS

The prevalence of zinc (Zn) insufficiency in humans is a growing worldwide health concern, impacting almost two billion individuals globally.In impoverished nations, a primary cause of economic losses is inadequate intake of micronutrients, particularly zinc. When people's health deteriorates, the expense of caring for them rises, and their reduced productivity damages the economy of the nation, (Gibson, 2006). Zinc deficiency and malnutrition are common in these nations because a large portion of the population consumes diets high in grains, which lack zinc. 3 to16 milligrams of zinc should be consumed daily by the average individual, (Moser-Veillon, 1990). People who do not receive enough zinc may have a wide range of health issues. The skin, digestive system, brain, immune system, bones, and reproductive system are among the organ systems in the body that are impacted by a severe zinc shortage, (Chasapis et al., 2020). Our body's metabolic processes suffer when there is insufficient zinc, which affects all tissues. Before the advantages of zinc supplementation were known, persons with acrodermatitis enteropathica frequently passed away at an early age, (Krebs, 2013). It has proven difficult to identify the precise biochemical causes of the skin lesions and other symptoms associated with this illness.

4.1 Milder Cases of Zinc Deficiency

Less severe cases of zinc insufficiency may manifest with discreet symptoms that can often be overlooked or attributed to other causes. Some signs and symptoms of mild zinc deficiency include:

1) **Diminished Immune Function:** Zinc plays a vital role in the functioning of the immune system. A mild deficiency has the potential to result in increased susceptibility to infections or delayed recuperation from illness, (Dardenne, 2002).
2) **Skin Issues:** A mild shortage in zinc can lead to the development of dry, flaky skin or minor skin irritations, (Schwartz, Marsh, & Draelos, 2005).
3) **Decreased Appetite:** Zinc deficiency can affect taste and smell, leading to a reduced appetite. Zinc deficiency has the potential to impact gustatory and olfactory perception, resulting in a diminished desire to consume food, (Yagi et al., 2013).
4) **Hair Loss:** Although hair loss is more frequently linked to severe zinc insufficiency, minor deficiency can still lead to thinning hair or delayed hair development, (Kil, Kim, & Kim, 2013).
5) **Mood Alterations:** Zinc is involved in the modulation of neurotransmitters; hence a slight shortage may result in mood fluctuations, irritation, or moderate depression, (Marger, Schubert, & Bertrand, 2014).
6) **Decreased Wound Healing:** Zinc is important for wound healing, so mild deficiency may result in slower healing of minor cuts or scrapes, (Marger, Schubert, & Bertrand, 2014).

7) **Poor Night Vision:** Zinc is involved in the metabolism of vitamin A, which is essential for good vision. Mild deficiency may lead to difficulty adjusting to darkness or poor night vision, (Koop et al., 2018).
8) **Decreased Fertility:** Zinc is necessary for reproductive health in both men and women. Mild deficiency may lead to suboptimal fertility, (Fallah, Mohammad-Hasani, & Colagar, 2018).

4.2 Severe Cases of Zinc Deficiency

The body may experience more pronounced and even life-threatening effects in cases of severe zinc deficiency. Several indicators and manifestations of severe zinc insufficiency include:

1) **Delayed Growth and Development:** Zinc is crucial for growth and development, particularly in children. Severe deficiency can lead to stunted growth, delayed sexual maturation, and developmental delays, (Sorokman et al., 2019).
2) **Impaired Immune Function:** Severe zinc deficiency compromises immune system function, leading to an increased susceptibility to infections and illnesses. This can manifest as recurrent infections or severe infections that are difficult to treat, (Wessels, Fischer, & Rink, 2021).
3) **Severe Dermatological Issues:** Skin problems associated with severe zinc deficiency can include severe dermatitis, eczema-like rashes, or ulcerations. The skin may become extremely dry, flaky, and prone to infections, (Ogawa et al., 2018).
4) **Loss of Appetite and Weight Loss:** Severe zinc deficiency can cause a complete loss of appetite, leading to significant weight loss and malnutrition, (Chao, Chang, & Huang, 2018).
5) **Hair Loss and Nail Problems:** Hair loss may become more severe in cases of profound zinc deficiency, and nails may become brittle and prone to splitting or peeling, (Kil, Kim, & Kim, 2013) (Muddasani et al., 2021).
6) **Neurological Symptoms:** Severe zinc deficiency can affect neurological function, leading to symptoms such as lethargy, weakness, tremors, and difficulty concentrating. In extreme cases, it can lead to seizures or other neurological complications, (Mezzaroba et al., 2019).
7) **Impaired Wound Healing:** Zinc is essential for wound healing, and severe deficiency can lead to slow wound healing, increased risk of infection, and the development of chronic ulcers, (Chen et al., 2022).
8) **Hypogonadism:** In males, severe zinc deficiency can lead to hypogonadism, characterized by decreased testosterone levels, impaired sperm production, and infertility, (Santos & Teixeira, 2019).

9) **Compromised Vision:** Severe zinc deficiency can affect vision, leading to night blindness, impaired dark adaptation, and other vision problems, (Gildbert et al., 2019).
10) **Increased Risk of Pregnancy Complications:** Severe zinc deficiency in pregnant women can increase the risk of complications such as low birth weight, preterm birth, and congenital abnormalities in the developing fetus, (Garner et al., 2021).

5. TREATMENT OF ZINC DEFICIENCY

Zinc deficiency is usually treated by taking zinc supplements and taking care of any underlying problems that are causing the lack. Here is a summary of the treatment plan:

- **Zinc Supplements:** Taking zinc supplements is the main way to treat zinc shortage. Zinc gluconate, zinc sulphate, and zinc acetate are some of the different types that these supplements, (Duan et al., 2023).
- **Changes to your diet:** In addition to taking supplements, eating more foods that are high in zinc can help fix the problem. Red meat, chicken, fish (like oysters and crab), nuts, seeds, legumes, and dairy products are all good sources of zinc. Including a mix of these foods in your diet can help you get enough zinc, (Muthukumar et al., 2020).
- **Taking Care of the Root Causes:** Zinc deficiency can be caused by several-reasons, such as not getting enough zinc in your food, problems with absorption, long-term illnesses, or some medications. For long-term management, it is important to find and treat any underlying diseases that are causing the deficiency, (Gupta, Brazier, & Lowe, 2020).
- **Monitoring:** It may be necessary to check zinc levels in the blood on a regular basis to see how well supplements are working and make sure levels stay in the right range. This tracking lets doctors change the amount of zinc supplements that people take as needed, (Larson-Meyer, Woolf, & Burke, 2018).
- **Taking Care of Symptoms:** Depending on how bad the deficiency is and what symptoms are happening, extra supportive steps may be needed to take care of some symptoms. For instance, people with serious skin problems may be given topical treatments, and people who are losing a lot of weight or not getting enough food may be given nutritional support, (Zou et al., 2023).
- **Follow-Up Care:** People who are getting treatment for zinc deficiency should keep in touch with their doctor to check on their progress, see how well the

treatment is working, and talk about any problems or concerns that may come up.

6. PHYTOCHEMICALS INVOLVEMENT IN ZINC DEFICIENCY IN HUMANS

Phytochemicals are produced by all types of plants, such as fruits, vegetables, legumes, and grains. They form a vital component of the plant's immune system, safeguarding it against viral, bacterial, fungal, and parasitic threats, (Oz & Kafkas, 2017). Phytochemicals can provide humans with a similar level of protection. Along with all other functions, they are important for maintaining healthy zinc levels in our bodies. They assist by facilitating the body's absorption of zinc, preventing other substances from obstructing zinc absorption, and enhancing the body's utilization of zinc, (Roohani et al., 2013). To put it simply, phytochemicals play a major role in the way our bodies utilize zinc. Consuming a variety of meals high in phytochemicals and foods high in zinc from plants can help prevent or treat zinc deficiency while maintaining our health. However, since each person's diet is unique, it is a good idea to see a physician or nutritionist for specific recommendations on how much zinc we should consume and whether we need take supplements or not.

6.1 Mechanism of Action of Phytochemicals Used to Combat Zinc Deficiency

The mechanisms of action of phytochemicals (compounds found in plants) used to combat zinc deficiency can vary depending on the specific phytochemical and how it interacts with the body's processes. Here are some common mechanisms through which phytochemicals can help alleviate zinc deficiency:

- **Aiding in Zinc Absorption:** By producing combinations that dissolve in the stomach, some plant compounds, such as polyphenols, flavonoids, and saponins, facilitate our bodies' absorption of zinc. Vitamin C, which is included in fruits and vegetables, also aids by keeping zinc from clumping together so that it cannot be absorbed, (Smith, 1991).
- **Stopping Zinc Blockers:** By causing zinc to clump together in the stomach, other plant compounds like phytates and tannins, which are included in grains, legumes, tea, and some fruits, can prevent zinc from being absorbed. Consuming these items in moderation lowers the risk of zinc insufficiency while maintaining a balanced diet, (Singh & Prasad, 2023) (Nissar et al., 2017).

- **Supporting Zinc Utilization**: By forming the protein metallothionein, which transports zinc throughout the body, vitamin A, which is present in orange and yellow fruits as well as leafy greens, helps our bodies utilize zinc. Many fruits and vegetables include carotenoids, which may also be beneficial since they maintain a healthy gut and reduce inflammation, both of which improve our absorption of zinc, (Tapiero & Tew, 2003) (Eroglu et al., 2023).

Table 1. Role of secondary metabolites in relation to zinc deficiency

S. No.	Phytochemicals	Mechanism of action of zinc deficiency	Food Sources	Use in zinc Deficiency	Ref.
1	Tannins	May bind to zinc to generate insoluble complexes that hinder absorption.	Wine, grapes, apples Tea, coffee	May prevent the absorption of zinc, but may also have other health advantages.	(Duan et al., 2023)
2	Flavonoids	Zinc can bind with certain flavonoids to facilitate absorption.	Red wine, tea, veggies, and fruits.	Certain flavonoids may improve the absorption of zinc.	(Duan et al., 2023)
3	Phytates	Forms insoluble compounds that impede the absorption of zinc.	Legumes, seeds, nuts, and whole grains	May prevent the absorption of zinc, while moderate intake can be advantageous.	(Mukhopadhyay et al., 2018)
4	Saponins	May increase the solubility of zinc by creating soluble complexes.	Legume crops (lentils, beans).	May improve absorption of zinc by combining with zinc to create complexes.	(Mukhopadhyay et al., 2018)
5	Polyphenols	Certain polyphenols can chelate zinc, improving absorption.	Wine, tea, veggies, and fruits.	Some polyphenols could improve the absorption of zinc.	(Lakey-Beitia et al., 2021)
6	Vitamin A	Promotes the metallothionein synthesis, which facilitates the absorption of zinc.	Leafy greens, orange, and yellow fruits	Helps the body absorb and use zinc	(Yanar, 2023)
7	Carotenoids	Certain carotenoids may help absorb zinc in an indirect way by promoting gut health and reducing inflammation.	Sweet potatoes, spinach, carrots, and other fruits	Certain carotenoids may help absorb zinc in an indirect way.	(Rinninella et al., 2018)
8	Vitamin C	Decreases zinc precipitation to improve absorption of zinc	Berries, citrus fruits, and a variety of veggies	When taken in combination, improves the absorption of zinc.	(Zhang et al., 2021)
9	Allyl Sulphides	Interactions with various physiological processes and components of the diet	garlic and onions	Enhancing zinc absorption	(Abniki, Azizi, & Panahi, 2021)

Table 2. List of some dietary phytochemicals known to modulate zinc levels

S. No	Dietary Phytochemical	Source	Effect on Zinc Signaling	Ref.
1	Quercetin	Onions, Apples, and Berries	Enhance zinc absorption by facilitating the formation of a complex between zinc and polyphenols	(Singh et al., 2021)
2	Epigallocatechin-3-gallate (EGCG)	Green tea	Facilitate Zn accumulation, suppress metallothioneins and ZnT1, promote ZIP1 and ZIP4	(Singh et al., 2021) (Borowska, Brzoska, & Tomczyk, 2018)
3.	Grape-seed procyanidin extract (GSPE)	Grape seeds	Suppress ZIP3, ZIP5, ZIP7, and ZIP11, while promoting ZIP6, ZIP10, and ZIP13	(Singh et al., 2021) (Wang et al., 2023)
4	Curcumin	Turmeric	Enhance the mobilization of Zn and augment the presence of Zn-binding ligands	(Prasad & Lall, 2022)
5	Phytic acid	Seeds, Grains, Legumes, and Nuts	Impede the assimilation of Zn by forming insoluble compounds with it	(Zhang et al., 2022)
6	Soybean extracts and soyasaponin Bb	Soyabean	Increase Zn uptake, enhance metallothioneins	(Chen et al., 2022)
7	Catechins	Green tea	Form complex with Zn ions in GIT, influence the expression of genes involved in zinc homeostasis	(Zhang et al., 2021)

6. CONCLUSION AND FUTURE PROSPECTS

Zinc is an essential mineral for all people, but it is especially critical for infants and expectant mothers as it aids in digestion, guards against infections, and wards against nutritionally linked illnesses. It supports the healthy function of enzymes and is essential for several bodily functions. Because low zinc damages cells, it can result in conditions including diabetes, cancer, and obesity. While plant-based diets can provide additional zinc, many individuals, particularly in impoverished nations, do not acquire enough zinc from their diets. With so many people, this is a major issue on a global scale.Enhancing food with additional minerals, such as zinc and biofortification, is an excellent strategy to guarantee that people consume adequate food, particularly as the population increases. Future studies will concentrate on addressing dietary issues such as deficiencies in certain micronutrients, such as zinc. We will also examine the role zinc plays in illness prevention, how to utilize zinc as a medicine, and how to increase the amount of zinc in crops for better health.

REFERENCES

Abniki, M., Azizi, Z., & Panahi, H. A. (2021). Design of 3-aminophenol-grafted polymer-modified zinc sulphide nanoparticles as drug delivery system. *IET Nanobiotechnology / IET*, *15*(8), 664–673. DOI: 10.1049/nbt2.12063 PMID: 34694721

Borowska, S., Brzoska, M. M., & Tomczyk, M. (2018). Complexation of bioelements and toxic metals by polyphenolic compounds–Implications for health. *Current Drug Targets*, *19*(14), 1612–1638. DOI: 10.2174/1389450119666180403101555 PMID: 29611487

Chao, H. C., Chang, Y. J., & Huang, W. L. (2018). Cut-off serum zinc concentration affecting the appetite, growth, and nutrition status of undernourished children supplemented with zinc. *Nutrition in Clinical Practice*, *33*(5), 701–710. DOI: 10.1002/ncp.10079 PMID: 29603391

Chasapis, C. T., Ntoupa, P.-S. A., Spiliopoulou, C. A., & Stefanidou, M. E. (2020). Recent aspects of the effects of zinc on human health. *Archives of Toxicology*, *94*(5), 1443–1460. DOI: 10.1007/s00204-020-02702-9 PMID: 32394086

Chen, X., He, C., Zhang, K., Wang, J., Ding, X., Zeng, Q., Peng, H., Bai, J., Lv, L., Xuan, Y., & Bai, S. (2022). Comparison of zinc bioavailability in zinc-glycine and zinc-methionine chelates for broilers fed with a corn-soybean meal diet. *Frontiers in Physiology*, *13*, 983954. DOI: 10.3389/fphys.2022.983954 PMID: 36467690

Chen, Y., Cai, J., Liu, D., Liu, S., Lei, D., Zheng, L., Wei, Q., & Gao, M. (2022). Zinc-based metal organic framework with antibacterial and anti-inflammatory properties for promoting wound healing. *Regenerative Biomaterials*, *9*, rbac019. DOI: 10.1093/rb/rbac019 PMID: 35493287

Coleman, J. E. (1992). Zinc proteins: Enzymes, storage proteins, transcription factors, and replication proteins. *Annual Review of Biochemistry*, *61*(1), 897–946. DOI: 10.1146/annurev.bi.61.070192.004341 PMID: 1497326

Dardenne, M. (2002). Zinc and immune function. *European Journal of Clinical Nutrition*, *56*(3), S20–S23. DOI: 10.1038/sj.ejcn.1601479 PMID: 12142956

Duan, M., Li, T., Liu, B., Yin, S., Zang, J., Lv, C., Zhao, G., & Zhang, T. (2023). Zinc nutrition and dietary zinc supplements. *Critical Reviews in Food Science and Nutrition*, *63*(9), 1277–1292. DOI: 10.1080/10408398.2021.1963664 PMID: 34382897

Eroglu, A., Al'Abri, I. S., Kopec, R. E., Crook, N., & Bohn, T. (2023). Carotenoids and their health benefits as derived via their interactions with gut microbiota. *Advances in Nutrition*, *14*(2), 238–255. DOI: 10.1016/j.advnut.2022.10.007 PMID: 36775788

Fallah, A., Mohammad-Hasani, A., & Colagar, A. H. (2018). Zinc is an essential element for male fertility: A review of Zn roles in men's health, germination, sperm quality, and fertilization. *Journal of Reproduction & Infertility*, *19*(2), 69. PMID: 30009140

Frassinetti, S., Bronzetti, G. L., Caltavuturo, L., Cini, M., & Della Croce, C. (2006). The role of zinc in life: A review. *Journal of Environmental Pathology, Toxicology and Oncology*, *25*(3), 597–610. DOI: 10.1615/JEnvironPatholToxicolOncol.v25.i3.40 PMID: 17073562

Garner, T. B., Hester, J. M., Carothers, A., & Diaz, F. J. (2021). Role of zinc in female reproduction. *Biology of Reproduction*, *104*(5), 976–994. DOI: 10.1093/biolre/ioab023 PMID: 33598687

Gibson, R. S. (2006). Zinc: The missing link in combating micronutrient malnutrition in developing countries. *The Proceedings of the Nutrition Society*, *65*(1), 51–60. DOI: 10.1079/PNS2005474 PMID: 16441944

Gibson, R. S., Raboy, V., & King, J. C. (2018). Implications of phytate in plant-based foods for iron and zinc bioavailability, setting dietary requirements, and formulating programs and policies. *Nutrition Reviews*, *76*(11), 793–804. DOI: 10.1093/nutrit/nuy028 PMID: 30010865

Gilbert, R., Peto, T., Lengyel, I., & Emri, E. (2019). Zinc nutrition and inflammation in the aging retina. *Molecular Nutrition & Food Research*, *63*(15), 1801049. DOI: 10.1002/mnfr.201801049 PMID: 31148351

Gondal, A. H., Zafar, A., Zainab, D., Toor, M., Sohail, S., & Ameen, S.. (2021). A detailed review study of zinc involvement in animal, plant and human nutrition. *Indian Journal of Pure & Applied Biosciences*, *9*(2), 262–271. DOI: 10.18782/2582-2845.8652

Gonoodi, K., Moslem, A., Darroudi, S., Ahmadnezhad, M., Mazloum, Z., Tayefi, M., Zadeh, S. A. T., Eslami, S., Shafiee, M., Khashayarmanesh, Z., Haghighi, H. M., Ferns, G. A., & Ghayour-Mobarhan, M. (2018). Serum and dietary zinc and copper in Iranian girls. *Clinical Biochemistry*, *54*, 25–31. DOI: 10.1016/j.clinbiochem.2018.02.006 PMID: 29438682

Gupta, S., Brazier, A., & Lowe, N. (2020). Zinc deficiency in low- and middle-income countries: Prevalence and approaches for mitigation. *Journal of Human Nutrition and Dietetics*, *33*(5), 624–643. DOI: 10.1111/jhn.12791 PMID: 32627912

Hennigar, S. R., Lieberman, H. R., Fulgoni, V. L.III, & McClung, J. P. (2018). Serum zinc concentrations in the US population are related to sex, age, and time of blood draw but not dietary or supplemental zinc. *The Journal of Nutrition, 148*(8), 1341–1351. DOI: 10.1093/jn/nxy105 PMID: 29947812

Himoto, T., & Masaki, T. (2018). Associations between zinc deficiency and metabolic abnormalities in patients with chronic liver disease. *Nutrients, 10*(1), 88. DOI: 10.3390/nu10010088 PMID: 29342898

Hussain, A., Jiang, W., Wang, X., Shahid, S., Saba, N., Ahmad, M., Dar, A., Masood, S. U., Imran, M., & Mustafa, A. (2022). Mechanistic impact of zinc deficiency in human development. *Frontiers in Nutrition, 9*, 717064. DOI: 10.3389/fnut.2022.717064 PMID: 35356730

Khalid, M. S., Aljohani, M. M., Alomrani, N. A., Oyouni, A. A. A., Alzahrani, O., & Ahmad, M. A.. (2020). COVID-19 and immune function—"A significant" zinc. *Oriental Journal of Chemistry, 36*(6), 1026. DOI: 10.13005/ojc/360604

Khan, S. T., Malik, A., Alwarthan, A., & Shaik, M. R. (2022). The enormity of the zinc deficiency problem and available solutions: An overview. *Arabian Journal of Chemistry, 15*(3), 103668. DOI: 10.1016/j.arabjc.2021.103668

Kil, M. S., Kim, C. W., & Kim, S. S. (2013). Analysis of serum zinc and copper concentrations in hair loss. *Annals of Dermatology, 25*(4), 405. DOI: 10.5021/ad.2013.25.4.405 PMID: 24371385

Koop, A. H., Mousa, O. Y., Pham, L. E., Corral-Hurtado, J. E., Pungpapong, S., & Keaveny, A. P. (2018). An argument for vitamin D, A, and zinc monitoring in cirrhosis. *Annals of Hepatology, 17*(6), 920–932. DOI: 10.5604/01.3001.0012.7192 PMID: 30600288

Krebs, N. F. (2013). Update on zinc deficiency and excess in clinical pediatric practice. *Annals of Nutrition & Metabolism, 62*(Suppl. 1), 19–29. DOI: 10.1159/000348261 PMID: 23689110

Kumar, N., Krishnani, K. K., & Singh, N. P. (2018). Effect of dietary zinc-nanoparticles on growth performance, anti-oxidative and immunological status of fish reared under multiple stressors. *Biological Trace Element Research, 186*(1), 267–278. DOI: 10.1007/s12011-018-1285-2 PMID: 29524193

Lakey-Beitia, J., Burillo, A. M., La Penna, G., Hegde, M. L., & Rao, K. (2021). Polyphenols as potential metal chelation compounds against Alzheimer's disease. *Journal of Alzheimer's Disease, 82*(s1), S335–S357. DOI: 10.3233/JAD-200185 PMID: 32568200

Larson-Meyer, D. E., Woolf, K., & Burke, L. (2018). Assessment of nutrient status in athletes and the need for supplementation. *International Journal of Sport Nutrition and Exercise Metabolism*, *28*(2), 139–158. DOI: 10.1123/ijsnem.2017-0338 PMID: 29252049

Lassi, Z. S., Kurji, J., de Oliveira, C. S., Moin, A., & Bhutta, Z. A. (2020). Zinc supplementation for the promotion of growth and prevention of infections in infants less than six months of age. *Cochrane Database of Systematic Reviews*, *2020*(4). Advance online publication. DOI: 10.1002/14651858.CD010205.pub2 PMID: 32266964

Li, J., Cao, D., Huang, Y., Chen, B., Chen, Z., Wang, R., Dong, Q., Wei, Q., & Liu, L. (2022). Zinc intakes and health outcomes: An umbrella review. *Frontiers in Nutrition*, *9*, 798078. DOI: 10.3389/fnut.2022.798078 PMID: 35211497

Liu, E., Pimpin, L., Shulkin, M., Kranz, S., Duggan, C. P., Mozaffarian, D., & Fawzi, W. (2018). Effect of zinc supplementation on growth outcomes in children under 5 years of age. *Nutrients*, *10*(3), 377. DOI: 10.3390/nu10030377 PMID: 29558383

Marger, L., Schubert, C., & Bertrand, D. (2014). Zinc: An underappreciated modulatory factor of brain function. *Biochemical Pharmacology*, *91*(4), 426–435. DOI: 10.1016/j.bcp.2014.08.002 PMID: 25130547

Mezzaroba, L., Alfieri, D. F., Simão, A. N. C., & Reiche, E. M. V. (2019). The role of zinc, copper, manganese and iron in neurodegenerative diseases. *Neurotoxicology*, *74*, 230–241. DOI: 10.1016/j.neuro.2019.07.007 PMID: 31377220

Moser-Veillon, P. B. (1990). Zinc: Consumption patterns and dietary recommendations. *Journal of the American Dietetic Association*, *90*(8), 1089–1094. DOI: 10.1016/S0002-8223(21)01706-5 PMID: 2166098

Muddasani, S., Lin, G., Hooper, J., & Sloan, S. B. (2021). Nutrition and nail disease. *Clinics in Dermatology*, *39*(5), 819–828. DOI: 10.1016/j.clindermatol.2021.05.009 PMID: 34785009

Mukhopadhyay, S., Mukherjee, S., Hashim, M. A., Sahu, J. N., Martinez-Villegas, N., & Gupta, B. S. (2018). Zinc removal from soil by washing with saponin obtained from *Sapindus mukorossi*.*Journal of Environmental Analytical Chemistry*, *5*(4). Advance online publication. DOI: 10.4172/2380-2391.1000249

Muthukumar, J., Selvasekaran, P., Lokanadham, M., & Chidambaram, R. (2020). Food and food products associated with food allergy and food intolerance – An overview. *Food Research International*, *138*, 109780. DOI: 10.1016/j.foodres.2020.109780 PMID: 33288166

Nissar, J., Ahad, T., Naik, H., & Hussain, S. (2017). A review: Phytic acid—As antinutrient or nutraceutical. *Journal of Pharmacognosy and Phytochemistry*, *6*(6), 1554–1560.

Noulas, C., Tziouvalekas, M., & Karyotis, T. (2018). Zinc in soils, water and food crops. *Journal of Trace Elements in Medicine and Biology*, *49*, 252–260. DOI: 10.1016/j.jtemb.2018.02.009 PMID: 29472130

Ogawa, Y., Kinoshita, M., Shimada, S., & Kawamura, T. (2018). Zinc and skin disorders. *Nutrients*, *10*(2), 199. DOI: 10.3390/nu10020199 PMID: 29439479

Oz, A. T., & Kafkas, E. (2017). Phytochemicals in fruits and vegetables. In Waisundara, V. (Ed.), *Superfood and functional food* (pp. 175–184). IntechOpen.

Prasad, S., & Lall, R. (2022). Zinc-curcumin based complexes in health and diseases: An approach in chemopreventive and therapeutic improvement. *Journal of Trace Elements in Medicine and Biology*, *73*, 127023. DOI: 10.1016/j.jtemb.2022.127023 PMID: 35780653

Rinninella, E., Mele, M. C., Merendino, N., Cintoni, M., Anselmi, G., Caporossi, A., Gasbarrini, A., & Minnella, A. M. (2018). The role of diet, micronutrients and the gut microbiota in age-related macular degeneration: New perspectives from the gut–retina axis. *Nutrients*, *10*(11), 1677. DOI: 10.3390/nu10111677 PMID: 30400586

Roohani, N., Hurrell, R., Kelishadi, R., & Schulin, R. (2013). Zinc and its importance for human health: An integrative review. *Journal of Research in Medical Sciences : the Official Journal of Isfahan University of Medical Sciences*, *18*(2), 144. PMID: 23914218

Santos, H. O., & Teixeira, F. J. (2019). Use of medicinal doses of zinc as a safe and efficient coadjutant in the treatment of male hypogonadism. *The Aging Male*. PMID: 30767598

Schwartz, J. R., Marsh, R. G., & Draelos, Z. D. (2005). Zinc and skin health: Overview of physiology and pharmacology. *Dermatologic Surgery*, *31*(s1), 837–847. DOI: 10.1111/j.1524-4725.2005.31729 PMID: 16029676

Shah, D., & Sachdev, H. (2006). Zinc deficiency in pregnancy and fetal outcome. *Nutrition Reviews*, *64*(1), 15–30. DOI: 10.1111/j.1753-4887.2006.tb00169.x PMID: 16491666

Singh, C. K., Chhabra, G., Patel, A., Chang, H., & Ahmad, N. (2021). Dietary phytochemicals in zinc homeostasis: A strategy for prostate cancer management. *Nutrients*, *13*(6), 1867. DOI: 10.3390/nu13061867 PMID: 34070833

Singh, P., & Prasad, S. (2023). A review on iron, zinc and calcium biological significance and factors affecting their absorption and bioavailability. *Journal of Food Composition and Analysis, 114*, 105529. DOI: 10.1016/j.jfca.2023.105529

Skrajnowska, D., & Bobrowska-Korczak, B. (2019). Role of zinc in immune system and anti-cancer defense mechanisms. *Nutrients, 11*(10), 2273. DOI: 10.3390/nu11102273 PMID: 31546724

Smith, L. H. (1991). *Clinical guide to the use of vitamin C.* SEANET Corporation–Internet Services for the Puget Sound Region. https://www.seanet.com/~alexs/ascorbate/198x/smith-lh-clinical_guide_1988.htm

Sorokman, T., Sokolnyk, S., Popelyuk, A.-M., Makarova, O., Bezruk, T., & Moldovan, P. (2019). Zinc level in children with short stature. *Romanian Journal of Pediatrics, 68*(4), 248–254. DOI: 10.37897/RJP.2019.4.4

Tapiero, H., & Tew, K. D. (2003). Trace elements in human physiology and pathology: Zinc and metallothioneins. *Biomedicine and Pharmacotherapy, 57*(9), 399–411. DOI: 10.1016/S0753-3322(03)00081-7 PMID: 14652165

Wang, J., Li, Y., Yang, Y., Xiao, C., Ruan, Q., Li, P., Zhou, Q., Sheng, M., Hao, X., & Kai, G. (2023). Comprehensive analysis of OpHD-ZIP transcription factors related to the regulation of camptothecin biosynthesis in *Ophiorrhiza pumila.International Journal of Biological Macromolecules, 242*, 124910. DOI: 10.1016/j.ijbiomac.2023.124910 PMID: 37217041

Wessels, I., Fischer, H. J., & Rink, L. (2021). Dietary and physiological effects of zinc on the immune system. *Annual Review of Nutrition, 41*(1), 133–175. DOI: 10.1146/annurev-nutr-122019-120635 PMID: 34255547

Yagi, T., Asakawa, A., Ueda, H., Ikeda, S., Miyawaki, S., & Inui, A. (2013). The role of zinc in the treatment of taste disorders. *Recent Patents on Food, Nutrition & Agriculture, 5*(1), 44–51. DOI: 10.2174/2212798411305010007 PMID: 23305423

Yanar, K. (2023). Vitamin-associated elements. In *A guide to vitamins and their effects on diseases* (p. 164).

Zhang, Y., Li, X., Li, J., Khan, M. Z. H., Ma, F., & Liu, X. (2021). A novel zinc complex with antibacterial and antioxidant activity. *BMC Chemistry, 15*(1), 1–12. DOI: 10.1186/s13065-021-00745-2 PMID: 33722300

Zhang, Y., Peng, C., Zeng, Z., Zhang, X., Zhang, L., Ma, Y., & Wang, Z. (2022). Sustainable phytic acid–zinc anticorrosion interface for highly reversible zinc metal anodes. *ACS Applied Materials & Interfaces, 14*(8), 10419–10427. DOI: 10.1021/acsami.1c24288 PMID: 35179367

Zhang, Y. Y., Stockmann, R., Ng, K., & Ajlouni, S. (2021). Opportunities for plant-derived enhancers for iron, zinc, and calcium bioavailability: A review. *Comprehensive Reviews in Food Science and Food Safety*, *20*(1), 652–685. DOI: 10.1111/1541-4337.12669 PMID: 33443794

Zou, P., Du, Y., Yang, C., & Cao, Y. (2023). Trace element zinc and skin disorders. *Frontiers in Medicine*, *9*, 1093868. DOI: 10.3389/fmed.2022.1093868 PMID: 36733937

Chapter 9
Various Strategies to Alleviate Zinc Deficiency and Its Management

Hrithik Dey
https://orcid.org/0009-0000-6196-1911
Lloyd Institute of Management and Technology, India

Surovi Paul
https://orcid.org/0009-0000-6972-331X
Lloyd Institute of Management and Technology, India

Meenakshi Kaira
Lloyd Institute of Management and Technology, India

ABSTRACT

Zinc deficiency is a global health issue, especially in developing countries where diets often lack diversity and essential nutrients. Alleviating zinc deficiency requires a multifaceted approach involving dietary diversification, biofortification, and zinc supplementation. Dietary diversification, with a varied diet rich in zinc-containing foods like meat, seafood, dairy, legumes, nuts, seeds, and whole grains, is essential for meeting zinc requirements and mitigating health effects. Biofortification, which enhances the zinc content of staple crops through breeding or biotechnology, offers a sustainable solution to improve zinc intake and address deficiency-related health issues. Zinc supplementation provides targeted interventions for vulnerable populations, supporting growth, immune function, and overall well-being, and helps manage diseases like acute respiratory infections and Wilson's disease. By integrating dietary diversification, biofortification, and supplementation, we can effectively manage zinc deficiency and improve global health outcomes.

DOI: 10.4018/979-8-3693-5355-4.ch009

INTRODUCTION

Zinc deficiency is a widespread global health concern, affecting around one-third of the world's population, with a particularly high prevalence in developing countries. (Caulfield & Black, 2004) Zinc is a vital trace element necessary for numerous physiological processes, including immune system function, DNA synthesis, cell division, and protein production. (Stefanidou et al., 2006) A zinc deficiency can lead to significant health problems such as stunted growth in children, (Black, 1998) impaired immune function, (Dardenne, 2002) skin disorders, (Ogawa et al., 2016) cognitive impairments, (Sun et al., 2022), and increased susceptibility to infections and chronic diseases. (Walker & Black, 2004) To effectively address zinc deficiency, a multifaceted approach is required. (Lowe et al., 2024) Dietary strategies are crucial, focusing on increasing the intake of zinc-rich foods such as meat, seafood, and dairy products, (Roohani et al., 2013) as well as enhancing the bioavailability of zinc from plant-based sources through dietary diversification and food fortification. (Gibson & Hotz, 2001; McClements & McClements, 2023) Supplementation is another key strategy, involving the use of zinc supplements like zinc sulfate, zinc gluconate, and zinc acetate to quickly boost zinc levels in at-risk individuals. (Duan et al., 2023) This approach must be carefully managed to ensure appropriate dosages and administration protocols tailored to different age groups and physiological needs, ensuring both efficacy and safety. (Wang et al., 2019) Public health interventions play a vital role in managing zinc deficiency on a larger scale. (Penny, 2013) Organizations such as the World Health Organization (WHO) and UNICEF lead initiatives aimed at reducing the prevalence of zinc deficiency through community-based programs, education campaigns, and policy development. (Organization, 2007; Videira, 2020) These initiatives often include promoting zinc supplementation and fortification programs, as well as educating communities about the importance of zinc in the diet. (Gibson & Ferguson, 1998; Rodríguez-Carmona et al., 2020) Agricultural innovations offer long-term solutions to zinc deficiency. (G. Singh & Pal, 2024; Takkar, 1996) Biofortification, which involves breeding crops to have higher zinc content, and soil enrichment practices are key strategies to increase the zinc content in staple crops. (Cakmak, 2008; Praharaj et al., 2021) Effective management of zinc deficiency requires the integration of these diverse strategies into comprehensive public health policies. (Gibson, 2012b) National nutrition programs, community education campaigns, and collaborative efforts between governments, non-governmental organizations, and health institutions are critical. (Picolo et al., 2019; Swart et al., 2008) These initiatives must be tailored to address the specific needs of vulnerable populations, such as children, pregnant women, and the elderly, to ensure sustainable improvements in zinc nutrition. (Prasad, 1996; Yasuda & Tsutsui, 2016)

CAUSES OF ZINC DEFICIENCY

Figure 1. Causes of zinc deficiency

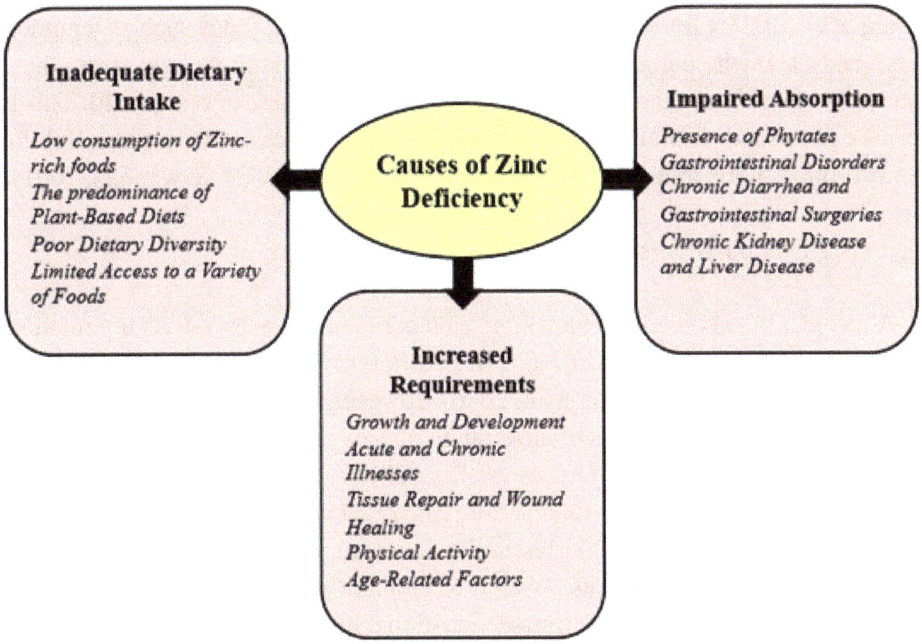

Inadequate Dietary Intake

- ***Low consumption of Zinc-rich foods***

One of the primary causes of zinc deficiency is the insufficient intake of foods that are high in zinc. (Hambidge & Krebs, 2007) Animal-based foods, including meat, seafood, and dairy products, are among the best sources of bioavailable zinc. (Gibson, 2012a; Mwangi et al., 2018) These foods contain zinc in forms that the body can easily absorb and utilize. (O'dell et al., 1972) Red meat and shellfish, such as oysters, are particularly rich in zinc. (Bilandžić et al., 2014) However, in many parts of the world, access to these foods is limited due to economic, cultural, or geographical reasons. (Bailey et al., 2015; Kumssa et al., 2015) In low-income countries, diets often rely heavily on staple crops like rice, maize, and wheat. These staples are poor sources of zinc and do not meet the nutritional requirements for zinc when consumed in isolation or large quantities as the main component of the diet. (Kiran et al., 2022)

- ***The predominance of Plant-Based Diets***

Plant-based diets, which are increasingly popular for ethical, environmental, and health reasons, can also contribute to zinc deficiency if not properly managed. (Craig et al., 2021; Gibson & Ferguson, 1998) While plant foods such as legumes, nuts, seeds, and whole grains do contain zinc, the bioavailability of zinc from these sources is often lower than from animal-based foods. (Rousseau et al., 2020) This is because plant foods contain compounds like phytates, which bind to zinc and inhibit its absorption in the intestines. (Gibson et al., 2018; WEAVER & Kannan, 2001)

- ***Poor Dietary Diversity***

A diet lacking in diversity can lead to zinc deficiency. Dietary diversity refers to the inclusion of a wide variety of foods from different food groups, ensuring that all nutritional needs are met. (Nair et al., 2016) However, in many developing regions, people do not have access to a diverse range of foods due to economic constraints or food insecurity. (Freeland-Graves et al., 2020) Staple foods that form the bulk of such diets, like cereals and tubers, are typically low in zinc. (Hotz, 2009) Even though these staples provide calories and basic nutrition, they do not supply enough zinc to meet daily requirements. (Welch & Graham, 2004) Additionally, reliance on a few food items reduces the overall nutritional quality of the diet, exacerbating the risk of zinc deficiency. (Gibson & Ferguson, 1998)

- ***Limited Access to a Variety of Foods***

Economic and geographical factors play significant roles in zinc deficiency. (Kumssa et al., 2015) In many developing countries, poverty limits the ability to purchase a variety of foods, including zinc-rich animal products and diverse plant foods. (Lockyer et al., 2018) Geographical isolation, such as living in remote or rural areas, can further restrict access to markets that sell a variety of foods. (Ver Ploeg et al., 2009) In some regions, seasonal variations affect food availability, with certain zinc-rich foods only being available during specific times of the year. (Askari et al., 2019) Addressing inadequate dietary intake involves improving access to zinc-rich foods, enhancing dietary diversity, and educating communities about the importance of balanced nutrition. (S. Gupta et al., 2020) Strategies such as food fortification, community gardening, and economic support for vulnerable populations can help mitigate these challenges and reduce the prevalence of zinc deficiency. (Bhutta et al., 2013)

Impaired Absorption

- ***Presence of Phytates***

Phytates, or phytic acid, are naturally occurring compounds found in plant-based foods such as grains, legumes, nuts, and seeds. (Nissar et al., 2017) While these foods can be part of a healthy diet, they also contain high levels of phytates, which can significantly hinder zinc absorption in the human body. (B. O. Lönnerdal, 2000) Phytates bind to zinc in the gastrointestinal tract and form insoluble complexes that the body cannot absorb. (WEAVER & Kannan, 2001) This is particularly problematic in regions where diets are heavily reliant on staple crops that are rich in phytates and low in zinc, such as rice, maize, and wheat. (Shariatipour & Heidari, 2020) Efforts to reduce phytate content in the diet can include food processing techniques like soaking, fermenting, sprouting, and cooking, which help break down phytates and enhance zinc bioavailability. (R. K. Gupta et al., 2015) Additionally, promoting dietary diversification to include foods with lower phytate content can help improve zinc absorption. (Gibson & Hotz, 2001)

- ***Gastrointestinal Disorders***

Various gastrointestinal disorders can impair the body's ability to absorb zinc, leading to deficiency. (Krebs, 2000) Conditions such as Crohn's disease, celiac disease, and irritable bowel syndrome (IBS) cause inflammation and damage to the intestinal lining, which can hinder nutrient absorption. (Mentella et al., 2020) For example, Crohn's disease can cause ulcers and inflammation in the digestive tract, reducing the surface area available for nutrient absorption, including zinc. (Sturniolo et al., 2000) Individuals with celiac disease, an autoimmune disorder triggered by gluten, suffer from damage to the small intestine's villi, the tiny hair-like structures that absorb nutrients. (Tran et al., 2011) Similarly, IBS, characterized by chronic inflammation and irregular bowel movements, can disrupt the normal absorption processes. (Rezazadegan et al., 2022)

- ***Chronic Diarrhea and Gastrointestinal Surgeries***

Chronic diarrhea is another condition that can lead to zinc deficiency. Diarrhea increases the rate at which zinc is excreted from the body, reducing its availability for absorption. (Hambidge, 1992) Frequent or prolonged episodes of diarrhea can deplete the body's zinc stores and hinder the absorption of zinc from the diet. (Wapnir, 2000) Gastrointestinal surgeries, such as bariatric surgery for weight loss, can also impair zinc absorption. These surgeries often involve resection or bypass of parts of the small intestine, which can significantly reduce the area available for nutrient absorption. (Sallé et al., 2010) Post-surgery, patients may experience deficiencies in several micronutrients, including zinc, and require ongoing nutritional monitoring and supplementation. (Gasmi et al., 2022)

- ***Chronic Kidney Disease and Liver Disease***

Chronic kidney disease (CKD) and liver disease are other health conditions that can lead to impaired zinc absorption and increased zinc loss. (Katayama et al., 2018) In CKD, the kidneys' ability to filter and reabsorb essential nutrients is compromised, resulting in increased urinary excretion of zinc. (Cummings & Kovacic, 2009) Patients with CKD often have to adhere to specific dietary restrictions that may limit their zinc intake further. (Joo et al., 2021) Liver disease, such as cirrhosis, affects the liver's ability to store and metabolize zinc. (Grüngreiff et al., 2016) The liver plays a crucial role in regulating zinc levels in the body, and damage to this organ can lead to zinc imbalances. (Mohammad et al., 2012) Additionally, liver disease can interfere with the production of bile, which is necessary for the proper digestion and absorption of fats and fat-soluble vitamins, indirectly affecting zinc absorption. (B. Lönnerdal, 1989)

- ***Other Factors Affecting Absorption***

Certain lifestyle and dietary factors can also impair zinc absorption. (Roohani et al., 2013) High calcium and iron intake can compete with zinc for absorption sites in the intestines. While calcium and iron are essential nutrients, their excessive consumption, particularly from supplements, can reduce the efficiency of zinc absorption. (Powell et al., 1999) Alcoholism is another factor that significantly affects zinc absorption. Chronic alcohol consumption can damage the gastrointestinal lining, impairing nutrient absorption. Alcohol also increases urinary excretion of zinc, leading to further depletion. (Dinsmore et al., 1985)

Increased Requirements

- ***Growth and Development***

During certain life stages, the body's requirement for zinc increases significantly to support growth and development. Infants, children, and adolescents experience rapid growth and developmental changes that necessitate higher zinc intake. Zinc is crucial for cell division, protein synthesis, and overall growth. For example, during infancy and childhood, zinc supports the development of the brain, immune system, and skeletal structure. Insufficient zinc intake during these critical periods can lead to stunted growth, weakened immune function, and delayed cognitive development. (Urbano et al., 2002) Pregnant and lactating women also have increased zinc requirements. During pregnancy, zinc is vital for the growth and development of the fetus, including cell growth, DNA synthesis, and proper immune function. (Kumari et al., 2022) A deficiency in zinc during pregnancy can lead to adverse outcomes such as low birth weight, premature delivery, and congenital abnormalities. (Shah & Sachdev, 2001) Lactating women need additional zinc to ensure adequate zinc content in breast milk, which is essential for the growth and development of the nursing infant. (Dumrongwongsiri et al., 2015) Children and pregnant women are especially vulnerable to zinc deficiency due to their high physiological demands.

- ***Acute and Chronic Illnesses***

The body's demand for zinc increases during periods of illness, particularly in cases of acute infections and chronic diseases. (Bhowmik et al., 2010) Zinc plays a pivotal role in immune function, aiding in the production and function of immune cells, reducing oxidative stress, and enhancing the body's ability to fight infections. (Maggini et al., 2017) During an illness, the immune system's activity intensifies, and the body's zinc reserves are depleted more rapidly. This necessitates an increased dietary intake of zinc to support the immune response and facilitate recovery. (Skrajnowska & Bobrowska-Korczak, 2019)

- ***Tissue Repair and Wound Healing***

Zinc is essential for tissue repair and wound healing. It plays a critical role in collagen synthesis, cell proliferation, and inflammatory response modulation. (Lin et al., 2017) During periods of significant tissue repair, such as after surgery, injury, or burns, the body's zinc requirements increase to facilitate these processes. (Żwierełło et al., 2020) Inadequate zinc intake during these periods can lead to delayed wound healing, increased susceptibility to infections, and prolonged recovery times. (Livingstone, 2015)

- ***Physical Activity***

High levels of physical activity can also increase the body's zinc requirements. Athletes and individuals engaged in intense physical labor may lose significant amounts of zinc through sweat. (Speich et al., 2001) Moreover, physical exercise induces metabolic changes that elevate the body's demand for zinc to support energy production, muscle repair, and immune function. Failure to compensate for these losses through diet can result in zinc deficiency, which may impair physical performance and recovery. (Shao et al., 2021)

- ***Age-Related Factors***

Elderly individuals may have increased zinc requirements due to several factors, including decreased dietary intake, impaired absorption, and increased needs associated with age-related health conditions. (Mocchegiani et al., 2013) As people age, their ability to absorb nutrients can decline due to changes in gastrointestinal function, such as reduced stomach acid production. (Russell, 1992) Additionally, the elderly often have higher rates of chronic diseases that can impact zinc metabolism and increase requirements. (Mocchegiani et al., 2013) To address the increased requirements for zinc during these life stages and health conditions, tailored dietary recommendations and supplementation strategies are essential. (Maggini et al., 2018) Public health initiatives and clinical guidelines should focus on these vulnerable groups to prevent and manage zinc deficiency effectively. (Gibson, 2012b)

VARIOUS STRATEGIES TO ALLEVIATE ZINC DEFICIENCY

Figure 2. Various strategies to alleviate zinc deficiency

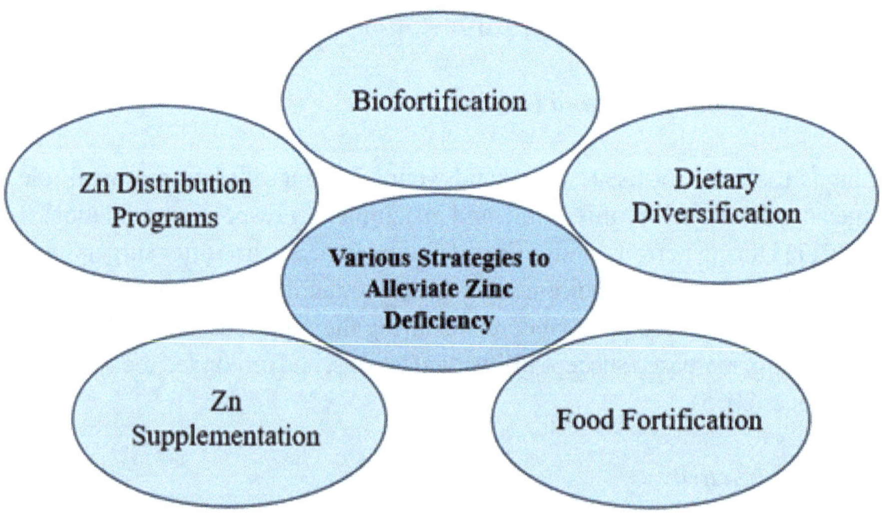

Dietary Diversification

Dietary diversification is a fundamental strategy for combating zinc deficiency, aiming to increase zinc intake by promoting the consumption of a wide range of foods rich in this essential mineral. The strategy recognizes that zinc is present in varying amounts and forms across different food groups, and a diverse diet provides the best opportunity to meet zinc requirements. (Nair et al., 2016)

- ***Animal-Based Foods***

Animal-based foods such as meat, seafood, and dairy products are among the most bioavailable sources of zinc due to their high zinc content and the absence of anti-nutritional factors that inhibit zinc absorption. (Sangeetha et al., 2022) Red meat, particularly beef and lamb, contains significant amounts of zinc, with the beef liver being one of the richest sources. (Williams, 2007) Seafood, especially shellfish like oysters, crab, and shrimp, is also highly concentrated in zinc. (Venugopal & Gopakumar, 2017) Furthermore, dairy products such as milk, cheese, and yogurt contribute to dietary zinc intake, with cheese being a notable source. (Shkembi & Huppertz, 2021)

- ***Plant-Based Foods***

While plant-based foods generally contain lower amounts of zinc compared to animal-based foods, they contribute substantially to overall zinc intake, especially in vegetarian and vegan diets. (Neufingerl & Eilander, 2021) Whole grains like wheat, rice, and oats contain zinc, albeit in lower amounts, and are often fortified with zinc in some regions. (Shelenga et al., 2021) Legumes such as beans, lentils, and chickpeas are valuable sources of zinc, although they also contain phytates, which can inhibit zinc absorption. (Parca et al., 2018) Nuts and seeds, including pumpkin seeds, sesame seeds, and almonds, provide zinc along with healthy fats and protein. (De, 2020)

- ***Dietary Practices to Enhance Zinc Absorption***

Incorporating dietary practices that enhance zinc absorption can maximize the bioavailability of zinc from plant-based sources. Pairing zinc-rich plant foods with enhancers of zinc absorption, such as animal protein or vitamin C-rich foods, can improve zinc uptake. (Gibson et al., 2018) For example, combining beans with meat or fish in a meal can enhance zinc absorption due to the presence of sulfur-containing amino acids from animal protein. (Sandström et al., 1989) Similarly, consuming foods rich in vitamin C, such as citrus fruits, strawberries, or bell peppers, alongside plant-based sources of zinc can increase zinc absorption by reducing the inhibitory effects of phytates. (Vicente et al., 2022)

- ***Cultural and Regional Considerations***

Dietary diversification strategies must also consider cultural preferences, regional availability of foods, and socioeconomic factors. Traditional diets in different cultures often provide unique combinations of foods that contribute to zinc intake. (S. Gupta et al., 2020) For example, diets in Mediterranean countries include a variety of plant-based foods, seafood, and dairy products, offering ample opportunities for zinc intake. (Alcorta et al., 2021) In regions where animal-based foods are scarce or expensive, promoting alternative zinc-rich plant foods and fortifying staple crops becomes particularly important. (Shams Tabrez & Malik, 2021)

- ***Challenges and Opportunities***

Despite the benefits of dietary diversification, challenges such as food insecurity, poverty, and limited access to diverse foods persist, especially in low-income communities. (Kahane et al., 2013) Addressing these challenges requires holistic approaches that encompass education, economic empowerment, agricultural development, and food policy interventions. (Pereznieto & Taylor, 2014) Empowering individuals and communities to make informed dietary choices and advocating for policies that support food security and nutrition are essential components of successful dietary diversification strategies. (Brouwer et al., 2021; Sampson et al., 2021)

Food Fortification

Food fortification is a targeted approach to combating zinc deficiency by enriching staple foods with additional zinc. This strategy aims to reach large populations, particularly in regions where access to diverse and nutrient-rich foods is limited. (García-Bañuelos et al., 2014) By fortifying commonly consumed foods with zinc, food fortification programs can effectively increase zinc intake across entire populations, thereby addressing widespread deficiencies. (Hall & King, 2022)

- ***Targeted Foods for Fortification***

Staple foods such as cereals, grains, and condiments are often chosen as vehicles for zinc fortification due to their widespread consumption and ability to reach diverse population groups. (Kiran et al., 2022) Wheat flour, maize meal, rice, and salt are commonly fortified with zinc in various countries. (Pachón et al., 2021) Fortifying these foods does not require significant changes in dietary habits or consumer behavior, making them suitable candidates for large-scale fortification programs. (Lotfi et al., 1996)

- ***Fortification Technologies and Methods***

Zinc can be added to foods through various fortification technologies and methods. For dry staple foods like flour, maize meal, and rice, zinc compounds such as zinc sulfate, zinc oxide, or zinc gluconate are often used as fortificants. (Ohanenye et al., 2021) In some cases, double fortification with iron and zinc is implemented to address both iron and zinc deficiencies simultaneously. (Ma et al., 2008) For liquid foods like beverages or dairy products, soluble forms of zinc, such as zinc sulfate or zinc acetate, may be used as fortificants. These forms of zinc dissolve easily and are evenly distributed in the liquid, ensuring uniform fortification throughout the product. (Ahmad & Ahmed, 2019)

- ***Types of Food Fortification***

a) Mass Fortification

In mass fortification, zinc is added to widely consumed staple foods at the industrial level during processing. Common vehicles for mass fortification include wheat flour, maize meal, rice, and salt. These fortified foods are then distributed through existing supply chains to reach large segments of the population. (Das, Kumar, et al., 2013)

b) Targeted Fortification

Targeted fortification involves adding zinc to specific food products or supplements that are intended for vulnerable populations, such as pregnant women, infants, or young children. Examples include zinc-fortified infant formula, complementary foods, and prenatal supplements. (Hess & Brown, 2009)

c) Market-Based Fortification

Market-based fortification involves encouraging food producers to voluntarily fortify their products with zinc and market them as fortified foods. This approach relies on consumer demand for fortified products and may involve labeling initiatives to inform consumers about the added nutritional benefits. (Detzel & Klassen-Wigger, 2020; Hall & King, 2022)

- ***Advantages of Food Fortification***

Food fortification offers a multitude of advantages in addressing zinc deficiency. Firstly, it has a broad population impact, reaching vulnerable groups like pregnant women and children by fortifying widely consumed staple foods. (Das, Salam, et al., 2013) Secondly, it is cost-effective compared to other interventions, with minimal incremental costs for adding zinc to foods. (Adams et al., 2023) Thirdly, once implemented, fortification programs are sustainable over time, becoming integrated into regular food distribution channels. (Darnton-Hill & Nalubola, 2002) Fourthly, fortified foods provide a reliable and consistent source of zinc, allowing for precise control over nutritional quality and safety. (Gharibzahedi & Jafari, 2017)

Biofortification

Biofortification is a sustainable agricultural strategy aimed at increasing the nutritional content of crops, including their zinc content, through conventional breeding techniques or genetic engineering. By enhancing the zinc content of staple crops, biofortification offers a long-term solution to addressing zinc deficiency, particularly in regions where access to diverse diets and nutrient-rich foods is limited. (Shariatipour & Heidari, 2020) For example, in Guatemala, zinc-fortified sugar significantly improved serum zinc levels in rural populations (Rodríguez-Carmona et al., 2020). Similarly, HarvestPlus-led initiatives in India and Bangladesh successfully introduced zinc-enriched rice and wheat varieties, demonstrating measurable improvements in zinc status among children and women (Inabangan-Asilo et al., 2019).

- ***Conventional Breeding Approaches***

Conventional breeding methods involve selecting and crossbreeding plant varieties with naturally higher zinc content or better zinc uptake from the soil. (Sadeghzadeh, 2013) Breeders focus on traits such as high zinc concentration in grains, improved zinc uptake and translocation within the plant, and agronomic characteristics suited to local growing conditions. (Swamy et al., 2016)

- ***Genetic Engineering Techniques***

Genetic engineering allows for more targeted and rapid manipulation of crop genomes to increase zinc content. Scientists can introduce genes responsible for zinc uptake, transport, and accumulation into crop plants to enhance their zinc biofortification potential. (Kamaral et al., 2022) Genetic modification may also involve silencing genes that inhibit zinc absorption or altering the expression of genes involved in zinc metabolism. (N. Gupta et al., 2016)

- ***Target Crops for Biofortification***

Biofortification efforts primarily target staple crops that serve as dietary staples for large populations, such as rice, wheat, maize, beans, and legumes. These crops are often consumed in significant quantities, particularly by low-income and food-insecure communities, making them ideal candidates for biofortification initiatives. (Blair, 2013) Additionally, targeting crops that are culturally important and widely cultivated ensures that biofortified varieties are readily adopted and integrated into existing farming systems. (Nestel et al., 2006)

- ***Advantages of Biofortification***

Biofortification offers numerous advantages in combating zinc deficiency. Firstly, it provides a sustainable solution by integrating increased zinc content directly into staple crops, ensuring long-term access to essential nutrients without the need for ongoing interventions. (Kiran et al., 2022) Secondly, biofortified crops not only boost zinc intake but also offer additional nutritional benefits, including improved iron, vitamin A, and protein content, addressing multiple nutrient deficiencies simultaneously. (Avnee et al., 2023) Thirdly, biofortified crop varieties empower farmers by enhancing crop yields and market value, thereby improving livelihoods and food security in agricultural communities. (Yadava et al., 2018) Additionally, biofortified crops are developed to retain the taste, texture, and cooking qualities of conventional varieties, ensuring cultural acceptance and widespread adoption. (Siwela et al., 2020)

- **Challenges and Considerations**

Despite its many advantages, biofortification faces several challenges, including technical constraints, regulatory requirements, and public acceptance. Developing biofortified crop varieties with optimal agronomic performance, nutritional quality, and consumer acceptance requires significant research and investment. Moreover, ensuring equitable access to biofortified crops and addressing socio-economic barriers to adoption are critical for maximizing the impact of biofortification initiatives. (U. Singh et al., 2016; Van Der Straeten et al., 2017)

Zinc Supplementation

- ***Effectiveness of Zinc Supplementation***

Zinc supplementation is highly effective in improving zinc status and addressing deficiency-related health issues. Studies consistently demonstrate its ability to reduce the incidence and severity of diarrhea in children, lower the risk of respiratory infections, promote growth, enhance immune function, and mitigate adverse pregnancy outcomes such as preterm birth and low birth weight. Additionally, zinc supplementation has shown promise in improving cognitive function, wound healing, and overall well-being across various age groups. (Prasad, 1998, 2008; Roohani et al., 2013) While supplementation is beneficial, excessive zinc intake can pose health risks such as copper deficiency, nausea, and immune suppression. The tolerable upper intake level (UL) varies by age and must be observed in policy and clinical practice to prevent adverse outcomes (Schoofs et al., 2024). A Cochrane systematic review included 96 studies with over 219,000 children aged 6 months to 12 years. It found that zinc supplementation might help prevent episodes of diarrhea and slightly improve growth, especially in regions with high zinc deficiency prevalence (Mayo-Wilson et al., 2014).

- ***Dosage Considerations***

Dosage recommendations for zinc supplementation vary based on age, sex, physiological status, and the severity of deficiency. Infants, children, pregnant and lactating women, and individuals with specific medical conditions may require different dosages. (Corbo & Lam, 2013) Common forms of zinc supplements include tablets, capsules, syrups, and dispersible powders, with formulations tailored to meet the needs of diverse populations. (Islam et al., 2018)

- ***Challenges and Considerations***

Despite its effectiveness, zinc supplementation may face challenges related to access, affordability, supply chain management, and cultural beliefs. Limited availability of supplements, inadequate awareness of zinc deficiency, and competing health priorities may hinder program uptake, particularly in resource-constrained settings. (Chinni et al., 2021; Maret & Sandstead, 2006)

CONCLUSION

This chapter has outlined various strategies to tackle zinc deficiency and manage its impacts. From understanding its causes to exploring solutions like dietary adjustments, fortification, and supplementation, we've uncovered practical ways to address this nutritional challenge. By implementing these strategies with diligence and collaboration, we can make significant strides toward improving zinc nutrition and overall health outcomes. However, challenges such as access to resources, awareness, and sustainability remain pertinent. Hence, concerted efforts are needed from governments, NGOs, healthcare providers, and communities to ensure the effective implementation and scaling-up of these interventions. Moreover, ongoing research and evaluation are essential to refine existing approaches and develop innovations.

FUTURE PERSPECTIVES

Zinc deficiency management holds promise for continued innovation and progress. As research advances, there is a growing recognition of the interconnectedness between nutrition, health, and sustainable development, underscoring the importance of addressing nutritional deficiencies like zinc inadequacy. Emerging technologies such as precision agriculture and genetic engineering offer opportunities for further enhancing the bioavailability of zinc in staple crops, thereby bolstering food security and nutrition at the global level. Moreover, advancements in public health infrastructure and policy frameworks can facilitate the integration of zinc deficiency management into broader health and development agendas, ensuring equitable access to interventions and sustained improvements in population health. By embracing a holistic approach that encompasses scientific innovation, multisectoral collaboration, and evidence-based policy-making, we can pave the way for a future where zinc deficiency is effectively addressed, and individuals worldwide thrive with optimal health and well-being. Future research should explore the interplay between zinc and gut microbiota, the development of personalized supplementation strategies using genetic and biomarker profiling, and the long-term effectiveness of integrated food system interventions. Moreover, scalable, cost-effective monitoring technologies for zinc status in community settings remain a research priority.

REFERENCES

Adams, K. P., Jarvis, M., Vosti, S. A., Manger, M. S., Tarini, A., Somé, J. W., Somda, H., & McDonald, C. M. (2023). Estimating the cost and cost-effectiveness of adding zinc to, and improving the performance of, Burkina Faso's mandatory wheat flour fortification programme. *Maternal and Child Nutrition, 19*(3), e13515. DOI: 10.1111/mcn.13515 PMID: 37021818

Ahmad, A., & Ahmed, Z. (2019). Fortification in beverages. In *Production and management ofbeverages* (pp. 85–122). Elsevier., https://www.sciencedirect.com/science/article/pii/B9780128152607000031 DOI: 10.1016/B978-0-12-815260-7.00003-1

Alcorta, A., Porta, A., Tárrega, A., Alvarez, M. D., & Vaquero, M. P. (2021). Foods for plant-based diets: Challenges and innovations. *Foods, 10*(2), 293. DOI: 10.3390/foods10020293 PMID: 33535684

Askari, S., Asghari, G., Farhadnejad, H., Ghanbarian, A., Mirmiran, P., & Azizi, F. (2019). Seasonal variations of serum zinc concentration in adult population: Tehran lipid and glucose study. *Iranian Journal of Public Health, 48*(8), 1496. PMID: 32292733

Avnee, S., Sood, S., Chaudhary, D. R., Jhorar, P., & Rana, R. S. (2023). Biofortification: An approach to eradicate micronutrient deficiency. *Frontiers in Nutrition, 10*, 1233070. DOI: 10.3389/fnut.2023.1233070 PMID: 37789898

Bailey, R. L., West, K. P.Jr, & Black, R. E. (2015). The epidemiology of global micronutrient deficiencies. *Annals of Nutrition & Metabolism, 66*(Suppl. 2), 22–33. DOI: 10.1159/000371618 PMID: 26045325

Bhowmik, D., Chiranjib, K., & Kumar, S. (2010). A potential medicinal importance of zinc in human health and chronic. *Int J Pharm, 1*(1), 05–11.

Bhutta, Z. A., Salam, R. A., & Das, J. K. (2013). Meeting the challenges of micronutrient malnutrition in the developing world. *British Medical Bulletin, 106*(1), 7–17. DOI: 10.1093/bmb/ldt015 PMID: 23645843

Bilandžić, N., Sedak, M., Đokić, M., Varenina, I., Solomun Kolanović, B., Božić, Đ., Brstilo, M., & Šimić, B. (2014). Determination of zinc concentrations in foods of animal origin, fish and shellfish from Croatia and assessment of their contribution to dietary intake. *Journal of Food Composition and Analysis, 35*(2), 61–66. DOI: 10.1016/j.jfca.2014.04.006

Black, M. M. (1998). Zinc deficiency and child development. *The American Journal of Clinical Nutrition, 68*(2), 464S–469S. DOI: 10.1093/ajcn/68.2.464S PMID: 9701161

Blair, M. W. (2013). Mineral biofortification strategies for food staples: The example of common bean. *Journal of Agricultural and Food Chemistry, 61*(35), 8287–8294. DOI: 10.1021/jf400774y PMID: 23848266

Brouwer, I. D., Van Liere, M. J., De Brauw, A., Dominguez-Salas, P., Herforth, A., Kennedy, G., Lachat, C., Omosa, E. B., Talsma, E. F., Vandevijvere, S., Fanzo, J., & Ruel, M. (2021). Reverse thinking: Taking a healthy diet perspective towards food systems transformations. *Food Security, 13*(6), 1497–1523. DOI: 10.1007/s12571-021-01204-5

Cakmak, I. (2008). Enrichment of cereal grains with zinc: Agronomic or genetic biofortification? *Plant and Soil, 302*(1-2), 1–17. DOI: 10.1007/s11104-007-9466-3

Caulfield, L. E., & Black, R. E. (2004). Zinc deficiency. *Comparative Quantification of Health Risks: Global and Regional Burden of Disease Attributable to Selected Major Risk Factors, 1*, 257–280. PMID: 15100497

Chinni, V., El-Khoury, J., Perera, M., Bellomo, R., Jones, D., Bolton, D., Ischia, J., & Patel, O. (2021). Zinc supplementation as an adjunct therapy for COVID-19: Challenges and opportunities. *British Journal of Clinical Pharmacology, 87*(10), 3737–3746. DOI: 10.1111/bcp.14826 PMID: 33742473

Corbo, M. D., & Lam, J. (2013). Zinc deficiency and its management in the pediatric population: A literature review and proposed etiologic classification. *Journal of the American Academy of Dermatology, 69*(4), 616–624. DOI: 10.1016/j.jaad.2013.04.028 PMID: 23688650

Craig, W. J., Mangels, A. R., Fresán, U., Marsh, K., Miles, F. L., Saunders, A. V., Haddad, E. H., Heskey, C. E., Johnston, P., Larson-Meyer, E., & Orlich, M. (2021). The safe and effective use of plant-based diets with guidelines for health professionals. *Nutrients, 13*(11), 4144. DOI: 10.3390/nu13114144 PMID: 34836399

Cummings, J. E., & Kovacic, J. P. (2009). The ubiquitous role of zinc in health and disease. *Journal of Veterinary Emergency and Critical Care (San Antonio, Tex.), 19*(3), 215–240. DOI: 10.1111/j.1476-4431.2009.00418.x PMID: 19691507

Dardenne, M. (2002). Zinc and immune function. *European Journal of Clinical Nutrition, 56*(3), S20–S23. DOI: 10.1038/sj.ejcn.1601479 PMID: 12142956

Darnton-Hill, I., & Nalubola, R. (2002). Fortification strategies to meet micronutrient needs: Sucesses and failures. *The Proceedings of the Nutrition Society*, *61*(2), 231–241. DOI: 10.1079/PNS2002150 PMID: 12133205

Das, J. K., Kumar, R., Salam, R. A., & Bhutta, Z. A. (2013). Systematic review of zinc fortification trials. *Annals of Nutrition & Metabolism*, *62*(Suppl. 1), 44–56. DOI: 10.1159/000348262 PMID: 23689112

Das, J. K., Salam, R. A., Kumar, R., & Bhutta, Z. A. (2013). Micronutrient fortification of food and its impact on woman and child health: A systematic review. *Systematic Reviews*, *2*(1), 1–24. DOI: 10.1186/2046-4053-2-67 PMID: 23971426

De, L. C. (2020). Edible seeds and nuts in human diet for immunity development. *International Journal of Recent Scientific Research*, *6*(11), 38877–38881.

Detzel, P., & Klassen-Wigger, P. (2020). Market-driven food fortification to address dietary needs. *World Review of Nutrition and Dietetics*, *121*, 81–88. DOI: 10.1159/000507522 PMID: 33502376

Dinsmore, W., Callender, M. E., McMaster, D., Todd, J., & Love, A. H. (1985). Zinc absorption in alcoholics using zinc-65. *Digestion*, *32*(4), 238–242. DOI: 10.1159/000199243 PMID: 4065445

Duan, M., Li, T., Liu, B., Yin, S., Zang, J., Lv, C., Zhao, G., & Zhang, T. (2023). Zinc nutrition and dietary zinc supplements. *Critical Reviews in Food Science and Nutrition*, *63*(9), 1277–1292. DOI: 10.1080/10408398.2021.1963664 PMID: 34382897

Dumrongwongsiri, O., Suthutvoravut, U., Chatvutinun, S., Phoonlabdacha, P., Sangcakul, A., Siripinyanond, A., Thiengmanee, U., & Chongviriyaphan, N. (2015). Maternal zinc status is associated with breast milk zinc concentration and zinc status in breastfed infants aged 4-6 months. *Asia Pacific Journal of Clinical Nutrition*, *24*(2), 273–280. PMID: 26078244

Freeland-Graves, J. H., Sachdev, P. K., Binderberger, A. Z., & Sosanya, M. E. (2020). Global diversity of dietary intakes and standards for zinc, iron, and copper. *Journal of Trace Elements in Medicine and Biology*, *61*, 126515. DOI: 10.1016/j.jtemb.2020.126515 PMID: 32450495

García-Bañuelos, M. L., Sida-Arreola, J. P., & Sánchez, E. (2014). Biofortification-promising approach to increasing the content of iron and zinc in staple food crops. *Journal of Elementology*, *19*(3). https://agro.icm.edu.pl/agro/element/bwmeta1.element.agro-3c9e2e65-f373-4936-acd2-a5850e3e70b8

Gasmi, A., Bjørklund, G., Mujawdiya, P. K., Semenova, Y., Peana, M., Dosa, A., Piscopo, S., Gasmi Benahmed, A., & Costea, D. O. (2022). Micronutrients deficiences in patients after bariatric surgery. *European Journal of Nutrition*, *61*(1), 55–67. DOI: 10.1007/s00394-021-02619-8 PMID: 34302218

Gharibzahedi, S. M. T., & Jafari, S. M. (2017). The importance of minerals in human nutrition: Bioavailability, food fortification, processing effects and nanoencapsulation. *Trends in Food Science & Technology*, *62*, 119–132. DOI: 10.1016/j.tifs.2017.02.017

Gibson, R. S. (2012a). A historical review of progress in the assessment of dietary zinc intake as an indicator of population zinc status. *Advances in Nutrition*, *3*(6), 772–782. DOI: 10.3945/an.112.002287 PMID: 23153731

Gibson, R. S. (2012b). Zinc deficiency and human health: Etiology, health consequences, and future solutions. *Plant and Soil*, *361*(1-2), 291–299. DOI: 10.1007/s11104-012-1209-4

Gibson, R. S., & Ferguson, E. L. (1998). Nutrition intervention strategies to combat zinc deficiency in developing countries. *Nutrition Research Reviews*, *11*(1), 115–131. DOI: 10.1079/NRR19980008 PMID: 19087462

Gibson, R. S., & Hotz, C. (2001). Dietary diversification/modification strategies to enhance micronutrient content and bioavailability of diets in developing countries. *British Journal of Nutrition*, *85*(S2), S159–S166. DOI: 10.1079/BJN2001309 PMID: 11509105

Gibson, R. S., Raboy, V., & King, J. C. (2018). Implications of phytate in plant-based foods for iron and zinc bioavailability, setting dietary requirements, and formulating programs and policies. *Nutrition Reviews*, *76*(11), 793–804. DOI: 10.1093/nutrit/nuy028 PMID: 30010865

Grüngreiff, K., Reinhold, D., & Wedemeyer, H. (2016). The role of zinc in liver cirrhosis. *Annals of Hepatology*, *15*(1), 7–16. DOI: 10.5604/16652681.1184191 PMID: 26626635

Gupta, N., Ram, H., & Kumar, B. (2016). Mechanism of Zinc absorption in plants: Uptake, transport, translocation and accumulation. *Reviews in Environmental Science and Biotechnology*, *15*(1), 89–109. DOI: 10.1007/s11157-016-9390-1

Gupta, R. K., Gangoliya, S. S., & Singh, N. K. (2015). Reduction of phytic acid and enhancement of bioavailable micronutrients in food grains. *Journal of Food Science and Technology*, *52*(2), 676–684. DOI: 10.1007/s13197-013-0978-y PMID: 25694676

Gupta, S., Brazier, A. K. M., & Lowe, N. M. (2020). Zinc deficiency in low- and middle-income countries: Prevalence and approaches for mitigation. *Journal of Human Nutrition and Dietetics*, *33*(5), 624–643. DOI: 10.1111/jhn.12791 PMID: 32627912

Hall, A. G., & King, J. C. (2022). Zinc fortification: Current trends and strategies. *Nutrients*, *14*(19), 3895. DOI: 10.3390/nu14193895 PMID: 36235548

Hambidge, K. M. (1992). Zinc and diarrhea. *Acta Paediatrica (Oslo, Norway)*, *81*(s383), 82–86. DOI: 10.1111/j.1651-2227.1992.tb12377.x PMID: 1421947

Hambidge, K. M., & Krebs, N. F. (2007). Zinc Deficiency: A Special Challenge1. *The Journal of Nutrition*, *137*(4), 1101–1105. DOI: 10.1093/jn/137.4.1101 PMID: 17374687

Hess, S. Y., & Brown, K. H. (2009). Impact of zinc fortification on zinc nutrition. *Food and Nutrition Bulletin*, *30*(1, suppl1), S79–S107. DOI: 10.1177/15648265090301S106 PMID: 19472603

Hotz, C. (2009). The Potential to Improve Zinc Status through Biofortification of Staple Food Crops with Zinc. *Food and Nutrition Bulletin*, *30*(1, suppl1), S172–S178. DOI: 10.1177/15648265090301S109 PMID: 19472606

Inabangan-Asilo, M. A., Swamy, B. P. M., Amparado, A. F., Descalsota-Empleo, G. I., Arocena, E. C., & Reinke, R. (2019). Stability and G×E analysis of zinc-biofortified rice genotypes evaluated in diverse environments. *Euphytica*, *215*(3), 1–7. DOI: 10.1007/s10681-019-2384-7

Islam, M. M., McDonald, C. M., Krebs, N. F., Westcott, J., Rahman, A. E., El Arifeen, S., Ahmed, T., King, J. C., & Black, R. E. (2018). Study protocol for a randomized, double-blind, community-based efficacy trial of various doses of zinc in micronutrient powders or tablets in young Bangladeshi children. *Nutrients*, *10*(2), 132. DOI: 10.3390/nu10020132 PMID: 30720778

Joo, Y. S., Kim, H. W., Lee, S., Nam, K. H., Yun, H.-R., Jhee, J. H., Han, S. H., Yoo, T.-H., Kang, S.-W., & Park, J. T. (2021). Dietary zinc intake and incident chronic kidney disease. *Clinical Nutrition (Edinburgh, Lothian)*, *40*(3), 1039–1045. DOI: 10.1016/j.clnu.2020.07.005 PMID: 32753349

Kahane, R., Hodgkin, T., Jaenicke, H., Hoogendoorn, C., Hermann, M., Keatinge, J. D. H., d'Arros Hughes, J., Padulosi, S., & Looney, N. (2013). Agrobiodiversity for food security, health and income. *Agronomy for Sustainable Development*, *33*, 671–693. DOI: 10.1007/s13593-013-0147-8

Kamaral, C., Neate, S. M., Gunasinghe, N., Milham, P. J., Paterson, D. J., Kopittke, P. M., & Seneweera, S. (2022). Genetic biofortification of wheat with zinc: Opportunities to fine-tune zinc uptake, transport and grain loading. *Physiologia Plantarum, 174*(1), e13612. DOI: 10.1111/ppl.13612 PMID: 34970752

Katayama, K., Kawaguchi, T., Shiraishi, K., Ito, T., Suzuki, K., Koreeda, C., Ohtake, T., Iwasa, M., Tokumoto, Y., Endo, R., Kawamura, N., Shiraki, M., Hanai, T., Habu, D., Tsuruta, S., Sakai, H., Miwa, Y., Kawada, N., Kato, A., & Suzuki, K. (2018). The prevalence and implication of zinc deficiency in patients with chronic liver disease. *Journal of Clinical Medicine Research, 10*(5), 437–444. DOI: 10.14740/jocmr3374w PMID: 29581807

Kiran, A., Wakeel, A., Mahmood, K., Mubaraka, R., Hafsa, , & Haefele, S. M. (2022). Biofortification of staple crops to alleviate human malnutrition: Contributions and potential in developing countries. *Agronomy (Basel), 12*(2), 452. DOI: 10.3390/agronomy12020452

Krebs, N. F. (2000). Overview of zinc absorption and excretion in the human gastrointestinal tract. *The Journal of Nutrition, 130*(5), 1374S–1377S. DOI: 10.1093/jn/130.5.1374S PMID: 10801946

Kumari, D., Garg, S., & Bhawrani, P. (2022). Zinc homeostasis in immunity and its association with preterm births. *Scandinavian Journal of Immunology, 95*(4), e13142. DOI: 10.1111/sji.13142 PMID: 35007353

Kumssa, D. B., Joy, E. J., Ander, E. L., Watts, M. J., Young, S. D., Walker, S., & Broadley, M. R. (2015). Dietary calcium and zinc deficiency risks are decreasing but remain prevalent. *Scientific Reports, 5*(1), 10974. DOI: 10.1038/srep10974 PMID: 26098577

Lin, P.-H., Sermersheim, M., Li, H., Lee, P., Steinberg, S., & Ma, J. (2017). Zinc in Wound Healing Modulation. *Nutrients, 10*(1), 16. DOI: 10.3390/nu10010016 PMID: 29295546

Livingstone, C. (2015). Zinc: Physiology, Deficiency, and Parenteral Nutrition. *Nutrition in Clinical Practice, 30*(3), 371–382. DOI: 10.1177/0884533615570376 PMID: 25681484

Lockyer, S., White, A., & Buttriss, J. L. (2018). Biofortified crops for tackling micronutrient deficiencies – what impact are these having in developing countries and could they be of relevance within Europe? *Nutrition Bulletin, 43*(4), 319–357. DOI: 10.1111/nbu.12347

Lönnerdal, B. (1989). Intestinal Absorption of Zinc. In Mills, C. F. (Ed.), *Zinc in Human Biology* (pp. 33–55). Springer London., DOI: 10.1007/978-1-4471-3879-2_3

Lönnerdal, B. O. (2000). Dietary factors influencing zinc absorption. *The Journal of Nutrition, 130*(5), 1378S–1383S. DOI: 10.1093/jn/130.5.1378S PMID: 10801947

Lotfi, M., Venkatesh Mannar, M. G., Merx, R. J., & Naber-van den Heuvel, P. (1996). *Micronutrient fortification of foods: Current practices, research, and opportunities*. IDRC, Micronutrient Initiative., https://idl-bnc-idrc.dspacedirect.org/bitstream/handle/10625/14002/104386.pdf?sequence=1

Lowe, N. M., Hall, A. G., Broadley, M. R., Foley, J., Boy, E., & Bhutta, Z. A. (2024). Preventing and controlling zinc deficiency across the life course: A call to action. *Advances in Nutrition, 15*(3), 100181. DOI: 10.1016/j.advnut.2024.100181 PMID: 38280724

Ma, G., Jin, Y., Li, Y., Zhai, F., Kok, F. J., Jacobsen, E., & Yang, X. (2008). Iron and zinc deficiencies in China: What is a feasible and cost-effective strategy? *Public Health Nutrition, 11*(6), 632–638. DOI: 10.1017/S1368980007001085 PMID: 17894916

Maggini, S., Maldonado, P., Cardim, P., Fernandez Newball, C., & Sota Latino, E. (2017). Vitamins C, D and zinc: Synergistic roles in immune function and infections. *Vitam Miner, 6*(167), 2376–1318. DOI: 10.4172/2376-1318.1000167

Maggini, S., Pierre, A., & Calder, P. (2018). Immune Function and Micronutrient Requirements Change over the Life Course. *Nutrients, 10*(10), 1531. DOI: 10.3390/nu10101531 PMID: 30336639

Maret, W., & Sandstead, H. H. (2006). Zinc requirements and the risks and benefits of zinc supplementation. *Journal of Trace Elements in Medicine and Biology, 20*(1), 3–18. DOI: 10.1016/j.jtemb.2006.01.006 PMID: 16632171

Mayo-Wilson, E., Junior, J. A., Imdad, A., Dean, S., Chan, X. H., Chan, E. S., Jaswal, A., & Bhutta, Z. A. (2014). Zinc supplementation for preventing mortality, morbidity, and growth failure in children aged 6 months to 12 years of age. *Cochrane Database of Systematic Reviews, 2014*(5), CD009384. DOI: 10.1002/14651858.CD009384.pub2 PMID: 24826920

McClements, I. F., & McClements, D. J. (2023). Designing healthier plant-based foods: Fortification, digestion, and bioavailability. *Food Research International, 169*, 112853. DOI: 10.1016/j.foodres.2023.112853 PMID: 37254427

Mentella, M. C., Scaldaferri, F., Pizzoferrato, M., Gasbarrini, A., & Miggiano, G. A. D. (2020). Nutrition, IBD and gut microbiota: A review. *Nutrients, 12*(4), 944. DOI: 10.3390/nu12040944 PMID: 32235316

Mocchegiani, E., Romeo, J., Malavolta, M., Costarelli, L., Giacconi, R., Diaz, L.-E., & Marcos, A. (2013). Zinc: Dietary intake and impact of supplementation on immune function in elderly. *Age (Dordrecht, Netherlands), 35*(3), 839–860. DOI: 10.1007/s11357-011-9377-3 PMID: 22222917

Mohammad, M. K., Zhou, Z., Cave, M., Barve, A., & McClain, C. J. (2012). Zinc and Liver Disease. *Nutrition in Clinical Practice, 27*(1), 8–20. DOI: 10.1177/0884533611433534 PMID: 22307488

Mwangi, M. N., Oonincx, D. G., Stouten, T., Veenenbos, M., Melse-Boonstra, A., Dicke, M., & Van Loon, J. J. (2018). Insects as sources of iron and zinc in human nutrition. *Nutrition Research Reviews, 31*(2), 248–255. DOI: 10.1017/S0954422418000094 PMID: 30033906

Nair, M. K., Augustine, L. F., & Konapur, A. (2016). Food-Based Interventions to Modify Diet Quality and Diversity to Address Multiple Micronutrient Deficiency. *Frontiers in Public Health, 3*. Advance online publication. DOI: 10.3389/fpubh.2015.00277 PMID: 26779472

Nestel, P., Bouis, H. E., Meenakshi, J. V., & Pfeiffer, W. (2006). Biofortification of staple food crops. *The Journal of Nutrition, 136*(4), 1064–1067. DOI: 10.1093/jn/136.4.1064 PMID: 16549478

Neufingerl, N., & Eilander, A. (2021). Nutrient intake and status in adults consuming plant-based diets compared to meat-eaters: A systematic review. *Nutrients, 14*(1), 29. DOI: 10.3390/nu14010029 PMID: 35010904

Nissar, J., Ahad, T., Naik, H. R., & Hussain, S. Z. (2017). A review phytic acid: As antinutrient or nutraceutical. *Journal of Pharmacognosy and Phytochemistry, 6*(6), 1554–1560.

O'dell, B. L., Burpo, C. E., & Savage, J. E. (1972). Evaluation of zinc availability in foodstuffs of plant and animal origin. *The Journal of Nutrition, 102*(5), 653–660. DOI: 10.1093/jn/102.5.653 PMID: 5063219

Ogawa, Y., Kawamura, T., & Shimada, S. (2016). Zinc and skin biology. *Archives of Biochemistry and Biophysics, 611*, 113–119. DOI: 10.1016/j.abb.2016.06.003 PMID: 27288087

Ohanenye, I. C., Emenike, C. U., Mensi, A., Medina-Godoy, S., Jin, J., Ahmed, T., Sun, X., & Udenigwe, C. C. (2021). Food fortification technologies: Influence on iron, zinc and vitamin A bioavailability and potential implications on micronutrient deficiency in sub-Saharan Africa. *Scientific African, 11*, e00667. DOI: 10.1016/j.sciaf.2020.e00667

Pachón, H., Reynolds, B., Duong, M., Tsang, B. L., Childs, L., Luthringer, C. L., Kang, Y., Vasta, F. C., & Codling, K. (2021). The potential contribution of fortified maize flour, oil, rice, salt, and wheat flour to estimated average requirements and tolerable upper intake levels for 15 nutrients in 153 countries. *Nutrients, 13*(2), 579. DOI: 10.3390/nu13020579 PMID: 33572488

Parca, F., Koca, Y. O., & Unay, A. (2018). Nutritional and antinutritional factors of some pulses seed and their effects on human health. *International Journal of Secondary Metabolite, 5*(4), 331–342. DOI: 10.21448/ijsm.488651

Penny, M. E. (2013). Zinc Supplementation in Public Health. *Annals of Nutrition & Metabolism, 62*(Suppl. 1), 31–42. DOI: 10.1159/000348263 PMID: 23689111

Pereznieto, P., & Taylor, G. (2014). A review of approaches and methods to measure economic empowerment of women and girls. *Gender and Development, 22*(2), 233–251. DOI: 10.1080/13552074.2014.920976

Picolo, M., Barros, I., Joyeux, M., Gottwalt, A., Possolo, E., Sigauque, B., & Kavle, J. A. (2019). Rethinking integrated nutrition-health strategies to address micronutrient deficiencies in children under five in Mozambique. *Maternal and Child Nutrition, 15*(S1), e12721. DOI: 10.1111/mcn.12721 PMID: 30748114

Powell, J. J., Jugdaohsingh, R., & Thompson, R. P. H. (1999). The regulation of mineral absorption in the gastrointestinal tract. *The Proceedings of the Nutrition Society, 58*(1), 147–153. DOI: 10.1079/PNS19990020 PMID: 10343352

Praharaj, S., Skalicky, M., Maitra, S., Bhadra, P., Shankar, T., Brestic, M., Hejnak, V., Vachova, P., & Hossain, A. (2021). Zinc Biofortification in Food Crops Could Alleviate the Zinc Malnutrition in Human Health. *Molecules (Basel, Switzerland), 26*(12), 3509. DOI: 10.3390/molecules26123509 PMID: 34207649

Prasad, A. S. (1996). Zinc deficiency in women, infants and children. *Journal of the American College of Nutrition, 15*(2), 113–120. DOI: 10.1080/07315724.1996.10718575 PMID: 8778139

Prasad, A. S. (1998). Zinc in human health: An update. *The Journal of Trace Elements in Experimental Medicine, 11*(2–3), 63–87. DOI: 10.1002/(SICI)1520-670X(1998)11:2/3<63::AID-JTRA2>3.0.CO;2-5

Prasad, A. S. (2008). Zinc in Human Health: Effect of Zinc on Immune Cells. *Molecular Medicine (Cambridge, Mass.)*, *14*(5–6), 353–357. DOI: 10.2119/2008-00033.Prasad PMID: 18385818

Rezazadegan, M., Shahdadian, F., Soheilipour, M., Tarrahi, M. J., & Amani, R. (2022). Zinc nutritional status, mood states and quality of life in diarrhea-predominant irritable bowel syndrome: A case–control study. *Scientific Reports*, *12*(1), 11002. DOI: 10.1038/s41598-022-15080-2 PMID: 35768522

Rodríguez-Carmona, Y., Denova-Gutiérrez, E., Sánchez-Uribe, E., Muñoz-Aguirre, P., Flores, M., & Salmerón, J. (2020). Zinc supplementation and fortification in Mexican children. *Food and Nutrition Bulletin*, *41*(1), 89–101. DOI: 10.1177/0379572119877757 PMID: 31955593

Roohani, N., Hurrell, R., Kelishadi, R., & Schulin, R. (2013). Zinc and its importance for human health: An integrative review. *Journal of Research in Medical Sciences : the Official Journal of Isfahan University of Medical Sciences*, *18*(2), 144. PMID: 23914218

Rousseau, S., Kyomugasho, C., Celus, M., Hendrickx, M. E., & Grauwet, T. (2020). Barriers impairing mineral bioaccessibility and bioavailability in plant-based foods and the perspectives for food processing. *Critical Reviews in Food Science and Nutrition*, *60*(5), 826–843. DOI: 10.1080/10408398.2018.1552243 PMID: 30632768

Russell, R. M. (1992). Changes in gastrointestinal function attributed to aging. *The American Journal of Clinical Nutrition*, *55*(6), 1203S–1207S. DOI: 10.1093/ajcn/55.6.1203S PMID: 1590257

Sadeghzadeh, B. (2013). A review of zinc nutrition and plant breeding. *Journal of Soil Science and Plant Nutrition*, *13*(4), 905–927. DOI: 10.4067/S0718-95162013005000072

Sallé, A., Demarsy, D., Poirier, A. L., Lelièvre, B., Topart, P., Guilloteau, G., Bécouarn, G., & Rohmer, V. (2010). Zinc Deficiency: A Frequent and Underestimated Complication After Bariatric Surgery. *Obesity Surgery*, *20*(12), 1660–1670. DOI: 10.1007/s11695-010-0237-5 PMID: 20706804

Sampson, D., Cely-Santos, M., Gemmill-Herren, B., Babin, N., Bernhart, A., Bezner Kerr, R., Blesh, J., Bowness, E., Feldman, M., Gonçalves, A. L., James, D., Kerssen, T., Klassen, S., Wezel, A., & Wittman, H. (2021). Food sovereignty and rights-based approaches strengthen food security and nutrition across the globe: A systematic review. *Frontiers in Sustainable Food Systems*, *5*, 686492. DOI: 10.3389/fsufs.2021.686492

Sandström, B., Almgren, A., Kivistö, B., & Cederblad, Å. (1989). Effect of protein level and protein source on zinc absorption in humans. *The Journal of Nutrition, 119*(1), 48–53. DOI: 10.1093/jn/119.1.48 PMID: 2492337

Sangeetha, V. J., Dutta, S., Moses, J. A., & Anandharamakrishnan, C. (2022). Zinc nutrition and human health: Overview and implications. *eFood, 3*(5), e17. DOI: 10.1002/efd2.17

Schoofs, H., Schmit, J., & Rink, L. (2024). Zinc toxicity: Understanding the limits. *Molecules (Basel, Switzerland), 29*(13), 3130. DOI: 10.3390/molecules29133130 PMID: 38999082

Shah, D., & Sachdev, H. S. (2001). Effect of gestational zinc deficiency on pregnancy outcomes: Summary of observation studies and zinc supplementation trials. *British Journal of Nutrition, 85*(S2), S101–S108. DOI: 10.1079/BJN2000301 PMID: 11509097

Shams Tabrez, K., & Malik, A. (2021). *Microbial biofertilizers and micronutrient availability: The role of zinc in agriculture and human health.* Springer Nature. https://books.google.com/books?hl=en&lr=&id=andTEAAAQBAJ&oi=fnd&pg=PR8&dq=In+regions+where+animal-based+foods+are+scarce+or+expensive,+promoting+alternative+zinc-rich+plant+foods+and+fortifying+staple+crops+becomes+particularly+important.&ots=oYNloCTN6o&sig=jbrZnyMkop_tKH5Y8kaMZfDrrTI

Shao, T., Verma, H. K., Pande, B., Costanzo, V., Ye, W., Cai, Y., & Bhaskar, L. (2021). Physical activity and nutritional influence on immune function: An important strategy to improve immunity and health status. *Frontiers in Physiology, 12*, 751374. DOI: 10.3389/fphys.2021.751374 PMID: 34690818

Shariatipour, N., & Heidari, B. (2020). Genetic-Based Biofortification of Staple Food Crops to Meet Zinc and Iron Deficiency-Related Challenges. In Aftab, T., & Hakeem, K. R. (Eds.), *Plant Micronutrients* (pp. 173–223). Springer International Publishing., DOI: 10.1007/978-3-030-49856-6_8

Shelenga, T. V., Kerv, Y. A., Perchuk, I. N. E., Solovyeva, A., Khlestkina, E. K. G., Loskutov, I., & Konarev, A. V. (2021). The potential of small grains crops in enhancing biofortification breeding strategies for human health benefit. *Agronomy (Basel), 11*(7), 1420. DOI: 10.3390/agronomy11071420

Shkembi, B., & Huppertz, T. (2021). Influence of dairy products on bioavailability of zinc from other food products: A review of complementarity at a meal level. *Nutrients, 13*(12), 4253. DOI: 10.3390/nu13124253 PMID: 34959808

Singh, G., & Pal, V. (2024). Agronomic innovations for enhancement of zinc content in pulses: A review. *Indian Journal of Pulses Research*, *37*(1), 11–21. DOI: 10.59797/jfl.v37.i1.173

Singh, U., Praharaj, C. S., Chaturvedi, S. K., & Bohra, A. (2016). Biofortification: Introduction, Approaches, Limitations, and Challenges. In Singh, U., Praharaj, C. S., Singh, S. S., & Singh, N. P. (Eds.), *Biofortification of Food Crops* (pp. 3–18). Springer India., DOI: 10.1007/978-81-322-2716-8_1

Siwela, M., Pillay, K., Govender, L., Lottering, S., Mudau, F. N., Modi, A. T., & Mabhaudhi, T. (2020). Biofortified crops for combating hidden hunger in South Africa: Availability, acceptability, micronutrient retention and bioavailability. *Foods*, *9*(6), 815. DOI: 10.3390/foods9060815 PMID: 32575819

Skrajnowska, D., & Bobrowska-Korczak, B. (2019). Role of zinc in immune system and anti-cancer defense mechanisms. *Nutrients*, *11*(10), 2273. DOI: 10.3390/nu11102273 PMID: 31546724

Speich, M., Pineau, A., & Ballereau, F. (2001). Minerals, trace elements and related biological variables in athletes and during physical activity. *Clinica Chimica Acta*, *312*(1–2), 1–11. DOI: 10.1016/S0009-8981(01)00598-8 PMID: 11580904

Stefanidou, M., Maravelias, C., Dona, A., & Spiliopoulou, C. (2006). Zinc: A multipurpose trace element. *Archives of Toxicology*, *80*(1), 1–9. DOI: 10.1007/s00204-005-0009-5 PMID: 16187101

Sturniolo, G. C., Leo, V. D., Barollo, M., Fries, W., Mazzon, E., & Ferronato, A. (2000). The many functions of zinc in inflammatory conditions of the gastrointestinal tract. *The Journal of Trace Elements in Experimental Medicine*, *13*(1), 33–39. DOI: 10.1002/(SICI)1520-670X(2000)13:1<33::AID-JTRA5>3.0.CO;2-K

Sun, R., Wang, J., Feng, J., & Cao, B. (2022). Zinc in cognitive impairment and aging. *Biomolecules*, *12*(7), 1000. DOI: 10.3390/biom12071000 PMID: 35883555

Swamy, B. P. M., Rahman, M. A., Inabangan-Asilo, M. A., Amparado, A., Manito, C., Chadha-Mohanty, P., Reinke, R., & Slamet-Loedin, I. H. (2016). Advances in breeding for high grain Zinc in Rice. *Rice (New York, N.Y.)*, *9*(1), 49. DOI: 10.1186/s12284-016-0122-5 PMID: 27671163

Swart, R., Sanders, D., & McLachlan, M. (2008). Nutrition: A primary health care perspective: Primary health care: Programme areas. *South African Health Review*, *2008*(1), 129–147.

Takkar, P. N. (1996). Micronutrient research and sustainable agricultural productivity in India. *Journal of the Indian Society of Soil Science*, *44*(4), 562–581.

Tran, C. D., Katsikeros, R., Manton, N., Krebs, N. F., Hambidge, K. M., Butler, R. N., & Davidson, G. P. (2011). Zinc homeostasis and gut function in children with celiac disease. *The American Journal of Clinical Nutrition*, *94*(4), 1026–1032. DOI: 10.3945/ajcn.111.018093 PMID: 21865333

Urbano, M. R., Vitalle, M. S., Juliano, Y., & Amancio, O. M. (2002). Iron, copper and zinc in adolescents during pubertal growth spurt. *Jornal de Pediatria*, *78*(4), 327–334. DOI: 10.2223/JPED.868 PMID: 14647765

Van Der Straeten, D., Fitzpatrick, T. B., & De Steur, H. (2017). Editorial overview: Biofortification of crops: achievements, future challenges, socio-economic, health and ethical aspects. *Current Opinion in Biotechnology*, *44*, VII–X. DOI: 10.1016/j.copbio.2017.03.007 PMID: 28342725

Venugopal, V., & Gopakumar, K. (2017). Shellfish: Nutritive Value, Health Benefits, and Consumer Safety. *Comprehensive Reviews in Food Science and Food Safety*, *16*(6), 1219–1242. DOI: 10.1111/1541-4337.12312 PMID: 33371588

Ver Ploeg, M., Breneman, V., Farrigan, T., Hamrick, K., Hopkins, D., Kaufman, P., Lin, B.-H., Nord, M., Smith, T. A., & Williams, R. (2009). *Access to affordable and nutritious food: Measuring and understanding food deserts and their consequences: report to congress*. https://ageconsearch.umn.edu/record/292130/

Vicente, A. R., Manganaris, G. A., Darre, M., Ortiz, C. M., Sozzi, G. O., & Crisosto, C. H. (2022). Compositional determinants of fruit and vegetable quality and nutritional value. In *Postharvest handling* (pp. 565–619). Elsevier., https://www.sciencedirect.com/science/article/pii/B9780128228456000191 DOI: 10.1016/B978-0-12-822845-6.00019-1

Videira, C. P. F. (2020). *Effectiveness of nutrition and WASH/malaria educational community-based interventions in reducing anemia, malnutrition and micronutrients deficiencies in preschool children from Bengo, Angola*. https://repositorio-aberto.up.pt/bitstream/10216/129251/2/419837.pdf

Walker, C. F., & Black, R. E. (2004). Zinc and the risk for infectious disease. *Annual Review of Nutrition*, *24*(1), 255–275. DOI: 10.1146/annurev.nutr.23.011702.073054 PMID: 15189121

Wang, X., Wu, W., Zheng, W., Fang, X., Chen, L., Rink, L., Min, J., & Wang, F. (2019). Zinc supplementation improves glycemic control for diabetes prevention and management: A systematic review and meta-analysis of randomized controlled trials. *The American Journal of Clinical Nutrition*, *110*(1), 76–90. DOI: 10.1093/ajcn/nqz041 PMID: 31161192

Wapnir, R. A. (2000). Zinc deficiency, malnutrition and the gastrointestinal tract. *The Journal of Nutrition, 130*(5), 1388S–1392S. DOI: 10.1093/jn/130.5.1388S PMID: 10801949

Weaver, C. M., & Kannan, S. (2001). Phytate and mineral bioavailability. In *Food phytates* (pp. 227–240). CRC Press., https://www.taylorfrancis.com/chapters/edit/10.1201/9781420014419-15/phytate-mineral-bioavailability-connie-weaver-srimathi-kannan

Welch, R. M., & Graham, R. D. (2004). Breeding for micronutrients in staple food crops from a human nutrition perspective. *Journal of Experimental Botany, 55*(396), 353–364. DOI: 10.1093/jxb/erh064 PMID: 14739261

Williams, P. (2007). Nutritional composition of red meat. *Nutrition & Dietetics: the Journal of the Dietitians Association of Australia, 64*(s4), S113–S119. DOI: 10.1111/j.1747-0080.2007.00197.x

World Health Organization. (2007). Community-based management of severe acute malnutrition: A joint statement by the World Health Organization, the World Food Programme, the United Nations System Standing Committee on Nutrition and the United Nations Children's Fund

Yadava, D. K., Hossain, F., & Mohapatra, T. (2018). Nutritional security through crop biofortification in India: Status & future prospects. *The Indian Journal of Medical Research, 148*(5), 621–631. DOI: 10.4103/ijmr.IJMR_1893_18 PMID: 30666987

Yasuda, H., & Tsutsui, T. (2016). Infants and elderlies are susceptible to zinc deficiency. *Scientific Reports, 6*(1), 21850. DOI: 10.1038/srep21850 PMID: 26912464

Żwierełło, W., Styburski, D., Maruszewska, A., Piorun, K., Skórka-Majewicz, M., Czerwińska, M., Maciejewska, D., Baranowska-Bosiacka, I., Krajewski, A., & Gutowska, I. (2020). Bioelements in the treatment of burn injuries–The complex review of metabolism and supplementation (copper, selenium, zinc, iron, manganese, chromium and magnesium). *Journal of Trace Elements in Medicine and Biology, 62*, 126616. DOI: 10.1016/j.jtemb.2020.126616 PMID: 32739827

Compilation of References

Abdel Fattah, N. S., Atef, M. M., & Al-Qaradaghi, S. M. (2016). Evaluation of serum zinc level in patients with newly diagnosed and resistant alopecia areata. *International Journal of Dermatology*, *55*(1), 24–29. DOI: 10.1111/ijd.12769 PMID: 26147750

Abdollahi, M., Ajami, M., Abdollahi, Z., Kalantari, N., Houshiarrad, A., Fozouni, F., Fallahrokni, A., & Mazandarani, F. S. (2019). Zinc supplementation is an effective and feasible strategy to prevent growth retardation in 6 to 24 month children: A pragmatic double blind, randomized trial. *Heliyon*, *5*(11), e02581. DOI: 10.1016/j.heliyon.2019.e02581 PMID: 31720482

Abdu, A. O., De Groote, H., Joy, E. J. M., Kumssa, D. B., Broadley, M. R., & Gashu, D. (2022). Zinc agronomic biofortification of staple crops may be a cost-effective strategy to alleviate zinc deficiency in Ethiopia. *Frontiers in Nutrition*, *9*, 1037161. DOI: 10.3389/fnut.2022.1037161 PMID: 36438724

Abniki, M., Azizi, Z., & Panahi, H. A. (2021). Design of 3-aminophenol-grafted polymer-modified zinc sulphide nanoparticles as drug delivery system. *IET Nanobiotechnology / IET*, *15*(8), 664–673. DOI: 10.1049/nbt2.12063 PMID: 34694721

Abolurin, O. O., Oyelami, O. A., & Oseni, S. B. (2020). A comparative study of the prevalence of zinc deficiency among children with acute diarrhoea in SouthWestern Nigeria. *African Health Sciences*, *20*(1), 406–412. DOI: 10.4314/ahs.v20i1.47 PMID: 33402929

Ackerman, B. H., & Kasbekar, N. (1997). Disturbances of Taste and Smell Induced by Drugs. *Pharmacotherapy*, *17*(3), 482–496. DOI: 10.1002/j.1875-9114.1997.tb03058.x PMID: 9165552

Ackland, M. L., & Michalczyk, A. A. (2016). Zinc and infant nutrition. *Archives of Biochemistry and Biophysics*, *611*, 51–57. DOI: 10.1016/j.abb.2016.06.011 PMID: 27317042

Adams, K. P., Jarvis, M., Vosti, S. A., Manger, M. S., Tarini, A., Somé, J. W., Somda, H., & McDonald, C. M. (2023). Estimating the cost and cost-effectiveness of adding zinc to, and improving the performance of, Burkina Faso's mandatory wheat flour fortification programme. *Maternal and Child Nutrition, 19*(3), e13515. DOI: 10.1111/mcn.13515 PMID: 37021818

Agedew, E., Tsegaye, B., Bante, A., Zerihun, E., Aklilu, A., Girma, M., Kerebih, H., Wale, M. Z., & Yirsaw, M. T. (2022). Zinc deficiency and associated factors among pregnant women's attending antenatal clinics in public health facilities of Konso Zone, Southern Ethiopia. *PLoS One, 17*(7), e0270971. DOI: 10.1371/journal.pone.0270971 PMID: 35797387

Aggett, P. J., & Harries, J. T. (1979). Current status of zinc in health and disease states. *Archives of Disease in Childhood, 54*(12), 909–917. DOI: 10.1136/adc.54.12.909 PMID: 119488

Ahmad, A., & Ahmed, Z. (2019). Fortification in beverages. In *Production and management of beverages* (pp. 85–122). Elsevier., https://www.sciencedirect.com/science/article/pii/B9780128152607000031 DOI: 10.1016/B978-0-12-815260-7.00003-1

Ahmad, R., Shaju, R., Atfi, A., & Razzaque, M. S. (2024). Zinc and Diabetes: A Connection between Micronutrient and Metabolism. *Cells, 13*(16), 1359. DOI: 10.3390/cells13161359 PMID: 39195249

Ahsan, A. K., Tebha, S. S., Sangi, R., Kamran, A., Zaidi, Z. A., Haque, T., & Ali Hamza, M. S. (2021). Zinc Micronutrient Deficiency and Its Prevalence in Malnourished Pediatric Children as Compared to Well-Nourished Children: A Nutritional Emergency. *Global Pediatric Health, 8*, 2333794X2110503. DOI: 10.1177/2333794X211050316

Aiqing, Z., Zhang, L., Ning, P., Chen, Q., Wang, B., Zhang, F., Yang, X., & Zhang, Y. (2022). Zinc in cereal grains: Concentration, distribution, speciation, bioavailability, and barriers to transport from roots to grains in wheat. *Critical Reviews in Food Science and Nutrition, 62*(28), 7917–7928. DOI: 10.1080/10408398.2021.1920883 PMID: 34224281

Alcorta, A., Porta, A., Tárrega, A., Alvarez, M. D., & Vaquero, M. P. (2021). Foods for Plant-Based Diets: Challenges and Innovations. *Foods, 10*(2), 293. DOI: 10.3390/foods10020293 PMID: 33535684

Allai, F. M., Gul, K., Zahoor, I., Ganaie, T. A., Nasir, G., & Azad, Z. R. A. A. (2022). Malnutrition: Impact of Zinc on Child Development. In Khan, S. T., & Malik, A. (Eds.), *Microbial Biofertilizers and Micronutrient Availability* (pp. 83–100). Springer International Publishing., DOI: 10.1007/978-3-030-76609-2_4

Allen, L. (2006a). World Health Organization., & Food and Agriculture Organization of the United Nations. *Guidelines on food fortification with micronutrients*. World Health Organization.

Allen, L. (2006b). World Health Organization., & Food and Agriculture Organization of the United Nations. *Guidelines on food fortification with micronutrients*. World Health Organization.

Allouche-Fitoussi, D., & Breitbart, H. (2020). The role of zinc in male fertility. *International Journal of Molecular Sciences*, *21*(20), 7796. DOI: 10.3390/ijms21207796 PMID: 33096823

Almendros, P., González, D., Fernández, M. D., García-Gomez, C., & Obrador, A. (2022). Both Zn biofortification and nutrient distribution pattern in cherry tomato plants are influenced by the application of ZnO nanofertilizer. *Heliyon*, *8*(3), e09130. Advance online publication. DOI: 10.1016/j.heliyon.2022.e09130 PMID: 35846478

Almohanna, H. M., Ahmed, A. A., Tsatalis, J. P., & Tosti, A. (2019). The Role of Vitamins and Minerals in Hair Loss: A Review. *Dermatology and Therapy*, *9*(1), 51–70. DOI: 10.1007/s13555-018-0278-6 PMID: 30547302

Alshaikh, B., Abo Zeed, M., Yusuf, K., Guin, M., & Fenton, T. (2022). Effect of enteral zinc supplementation on growth and neurodevelopment of preterm infants: A systematic review and meta-analysis. *Journal of Perinatology*, *42*(4), 430–439. DOI: 10.1038/s41372-021-01094-7 PMID: 34006967

Álvarez-Barrios, A., Álvarez, L., García, M., Artime, E., Pereiro, R., & González-Iglesias, H. (2021). Antioxidant defenses in the human eye: A focus on metallothioneins. *Antioxidants*, *10*(1), 89. DOI: 10.3390/antiox10010089 PMID: 33440661

Amin, N., Clark, C. C. T., Taghizadeh, M., & Djafarnejad, S. (2020). Zinc supplements and bone health: The role of the RANKL-RANK axis as a therapeutic target. *Journal of Trace Elements in Medicine and Biology*, *57*, 126417. DOI: 10.1016/j.jtemb.2019.126417 PMID: 31653549

Amoadu, M., Abraham, S. A., Adams, A. K., Akoto-Buabeng, W., Obeng, P., & Hagan, J. E.Jr. (2024). Risk Factors of Malnutrition among In-School Children and Adolescents in Developing Countries: A Scoping Review. *Children (Basel, Switzerland)*, *11*(4), 476. DOI: 10.3390/children11040476 PMID: 38671693

Arafsha, S. M., Aslam, M. F., Ellis, P. R., Latunde-Dada, G. O., & Sharp, P. A. (2023). Strategies to increase the bio-accessibility and bio-availability of iron and zinc from cereal products. *Proceedings of the Nutrition Society,* 1-7. DOI: 10.1017/S0029665123003543

Arndt, M. B., Abate, Y. H., Abbasi-Kangevari, M., Abd ElHafeez, S., Abdelmasseh, M., Abd-Elsalam, S., Abdulah, D. M., Abdulkader, R. S., Abidi, H., Abiodun, O., Aboagye, R. G., Abolhassani, H., Abtew, Y. D., Abu-Gharbieh, E., Abu-Rmeileh, N. M., Acuna, J. M., Adamu, K., Adane, D. E., Addo, I. Y., & Reiner, R. C.Jr. (2024). Global, regional, and national progress towards the 2030 global nutrition targets and forecasts to 2050: A systematic analysis for the Global Burden of Disease Study 2021. *Lancet*, *404*(10471), 2543–2583. DOI: 10.1016/S0140-6736(24)01821-X PMID: 39667386

Askari, S., Asghari, G., Farhadnejad, H., Ghanbarian, A., Mirmiran, P., & Azizi, F. (2019). Seasonal variations of serum zinc concentration in adult population: Tehran lipid and glucose study. *Iranian Journal of Public Health*, *48*(8), 1496. PMID: 32292733

Avnee, S., Sood, S., Chaudhary, D. R., Jhorar, P., & Rana, R. S. (2023). Biofortification: An approach to eradicate micronutrient deficiency. *Frontiers in Nutrition*, *10*, 1233070. DOI: 10.3389/fnut.2023.1233070 PMID: 37789898

Aydemir, T. B., Liuzzi, J. P., McClellan, S., & Cousins, R. J. (2009). Zinc transporter ZIP8 (SLC39A8) and zinc influence IFN-γ expression in activated human T cells. *Journal of Leukocyte Biology*, *86*(2), 337–348. DOI: 10.1189/jlb.1208759 PMID: 19401385

Aziz, J., Rahman, M. T., & Vaithilingam, R. D. (2021). Dysregulation of metallothionein and zinc aggravates periodontal diseases. *Journal of Trace Elements in Medicine and Biology*, *66*, 126754. DOI: 10.1016/j.jtemb.2021.126754 PMID: 33831799

Baarz, B. R., & Rink, L. (2022). Rebalancing the unbalanced aged immune system–A special focus on zinc. *Ageing Research Reviews*, *74*, 101541. DOI: 10.1016/j.arr.2021.101541 PMID: 34915196

Bailey, R. L., West, K. P.Jr, & Black, R. E. (2015). The epidemiology of global micronutrient deficiencies. *Annals of Nutrition & Metabolism*, *66*(Suppl. 2), 22–33. DOI: 10.1159/000371618 PMID: 26045325

Bajait, C., & Thawani, V. (2011). Role of zinc in pediatric diarrhea. *Indian Journal of Pharmacology*, *43*(3), 232–235. DOI: 10.4103/0253-7613.81495 PMID: 21713083

Bakaloudi, D. R., Halloran, A., Rippin, H. L., Oikonomidou, A. C., Dardavesis, T. I., Williams, J., Wickramasinghe, K., Breda, J., & Chourdakis, M. (2021). Intake and adequacy of the vegan diet. A systematic review of the evidence. *Clinical Nutrition (Edinburgh, Lothian)*, *40*(5), 3503–3521. DOI: 10.1016/j.clnu.2020.11.035 PMID: 33341313

Baltaci, A. K., Mogulkoc, R., & Baltaci, S. B. (2019). Review: The role of zinc in the endocrine system. *Pakistan Journal of Pharmaceutical Sciences*, *32*(1), 231–239. PMID: 30772815

Baltaci, A. K., Mogulkoc, R., & Baltaci, S. B. (2019). The role of zinc in the endocrine system. *Pakistan Journal of Pharmaceutical Sciences*, *32*(1). https://www.researchgate.net/profile/Saltuk-Baltaci/publication/331438506_Review_The_role_of_zinc_in_the_endocrine_system/links/5e1ffc32458515ba208a861e/Review-The-role-of-zinc-in-the-endocrine-system.pdf PMID: 30772815

Barffour, M. A., Hinnouho, G.-M., Wessells, K. R., Kounnavong, S., Ratsavong, K., Sitthideth, D., Bounheuang, B., Sengnam, K., Chanhthavong, B., Arnold, C. D., Brown, K. H., Larson, C. P., & Hess, S. Y. (2020). Effects of therapeutic zinc supplementation for diarrhea and two preventive zinc supplementation regimens on the incidence and duration of diarrhea and acute respiratory tract infections in rural Laotian children: A randomized controlled trial. *Journal of Global Health*, *10*(1), 010424. DOI: 10.7189/jogh.10.010424 PMID: 32612816

Barman, A., Bera, A., Saha, P., Tiwari, H., Dey, S., Kumar, S., Patel, S., & Meena, D. K. (2023). Agronomic Zn Biofortification of Cereal Crops a Sustainable Way to Ensuring Nutritional Security: A Review. *International Journal of Environment and Climate Change*, *13*(3), 151–168. DOI: 10.9734/ijecc/2023/v13i31693

Barman, S., & Srinivasan, K. (2022). Diabetes and zinc dyshomeostasis: Can zinc supplementation mitigate diabetic complications? *Critical Reviews in Food Science and Nutrition*, *62*(4), 1046–1061. DOI: 10.1080/10408398.2020.1833178 PMID: 33938330

Barrie, S. A., Wright, J. V., Pizzorno, J. E., Kutter, E., & Barron, P. C. (1987). Comparative absorption of zinc picolinate, zinc citrate and zinc gluconate in humans. *Agents and Actions*, *21*(1-2), 223–228. DOI: 10.1007/BF01974946 PMID: 3630857

Bartlett, H., & Eperjesi, F. (2003). Age-related macular degeneration and nutritional supplementation: A review of randomised controlled trials. *Ophthalmic & Physiological Optics*, *23*(5), 383–399. DOI: 10.1046/j.1475-1313.2003.00130.x PMID: 12950886

Bashir, A., Khan, Q. U., Alem, A., Hendi, A. A., Zaman, U., Khan, S. U., Rehman, K., Khan, A. A., Ullah, I., Anwar, Y., & Abdelrahman, E. A. (2023). Zinc and potassium fertilizer synergizes plant nutrient availability and affects growth, yield, and quality of wheat genotypes. *Plants*, *12*(12), 2241. DOI: 10.3390/plants12122241 PMID: 37375867

Beal, T., White, J. M., Arsenault, J. E., Okronipa, H., Hinnouho, G.-M., Murira, Z., Torlesse, H., & Garg, A. (2021). Micronutrient gaps during the complementary feeding period in South Asia: A Comprehensive Nutrient Gap Assessment. *Nutrition Reviews, 79*(Supplement_1), 26–34. DOI: 10.1093/nutrit/nuaa144 PMID: 33693912

Beer, K., Singh, A., Ravi, S. C., Gupta, A. K., Kumar, A., & Sharma, M. M.Division of Postharvest Management. (2024). A comprehensive review on the role of Vitamin A on human health and nutrition. *Journal of Environmental Biology, 45*(6), 645–653. DOI: 10.22438/jeb/45/6/MRN-5339

Belay, A., Gashu, D., Joy, E. J. M., Lark, R. M., Chagumaira, C., Likoswe, B. H., Zerfu, D., Ander, E. L., Young, S. D., Bailey, E. H., & Broadley, M. R. (2021). Zinc deficiency is highly prevalent and spatially dependent over short distances in Ethiopia. *Scientific Reports, 11*(1), 6510. DOI: 10.1038/s41598-021-85977-x PMID: 33753836

Bel-Serrat, S., Stammers, A.-L., Warthon-Medina, M., Moran, V. H., Iglesia-Altaba, I., Hermoso, M., Moreno, L. A., & Lowe, N. M. (2014). Factors that affect zinc bioavailability and losses in adult and elderly populations. *Nutrition Reviews, 72*(5), 334–352. DOI: 10.1111/nure.12105 PMID: 24739133

Berendsen, A. A. M., Kramer, C. S., & de Groot, L. C. P. G. M. (2019). The Newly Developed Elderly Nutrient-Rich Food Score Is a Useful Tool to Assess Nutrient Density in European Older Adults. *Frontiers in Nutrition, 6*(August), 1–14. DOI: 10.3389/fnut.2019.00119 PMID: 31457017

Berg, J. M., & Shi, Y. (1996). The Galvanization of Biology: A Growing Appreciation for the Roles of Zinc. *Science, 271*(5252), 1081–1085. DOI: 10.1126/science.271.5252.1081 PMID: 8599083

Berhe, K., Gebrearegay, F., & Gebremariam, H. (2019). Prevalence and associated factors of zinc deficiency among pregnant women and children in Ethiopia: A systematic review and meta-analysis. *BMC Public Health, 19*(1), 1–11. DOI: 10.1186/s12889-019-7979-3 PMID: 31829213

Berti, C., & Socha, P. (2023). Infant and Young Child Feeding Practices and Health. *Nutrients, 15*(5), 1184. DOI: 10.3390/nu15051184 PMID: 36904182

Bhantana, P., Moussa, M. G., Malla, R., Khadka, D., Vista, S. P., Shrestha, R. K., & Hu, C. X. (2022). Foliar versus soil biofortification of Zn in citrus (citrus reticulata Blanco) effect on mineral nutrition and fruit yield and quality. *Biomedical Journal of Scientific & Technical Research, 41*(3), 32755–32568. DOI: 10.26717/BJSTR.2022.41.006612

Bhatnagar, P., & Suman, M. (2020). *A review on role of zinc deficiency in humans and its rectification through Horti-agro food supplements*. 447–451.

Bhatnagar, S., & Taneja, S. (2001). Zinc and cognitive development. *British Journal of Nutrition, 85*(S2), S139–S145. DOI: 10.1079/BJN2000306 PMID: 11509102

Bhat, Y. J., Manzoor, S., Khan, A. R., & Qayoom, S. (2009). Trace element levels in alopecia areata. *Indian Journal of Dermatology, Venereology and Leprology, 75*(1), 29–31. DOI: 10.4103/0378-6323.45216 PMID: 19172027

Bhowmik, D., Chiranjib, K., & Kumar, S. (2010). A potential medicinal importance of zinc in human health and chronic. *Int J Pharm, 1*(1), 05–11.

Bhutta, Z. A., Salam, R. A., & Das, J. K. (2013). Meeting the challenges of micronutrient malnutrition in the developing world. In *British Medical Bulletin* (Vol. 106, Issue 1, pp. 7–17). DOI: 10.1093/bmb/ldt015

Bhutta, Z. A., Black, R. E., Brown, K. H., Gardner, J. M., Gore, S., Hidayat, A., Khatun, F., Martorell, R., Ninh, N. X., Penny, M. E., Rosado, J. L., Roy, S. K., Ruel, M., Sazawal, S., & Shankar, A. (1999). Prevention of diarrhea and pneumonia by zinc supplementation in children in developing countries: Pooled analysis of randomized controlled trials. *The Journal of Pediatrics, 135*(6), 689–697. DOI: 10.1016/S0022-3476(99)70086-7 PMID: 10586170

Bilandžić, N., Sedak, M., Đokić, M., Varenina, I., Solomun Kolanović, B., Božić, Đ., Brstilo, M., & Šimić, B. (2014). Determination of zinc concentrations in foods of animal origin, fish and shellfish from Croatia and assessment of their contribution to dietary intake. *Journal of Food Composition and Analysis, 35*(2), 61–66. DOI: 10.1016/j.jfca.2014.04.006

Birhanie, M. W., Adekunle, A. O., Arowojolu, A. O., Dugul, T. T., & Mebiratie, A. L. (2020). Micronutrients Deficiency and Their Associations with Pregnancy Outcomes: A Review. *Nutrition and Dietary Supplements, 12*(Supplements), 237–254. DOI: 10.2147/NDS.S274646

Black, M. M. (1998). Zinc deficiency and child development. *The American Journal of Clinical Nutrition, 68*(2), 464S–469S. DOI: 10.1093/ajcn/68.2.464S PMID: 9701161

Blair, M. W. (2013). Mineral biofortification strategies for food staples: The example of common bean. *Journal of Agricultural and Food Chemistry, 61*(35), 8287–8294. DOI: 10.1021/jf400774y PMID: 23848266

Blanco-Rojo, R., & Vaquero, M. P. (2019). Iron bioavailability from food fortification to precision nutrition. A review. *Innovative Food Science & Emerging Technologies*, *51*, 126–138. DOI: 10.1016/j.ifset.2018.04.015

Blasiak, J., Pawlowska, E., Chojnacki, J., Szczepanska, J., Chojnacki, C., & Kaarniranta, K. (2020). Zinc and Autophagy in Age-Related Macular Degeneration. *International Journal of Molecular Sciences*, *21*(14), 4994. DOI: 10.3390/ijms21144994 PMID: 32679798

Bloom, A., Bloom, S., Silva, H., Nicoll, A. J., & Sawhney, R. (2021). Zinc supplementation and its benefits in the management of chronic liver disease: An in-depth literature review. *Annals of Hepatology*, *25*, 100549. DOI: 10.1016/j.aohep.2021.100549 PMID: 34614431

Borowska, S., Brzoska, M. M., & Tomczyk, M. (2018). Complexation of bioelements and toxic metals by polyphenolic compounds–Implications for health. *Current Drug Targets*, *19*(14), 1612–1638. DOI: 10.2174/1389450119666180403101555 PMID: 29611487

Bouis, H. E. (n.d.). *S32*. www.harvestplus.org

Bouranis, D. L., & Chorianopoulou, S. N. (2023). Foliar Application of Sulfur-Containing Compounds—Pros and Cons. *Plants*, *12*(22), 3794. DOI: 10.3390/plants12223794 PMID: 38005690

Brion, L. P., Heyne, R., Steven Brown, L., Lair, C. S., Edwards, A., Burchfield, P. J., & Caraig, M. (2020). Zinc deficiency limiting head growth to discharge in extremely low gestational age infants with insufficient linear growth: A cohort study. *Journal of Perinatology*, *40*(11), 1694–1704. DOI: 10.1038/s41372-020-00778-w PMID: 32788617

Brouwer, I. D., Van Liere, M. J., De Brauw, A., Dominguez-Salas, P., Herforth, A., Kennedy, G., Lachat, C., Omosa, E. B., Talsma, E. F., Vandevijvere, S., Fanzo, J., & Ruel, M. (2021). Reverse thinking: Taking a healthy diet perspective towards food systems transformations. *Food Security*, *13*(6), 1497–1523. DOI: 10.1007/s12571-021-01204-5

Brown, K. H., Peerson, J. M., & Allen, L. H. (1998). Effect of zinc supplementation on children's growth: A meta-analysis of intervention trials. *Bibliotheca Nutritio et Dieta*, *54*, 76–83. PMID: 9597173

Brown, K. H., Peerson, J. M., Rivera, J., & Allen, L. H. (2002). Effect of supplemental zinc on the growth and serum zinc concentrations of prepubertal children: A meta-analysis of randomized controlled trials. *The American Journal of Clinical Nutrition, 75*(6), 1062–1071. DOI: 10.1093/ajcn/75.6.1062 PMID: 12036814

Brown, K. H., Rivera, J. A., Bhutta, Z., Gibson, R. S., King, J. C., Lönnerdal, B., Ruel, M. T., Sandtröm, B., Wasantwisut, E., & Hotz, C. (2004). International Zinc Nutrition Consultative Group (IZiNCG) technical document #1. Assessment of the risk of zinc deficiency in populations and options for its control. *Food and Nutrition Bulletin, 25*(1, Suppl 2), S99–S203.

Bruins, M. J., Bird, J. K., Aebischer, C. P., & Eggersdorfer, M. (2018). Considerations for secondary prevention of nutritional deficiencies in high-risk groups in high-income countries. *Nutrients, 10*(1), 47. DOI: 10.3390/nu10010047 PMID: 29304025

Butte, N. F., Lopez-Alarcon, M. G., & Garza, C. (2002). *Nutrient adequacy of exclusive breastfeeding for the term infant during the first six months of life*. World Health Organization. https://apps.who.int/iris/bitstream/handle/10665/42519/9241562110.pdf

Cakmak, I. (2008). Enrichment of cereal grains with zinc: Agronomic or genetic biofortification? *Plant and Soil, 302*(1-2), 1–17. DOI: 10.1007/s11104-007-9466-3

Cakmak, I., McLaughlin, M. J., & White, P. (2017). Zinc for better crop production and human health. *Plant and Soil, 411*(1–2), 1–4. DOI: 10.1007/s11104-016-3166-9

Calder, P. C., & Jackson, A. A. (2000). Undernutrition, infection and immune function. *Nutrition Research Reviews, 13*(1), 3–29. DOI: 10.1079/095442200108728981 PMID: 19087431

Carazo, A., Macáková, K., Matoušová, K., Krčmová, L. K., Protti, M., & Mladěnka, P. (2021). Vitamin A update: Forms, sources, kinetics, detection, function, deficiency, therapeutic use and toxicity. *Nutrients, 13*(5), 1703. DOI: 10.3390/nu13051703 PMID: 34069881

Carducci, B., Keats, E. C., & Bhutta, Z. A. (2021). Zinc supplementation for improving pregnancy and infant outcome. *Cochrane Database of Systematic Reviews*, 3. PMID: 33724446

Caulfield, L. E., & Black, R. E. (2004). Zinc deficiency. *Comparative Quantification of Health Risks: Global and Regional Burden of Disease Attributable to Selected Major Risk Factors, 1*, 257–280. PMID: 15100497

Cavan, K. R., Gibson, R. S., Grazioso, C. F., Isalgue, A. M., Ruz, M., & Solomons, N. W. (1993). Growth and body composition of periurban Guatemalan children in relation to zinc status: A longitudinal zinc intervention trial. *The American Journal of Clinical Nutrition, 57*(3), 344–352. DOI: 10.1093/ajcn/57.3.344 PMID: 8438768

Chao, H. C., Chang, Y. J., & Huang, W. L. (2018). Cut-off serum zinc concentration affecting the appetite, growth, and nutrition status of undernourished children supplemented with zinc. *Nutrition in Clinical Practice, 33*(5), 701–710. DOI: 10.1002/ncp.10079 PMID: 29603391

Chao, H.-C. (2023). Zinc Deficiency and Therapeutic Value of Zinc Supplementation in Pediatric Gastrointestinal Diseases. *Nutrients, 15*(19), 4093. DOI: 10.3390/nu15194093 PMID: 37836377

Chardigny, J.-M., & Walrand, S. (2016). Plant protein for food: Opportunities and bottlenecks. *OCL Oilseeds and Fats Crops and Lipids, 23*(4), 6-p.

Chasapis, C. T., Ntoupa, P.-S. A., Spiliopoulou, C. A., & Stefanidou, M. E. (2020). Recent aspects of the effects of zinc on human health. *Archives of Toxicology, 94*(5), 1443–1460. DOI: 10.1007/s00204-020-02702-9 PMID: 32394086

Chaudhary, V., Saraswathy, K. N., & Sarwal, R. (2022). Dietary diversity as a sustainable approach towards micronutrient deficiencies in India. *The Indian Journal of Medical Research, 156*(1), 31–45. DOI: 10.4103/ijmr.ijmr_3314_21 PMID: 36510896

Chekol Abebe, E., Asmamaw Dejenie, T., Mengie Ayele, T., Dagnew Baye, N., Agegnehu Teshome, A., & Tilahun Muche, Z. (2021). The role of regulatory B cells in health and diseases: A systemic review. *Journal of Inflammation Research, 14*, 75–84. DOI: 10.2147/JIR.S286426 PMID: 33469337

Chen, B., Yu, P., Chan, W. N., Xie, F., Zhang, Y., Liang, L., Leung, K. T., Lo, K. W., Yu, J., Tse, G. M. K., Kang, W., & To, K. F. (2024). Cellular zinc metabolism and zinc signaling: From biological functions to diseases and therapeutic targets. *Signal Transduction and Targeted Therapy, 9*(1), 6. DOI: 10.1038/s41392-023-01679-y PMID: 38169461

Chen, J. C., Chuang, C. H., Wang, J. D., & Wang, C. W. (2015). Combination therapy using chelating agent and zinc for Wilson's disease. *Journal of Medical and Biological Engineering, 35*(6), 697–708. DOI: 10.1007/s40846-015-0087-7 PMID: 26692828

Chen, X., He, C., Zhang, K., Wang, J., Ding, X., Zeng, Q., Peng, H., Bai, J., Lv, L., Xuan, Y., & Bai, S. (2022). Comparison of zinc bioavailability in zinc-glycine and zinc-methionine chelates for broilers fed with a corn-soybean meal diet. *Frontiers in Physiology*, *13*, 983954. DOI: 10.3389/fphys.2022.983954 PMID: 36467690

Chen, Y., Cai, J., Liu, D., Liu, S., Lei, D., Zheng, L., Wei, Q., & Gao, M. (2022). Zinc-based metal organic framework with antibacterial and anti-inflammatory properties for promoting wound healing. *Regenerative Biomaterials*, *9*, rbac019. DOI: 10.1093/rb/rbac019 PMID: 35493287

Chinnasamy, E., Arulmani, S., Deepa, K., Kumar, D. S., Madhavan, J., & Senthil, S. (2019). Growth, Spectral, Optical, Studies of A Zinc Picolinate Dihydrate NLO Single Crystal. *Materials Today: Proceedings*, *8*, 264–270. DOI: 10.1016/j.matpr.2019.02.110

Chinni, V., El-Khoury, J., Perera, M., Bellomo, R., Jones, D., Bolton, D., Ischia, J., & Patel, O. (2021). Zinc supplementation as an adjunct therapy for COVID-19: Challenges and opportunities. *British Journal of Clinical Pharmacology*, *87*(10), 3737–3746. DOI: 10.1111/bcp.14826 PMID: 33742473

Chitekwe, S., Parajuli, K. R., Paudyal, N., Haag, K. C., Renzaho, A., Issaka, A., & Agho, K. (2022). Individual, household and national factors associated with iron, vitamin A and zinc deficiencies among children aged 6–59 months in Nepal. *Maternal and Child Nutrition*, *18*(S1), 1–11. DOI: 10.1111/mcn.13305 PMID: 34897980

Choi, S., Liu, X., & Pan, Z. (2018). Zinc deficiency and cellular oxidative stress: Prognostic implications in cardiovascular diseases. *Acta Pharmacologica Sinica*, *39*(7), 1120–1132. DOI: 10.1038/aps.2018.25 PMID: 29926844

Ciampo, L. A. D., & Ciampo, I. R. L. D. (2024). Zinc: A Critical Micronutrient for Children's Health. *Archives of Current Research International*, *24*(10), 251–256. DOI: 10.9734/acri/2024/v24i10928

Classen, H.-G., Gröber, U., Löw, D., Schmidt, J., & Stracke, H. (2011). Zinc deficiency. Symptoms, causes, diagnosis and therapy. *Medizinische Monatsschrift fur Pharmazeuten*, *34*(3), 87–95. PMID: 21736013

Coleman, J. E. (1992). Zinc proteins: Enzymes, storage proteins, transcription factors, and replication proteins. *Annual Review of Biochemistry*, *61*(1), 897–946. DOI: 10.1146/annurev.bi.61.070192.004341 PMID: 1497326

Colvin, R. A., Lai, B., Holmes, W. R., & Lee, D. (2015). Understanding metal homeostasis in primary cultured neurons. Studies using single neuron subcellular and quantitative metallomics. *Metallomics*, *7*(7), 1111–1123. DOI: 10.1039/c5mt00084j PMID: 25894020

Conti, P. R. O. N. C. O. N. I., Ronconi, G., Caraffa, A. L., Gallenga, C. E., Ross, R., Frydas, I., & Kritas, S. K. (2020). Induction of pro-inflammatory cytokines (IL-1 and IL-6) and lung inflammation by Coronavirus-19 (COVI-19 or SARS-CoV-2): Anti-inflammatory strategies. *Journal of Biological Regulators and Homeostatic Agents*, *34*(2), 327–331.

Cope, E. C., Morris, D. R., Scrimgeour, A. G., & Levenson, C. W. (2012). Use of zinc as a treatment for traumatic brain injury in the rat: Effects on cognitive and behavioral outcomes. *Neurorehabilitation and Neural Repair*, *26*(7), 907–913. DOI: 10.1177/1545968311435337 PMID: 22331212

Corbo, M. D., & Lam, J. (2013). Zinc deficiency and its management in the pediatric population: A literature review and proposed etiologic classification. *Journal of the American Academy of Dermatology*, *69*(4), 616–624. DOI: 10.1016/j.jaad.2013.04.028 PMID: 23688650

Costa, M. I., Sarmento-Ribeiro, A. B., & Gonçalves, A. C. (2023). Zinc: From Biological Functions to Therapeutic Potential. *International Journal of Molecular Sciences*, *24*(5), 4822. DOI: 10.3390/ijms24054822 PMID: 36902254

Cousins, R. J. (1985). *Absorption, Transport, and Hepatic Metabolism of Copper and Zinc: Special Reference to Metallothionein and Ceruloplasmin*. www.physiology.org/journal/physrev

Cousins, R. J. (2010). Gastrointestinal Factors Influencing Zinc Absorption and Homeostasis. *International Journal for Vitamin and Nutrition Research*, *80*(45), 243–248. DOI: 10.1024/0300-9831/a000030 PMID: 21462106

Craig, W. J., Mangels, A. R., Fresán, U., Marsh, K., Miles, F. L., Saunders, A. V., Haddad, E. H., Heskey, C. E., Johnston, P., Larson-Meyer, E., & Orlich, M. (2021). The safe and effective use of plant-based diets with guidelines for health professionals. *Nutrients*, *13*(11), 4144. DOI: 10.3390/nu13114144 PMID: 34836399

Cummings, J. E., & Kovacic, J. P. (2009). The ubiquitous role of zinc in health and disease. *Journal of Veterinary Emergency and Critical Care (San Antonio, Tex.)*, *19*(3), 215–240. DOI: 10.1111/j.1476-4431.2009.00418.x PMID: 19691507

Cunha, T. A., Vermeulen-Serpa, K. M., Grilo, E. C., Leite-Lais, L., Brandão-Neto, J., & Vale, S. H. (2022). Association between zinc and body composition: An integrative review. *Journal of Trace Elements in Medicine and Biology*, *71*, 126940. DOI: 10.1016/j.jtemb.2022.126940 PMID: 35121408

Damianaki, K., Lourenco, J. M., Braconnier, P., Ghobril, J.-P., Devuyst, O., Burnier, M., Lenglet, S., Augsburger, M., Thomas, A., & Pruijm, M. (2020). Renal handling of zinc in chronic kidney disease patients and the role of circulating zinc levels in renal function decline. *Nephrology, Dialysis, Transplantation*, *35*(7), 1163–1170. DOI: 10.1093/ndt/gfz065 PMID: 31006015

Dardenne, M. (2002). Zinc and immune function. *European Journal of Clinical Nutrition*, *56*(3), S20–S23. DOI: 10.1038/sj.ejcn.1601479 PMID: 12142956

Darnton-Hill, I., & Nalubola, R. (2002). Fortification strategies to meet micronutrient needs: Sucesses and failures. *The Proceedings of the Nutrition Society*, *61*(2), 231–241. DOI: 10.1079/PNS2002150 PMID: 12133205

Das, J. K., Achakzai, A. B. K., & Bhutta, Z. A. (2016). Stop stunting: Pakistan perspective on how this could be realized. *Maternal and Child Nutrition*, *12*(S1, Suppl 1), 253–256. DOI: 10.1111/mcn.12285 PMID: 27187923

Das, J. K., Kumar, R., Salam, R. A., & Bhutta, Z. A. (2013). Systematic review of zinc fortification trials. *Annals of Nutrition & Metabolism*, *62*(Suppl. 1), 44–56. DOI: 10.1159/000348262 PMID: 23689112

Das, J. K., Salam, R. A., Kumar, R., & Bhutta, Z. A. (2013). Micronutrient fortification of food and its impact on woman and child health: A systematic review. *Systematic Reviews*, *2*(1), 1–24. DOI: 10.1186/2046-4053-2-67 PMID: 23971426

De La Cruz-Góngora, V., Palazuelos-González, R., & Domínguez-Flores, O. (2024). Micronutrient Deficiencies in Older Adults in Latin America: A Narrative Review. *Food and Nutrition Bulletin*, *45*(2, suppl), S26–S38. DOI: 10.1177/03795721231214587 PMID: 38146136

De, L. C. (2020). Edible seeds and nuts in human diet for immunity development. *International Journal of Recent Scientific Research*, *6*(11), 38877–38881.

Dembedza, M. P., Chopera, P., & Matsungo, T. M. (2024). Risk of zinc deficiency among children aged 0–59 months in sub-Saharan Africa: A narrative review. *The South African Journal of Clinical Nutrition : SAJCN : the Official Journal of the South African Society of Parenteral and Enteral Nutrition and the Association for Dietetics in South Africa*, *37*(2), 69–76. DOI: 10.1080/16070658.2023.2275932

Deshpande, J., Joshi, M., & Giri, P. (2013). Zinc: The trace element of major importance in human nutrition and health. *International Journal of Medical Science and Public Health, 2*(1), 1. DOI: 10.5455/ijmsph.2013.2.1-6

Detzel, P., & Klassen-Wigger, P. (2020). Market-driven food fortification to address dietary needs. *World Review of Nutrition and Dietetics, 121*, 81–88. DOI: 10.1159/000507522 PMID: 33502376

Dhaliwal, S., Nguyen, M., Vaughn, A. R., Notay, M., Chambers, C. J., & Sivamani, R. K. (2020). Effects of Zinc Supplementation on Inflammatory Skin Diseases: A Systematic Review of the Clinical Evidence. *American Journal of Clinical Dermatology, 21*(1), 21–39. DOI: 10.1007/s40257-019-00484-0 PMID: 31745908

Dhanyalakshmi, K. H., Mohan, R., Behera, S., Jha, U. C., Moharana, D., Behera, A., & Beena, R. (2024). Next Generation Nutrition: Genomic and Molecular Breeding Innovations for Iron and Zinc Biofortification in Rice. *Rice Science, 31*(5), 526–544. Advance online publication. DOI: 10.1016/j.rsci.2024.04.008

Dinsmore, W., Callender, M. E., McMaster, D., Todd, J., & Love, A. H. (1985). Zinc absorption in alcoholics using zinc-65. *Digestion, 32*(4), 238–242. DOI: 10.1159/000199243 PMID: 4065445

Djoumessi, Y. F. (2022). The impact of malnutrition on infant mortality and life expectancy in Africa. *Nutrition (Burbank, Los Angeles County, Calif.), 103*, 111760. DOI: 10.1016/j.nut.2022.111760 PMID: 35843043

Donaldson, M., & Touger-Decker, R. (2014). Vitamin and mineral supplements: Friend or foe when combined with medications? *The Journal of the American Dental Association, 145*(11), 1153–1158. DOI: 10.14219/jada.2014.78 PMID: 25359648

Dsouza, M. B. P.Mrs Barthalomea Prathibha Dsouza. (2023). A Study On The Health And Nutrition Education For Teenagers. [IJMR]. *EPRA International Journal of Multidisciplinary Research, 9*(9), 68–71. DOI: 10.36713/epra14326

Duan, M., Li, T., Liu, B., Yin, S., Zang, J., Lv, C., Zhao, G., & Zhang, T. (2023). Zinc nutrition and dietary zinc supplements. *Critical Reviews in Food Science and Nutrition, 63*(9), 1277–1292. DOI: 10.1080/10408398.2021.1963664 PMID: 34382897

Dumrongwongsiri, O., Chongviriyaphan, N., Chatvutinun, S., Phoonlabdacha, P., Sangcakul, A., Siripinyanond, A., & Suthutvoravut, U. (2021). Dietary intake and milk micro-nutrient levels in lactating women with full and partial breastfeeding. *Maternal and Child Health Journal, 25*(6), 991–997. DOI: 10.1007/s10995-020-03049-4 PMID: 33230681

Dumrongwongsiri, O., Suthutvoravut, U., Chatvutinun, S., Phoonlabdacha, P., Sangcakul, A., Siripinyanond, A., Thiengmanee, U., & Chongviriyaphan, N. (2015). Maternal zinc status is associated with breast milk zinc concentration and zinc status in breastfed infants aged 4-6 months. *Asia Pacific Journal of Clinical Nutrition, 24*(2), 273–280. PMID: 26078244

Eckardt, N. A., Ainsworth, E. A., Bahuguna, R. N., Broadley, M. R., Busch, W., Carpita, N. C., Castrillo, G., Chory, J., DeHaan, L. R., Duarte, C. M., Henry, A., Jagadish, S. V. K., Langdale, J. A., Leakey, A. D. B., Liao, J. C., Lu, K.-J., McCann, M. C., McKay, J. K., Odeny, D. A., & Zhang, X. (2023). Climate change challenges, plant science solutions. *The Plant Cell, 35*(1), 24–66. DOI: 10.1093/plcell/koac303 PMID: 36222573

Efeovbokhan, N., Bhattacharya, S. K., Ahokas, R. A., Sun, Y., Guntaka, R. V., Gerling, I. C., & Weber, K. T. (2014). Zinc and the prooxidant heart failure phenotype. *Journal of Cardiovascular Pharmacology, 64*(4), 393–400. DOI: 10.1097/FJC.0000000000000125 PMID: 25291496

El Din, E. M. S., Rabah, T. M., Metwally, A. M., Nassar, M. S., Elabd, M. A., Shalaan, A., Kandeel, W., El Etreby, L. A., & Shaaban, S. Y. (2019). Potential Risk Factors of Developmental Cognitive Delay in the First Two Years of Life. *Open Access Macedonian Journal of Medical Sciences, 7*(12), 2024–2030. DOI: 10.3889/oamjms.2019.566 PMID: 31406549

El-Sayed Saad, A. M., El-Gebally, E.-S. I., El-Mashad, G. M., & El-Hefnawy, S. M. (2018). Effect of zinc supplementation on serum zinc and leptin levels in children on regular hemodialysis. *Menoufia Medical Journal, 31*(2), 664–670.

Erick, M. (2018). Breast milk is conditionally perfect. *Medical Hypotheses, 111*, 82–89. DOI: 10.1016/j.mehy.2017.12.020 PMID: 29407004

Eroglu, A., Al'Abri, I. S., Kopec, R. E., Crook, N., & Bohn, T. (2023). Carotenoids and their health benefits as derived via their interactions with gut microbiota. *Advances in Nutrition, 14*(2), 238–255. DOI: 10.1016/j.advnut.2022.10.007 PMID: 36775788

Escobedo-Monge, M. F., Torres-Hinojal, M. C., Barrado, E., Escobedo-Monge, M. A., & Marugán-Miguelsanz, J. M. (2021). Zinc nutritional status in a series of children with chronic diseases: A cross-sectional study. *Nutrients, 13*(4), 1121. DOI: 10.3390/nu13041121 PMID: 33805416

Faber, M., Berti, C., & Smuts, M. (2014). Prevention and control of micronutrient deficiencies in developing countries: Current perspectives. *Nutrition and Dietary Supplements, 41*, 41. Advance online publication. DOI: 10.2147/NDS.S43523

Fallah, A., Mohammad-Hasani, A., & Colagar, A. H. (2018). Zinc is an essential element for male fertility: A review of Zn roles in men's health, germination, sperm quality, and fertilization. *Journal of Reproduction & Infertility*, *19*(2), 69. PMID: 30009140

Fanzo, J., Hawkes, C., Udomkesmalee, E., Afshin, A., Allemandi, L., Assery, O., Baker, P., Battersby, J., Bhutta, Z., & Chen, K. (2018). *2018 Global Nutrition Report: Shining a light to spur action on nutrition*. 88149.

Farias, P. M., Marcelino, G., Santana, L. F., De Almeida, E. B., Guimarães, R. D. C. A., Pott, A., Hiane, P. A., & Freitas, K. D. C. (2020). Minerals in Pregnancy and Their Impact on Child Growth and Development. *Molecules (Basel, Switzerland)*, *25*(23), 5630. DOI: 10.3390/molecules25235630 PMID: 33265961

Fink, G., & Heitner, J. (2014). Evaluating the cost-effectiveness of preventive zinc supplementation. *BMC Public Health*, *14*(1), 852. DOI: 10.1186/1471-2458-14-852 PMID: 25128210

Finner, A. M. (2013). Nutrition and hair: Deficiencies and supplements. *Dermatol. Clin.*, *31*(1), 167-172. doi:10:1016/j.det.2012.08.015

Finzi, E., & Harrington, A. (2021). Zinc treatment of outpatient COVID-19: A retrospective review of 28 consecutive patients. *Journal of Medical Virology*, *93*(5), 2588–2590. DOI: 10.1002/jmv.26812 PMID: 33475170

Foster, M., & Samman, S. (2010). Zinc and Redox Signaling: Perturbations Associated with Cardiovascular Disease and Diabetes Mellitus. *Antioxidants & Redox Signaling*, *13*(10), 1549–1573. DOI: 10.1089/ars.2010.3111 PMID: 20568953

Frassinetti, S., Bronzetti, G. L., Caltavuturo, L., Cini, M., & Della Croce, C. (2006). The role of zinc in life: A review. *Journal of Environmental Pathology, Toxicology and Oncology*, *25*(3), 597–610. DOI: 10.1615/JEnvironPatholToxicolOncol.v25.i3.40 PMID: 17073562

Freeland-Graves, J. H., Sachdev, P. K., Binderberger, A. Z., & Sosanya, M. E. (2020). Global diversity of dietary intakes and standards for zinc, iron, and copper. *Journal of Trace Elements in Medicine and Biology*, *61*, 126515. DOI: 10.1016/j.jtemb.2020.126515 PMID: 32450495

Frittelli, A., Botticella, E., Palombieri, S., Masci, S., Celletti, S., Fontanella, M. C., Astolfi, S., De Vita, P., Volpato, M., & Sestili, F. (2023). The suppression of TdMRP3 genes reduces the phytic acid and increases the nutrient accumulation in durum wheat grain. *Frontiers in Plant Science*, *14*, 1079559. DOI: 10.3389/fpls.2023.1079559 PMID: 36743506

Fukuda, T., Civic, N., Furuichi, T., Shimoda, S., Mishima, K., Higashiyama, H., Idaira, Y., Asada, Y., Kitamura, H., Yamasaki, S., Hojyo, S., Nakayama, M., Ohara, O., Koseki, H., Santos, H. G. D., Bonafe, L., Ha-Vinh, R., Zankl, A., Unger, S., & Hirano, T. (2008). The zinc transporter SLC39A13/ZIP13 is required for connective tissue development; it's involvement in BMP/TGF-beta, signalling pathways. *PLoS One*, *3*(11), e3642. DOI: 10.1371/journal.pone.0003642 PMID: 18985159

Fukushima, T., Horike, H., Fujiki, S., Kitada, S., Sasaki, T., & Kashihara, N. (2009). Zinc deficiency anemia and effects of zinc therapy in maintenance hemodialysis patients. *Therapeutic Apheresis and Dialysis*, *13*(3), 213–219. DOI: 10.1111/j.1744-9987.2009.00656.x PMID: 19527468

Gaffney-Stomberg, E. (2019). The Impact of Trace Minerals on Bone Metabolism. *Biological Trace Element Research*, *188*(1), 26–34. DOI: 10.1007/s12011-018-1583-8 PMID: 30467628

García-Bañuelos, M. L., Sida-Arreola, J. P., & Sánchez, E. (2014). Biofortification-promising approach to increasing the content of iron and zinc in staple food crops. *Journal of Elementology*, *19*(3). https://agro.icm.edu.pl/agro/element/bwmeta1.element.agro-3c9e2e65-f373-4936-acd2-a5850e3e70b8

Garcia-Casal, M. N., Estevez, D., & De-Regil, L. M. (2018). Multiple micronutrient supplementş in pregnancy: Implementation considerations for integration as part of quality services in routine antenatal care. Objectives, results, and conclusions of the meeting. *Maternal and Child Nutrition*, *14*(S5), e12704. DOI: 10.1111/mcn.12704 PMID: 30585705

García-Maldonado, E., Gallego-Narbón, A., & Vaquero, M. (2019). ¿ Son las dietas vegetarianas nutricionalmente adecuadas? Una revisión de la evidencia científica. *Nutrición Hospitalaria*, *36*(4), 950–961. PMID: 31232583

Garner, T. B., Hester, J. M., Carothers, A., & Diaz, F. J. (2021). Role of zinc in female reproduction. *Biology of Reproduction*, *104*(5), 976–994. DOI: 10.1093/biolre/ioab023 PMID: 33598687

Gasmi, A., Bjørklund, G., Mujawdiya, P. K., Semenova, Y., Peana, M., Dosa, A., Piscopo, S., Gasmi Benahmed, A., & Costea, D. O. (2022). Micronutrients deficiences in patients after bariatric surgery. *European Journal of Nutrition*, *61*(1), 55–67. DOI: 10.1007/s00394-021-02619-8 PMID: 34302218

Gembillo, G., Visconti, L., Giuffrida, A. E., Labbozzetta, V., Peritore, L., Lipari, A., Calabrese, V., Piccoli, G. B., Torreggiani, M., Siligato, R., & Santoro, D. (2022). Role of zinc in diabetic kidney disease. *Nutrients*, *14*(7), 1353. DOI: 10.3390/nu14071353 PMID: 35405968

Gharibzahedi, S. M. T., & Jafari, S. M. (2017). The importance of minerals in human nutrition: Bioavailability, food fortification, processing effects and nanoencapsulation. *Trends in Food Science & Technology*, *62*, 119–132. DOI: 10.1016/j.tifs.2017.02.017

Ghishan, F. K. (1984). Transport of electrolytes, water, and glucose in zinc deficiency. *Journal of Pediatric Gastroenterology and Nutrition*, *3*, 608–612. PMID: 6090631

Gibbs, M. (2010). *Manufactured complementary foods for infant and young child feeding in Asia: Micronutrient adequacy and improvement* [PhD Thesis, University of Otago]. https://ourarchive.otago.ac.nz/handle/10523/369

Gibson, R. S. (1994). Zinc nutrition in developing countries. *Nutrition Research Reviews*, *7*(1), 151–173. DOI: 10.1079/NRR19940010 PMID: 19094296

Gibson, R. S. (2006). Zinc: The missing link in combating micronutrient malnutrition in developing countries. *The Proceedings of the Nutrition Society*, *65*(1), 51–60. DOI: 10.1079/PNS2005474 PMID: 16441944

Gibson, R. S. (2012). A historical review of progress in the assessment of dietary zinc intake as an indicator of population zinc status. *Advances in Nutrition*, *3*(6), 772–782. DOI: 10.3945/an.112.002287 PMID: 23153731

Gibson, R. S. (2012b). Zinc deficiency and human health: Etiology, health consequences, and future solutions. *Plant and Soil*, *361*(1-2), 291–299. DOI: 10.1007/s11104-012-1209-4

Gibson, R. S. (2015). Dietary-induced Zinc Deficiency in low Income Countries: Challenges and Solutions The Avanelle Kirksey Lecture at Purdue University. *Nutrition Today*, *50*(1), 49–55. DOI: 10.1097/NT.0000000000000070

Gibson, R. S., & Anderson, V. P. (2009). A review of interventions based on dietary diversification or modification strategies with the potential to enhance intakes of total and absorbable zinc. *Food and Nutrition Bulletin*, *30*(1_suppl1), S108–S143. DOI: 10.1177/15648265090301S107 PMID: 19472604

Gibson, R. S., & Ferguson, E. L. (1998). Nutrition intervention strategies to combat zinc deficiency in developing countries. *Nutrition Research Reviews*, *11*(1), 115–131. DOI: 10.1079/NRR19980008 PMID: 19087462

Gibson, R. S., & Hotz, C. (2001). Dietary diversification/modification strategies to enhance micronutrient content and bioavailability of diets in developing countries. *British Journal of Nutrition*, *85*(S2), S159–S166. DOI: 10.1079/BJN2001309 PMID: 11509105

Gibson, R. S., Raboy, V., & King, J. C. (2018). Implications of phytate in plant-based foods for iron and zinc bioavailability, setting dietary requirements, and formulating programs and policies. *Nutrition Reviews*, *76*(11), 793–804. DOI: 10.1093/nutrit/nuy028 PMID: 30010865

Gibson, R., Ferguson, E., & Lehrfeld, J. (1998). Complementary foods for infant feeding in developing countries: Their nutrient adequacy and improvement. *European Journal of Clinical Nutrition*, *52*(10), 764–770. DOI: 10.1038/sj.ejcn.1600645 PMID: 9805226

Gilbert, R., Peto, T., Lengyel, I., & Emri, E. (2019). Zinc nutrition and inflammation in the aging retina. *Molecular Nutrition & Food Research*, *63*(15), 1801049. DOI: 10.1002/mnfr.201801049 PMID: 31148351

Giunta, C., Elcioglu, N. H., Albrecht, B., Eich, G., Chambaz, C., Janecke, A. R., Yeowell, H., Weis, M., Eyre, D. R., Kraenzlin, M., & Steinmann, B. (2008). Spondylocheiro dysplastic form of the Ehlers -Danlos syndrome -An autosomal -recessive entity caused by mutation in the zinc transporter gene SLC39A13. *American Journal of Human Genetics*, *82*(6), 1290–1305. DOI: 10.1016/j.ajhg.2008.05.001 PMID: 18513683

Gohari, H., Khajavian, N., Mahmoudian, A., & Bilandi, R. R. (2023). Copper and zinc deficiency to the risk of preterm labor in pregnant women: A case-control study. *BMC Pregnancy and Childbirth*, *23*(1), 366. DOI: 10.1186/s12884-023-05625-2 PMID: 37208743

Golden, M. H., Jackson, A. A., & Golden, B. E. (1977). Effect of zinc on thymus of recently malnourished children. *Lancet*, *2*(8047), 1057–1059. DOI: 10.1016/S0140-6736(77)91888-8 PMID: 72960

Gombart, A. F., Pierre, A., & Maggini, S. (2020). A review of micronutrients and the immune system–working in harmony to reduce the risk of infection. *Nutrients*, *12*(1), 236. DOI: 10.3390/nu12010236 PMID: 31963293

Gondal, A. H., Zafar, A., Zainab, D., Toor, M., Sohail, S., Ameen, S., Ijaz, A. Ch. B., Hussain, I., & Haider, S. (2021). A detailed review study of zinc involvement in animal, plant and human nutrition. *Indian Journal of Pure & Applied Biosciences*, *9*(2), 262–271. DOI: 10.18782/2582-2845.8652

Gonoodi, K., Moslem, A., Darroudi, S., Ahmadnezhad, M., Mazloum, Z., Tayefi, M., Zadeh, S. A. T., Eslami, S., Shafiee, M., Khashayarmanesh, Z., Haghighi, H. M., Ferns, G. A., & Ghayour-Mobarhan, M. (2018). Serum and dietary zinc and copper in Iranian girls. *Clinical Biochemistry*, *54*, 25–31. DOI: 10.1016/j.clinbiochem.2018.02.006 PMID: 29438682

Gonzales, K. A. U., & Fuchs, E. (2017). Skin and it's regenerative powers: An alliance between stem cells and their niche. *Developmental Cell, 43*(4), 387–401. DOI: 10.1016/j.devcel.2017.10.001 PMID: 29161590

Gowda, N. N., Siliveru, K., Prasad, P. V., Bhatt, Y., Netravati, B. P., & Gurikar, C. (2022). Modern processing of Indian millets: A perspective on changes in nutritional properties. *Foods, 11*(4), 499. DOI: 10.3390/foods11040499 PMID: 35205975

Gower-Winter, S. D., & Levenson, C. W. (2012). Zinc in the central nervous system: From molecules to behavior. *BioFactors (Oxford, England), 38*(3), 186–193. DOI: 10.1002/biof.1012 PMID: 22473811

Goyena, E. A., Maniego, M. L. V., Ducay, A. J. D., Musa, M. C. A., & Angeles-Agdeppa, I. (2021). Dietary zinc intake and the underlying factors of serum zinc deficiency among preschool children in the Philippines. *Philippine Journal of Science, 150*(3), 799–812. DOI: 10.56899/150.03.16

Grabrucker, M, A., Rowan, M., & C Garner, C. (2011). Brain-delivery of zinc-ions as potential treatment for neurological diseases: Mini review. *Drug Delivery Letters, 1*(1), 13–23. PMID: 22102982

Grieger, J. A., & Clifton, V. L. (2014). A review of the impact of dietary intakes in human pregnancy on infant birthweight. *Nutrients, 7*(1), 153–178. DOI: 10.3390/nu7010153 PMID: 25551251

Grüngreiff, K., Reinhold, D., & Wedemeyer, H. (2016). The role of zinc in liver cirrhosis. *Annals of Hepatology, 15*(1), 7–16. DOI: 10.5604/16652681.1184191 PMID: 26626635

Grzeszczak, K., Kwiatkowski, S., & Kosik-Bogacka, D. (2020). The role of Fe, Zn, and Cu in pregnancy. *Biomolecules, 10*(8), 1176. DOI: 10.3390/biom10081176 PMID: 32806787

Gupta, D. N., Rajendran, K., Mondal, S. K., Ghosh, S., & Bhattacharya, S. K. (2007). Operational feasibility of implementing community-based zinc supplementation: Impact on childhood diarrheal morbidity. *The Pediatric Infectious Disease Journal, 26*(4), 306–310. DOI: 10.1097/01.inf.0000258692.65485.d9 PMID: 17414392

Gupta, M., Mahajan, V. K., Mehta, K. S., & Chauhan, P. S. (2014). Zinc therapy in dermatology: A review. *Dermatology Research and Practice, 2014*, 1–11. https://www.hindawi.com/journals/drp/2014/709152/abs/. DOI: 10.1155/2014/709152 PMID: 25120566

Gupta, N., Ram, H., & Kumar, B. (2016). Mechanism of Zinc absorption in plants: Uptake, transport, translocation and accumulation. *Reviews in Environmental Science and Biotechnology, 15*(1), 89–109. DOI: 10.1007/s11157-016-9390-1

Gupta, R. K., Gangoliya, S. S., & Singh, N. K. (2015). Reduction of phytic acid and enhancement of bioavailable micronutrients in food grains. *Journal of Food Science and Technology, 52*(2), 676–684. DOI: 10.1007/s13197-013-0978-y PMID: 25694676

Gupta, S., Brazier, A. K. M., & Lowe, N. M. (2020). Zinc deficiency in low- and middle-income countries: Prevalence and approaches for mitigation. *Journal of Human Nutrition and Dietetics, 33*(5), 624–643. DOI: 10.1111/jhn.12791 PMID: 32627912

Haase, H., & Rink, L. (2014). Multiple impacts of zinc on immune function. *Metallomics, 6*(7), 1175. DOI: 10.1039/c3mt00353a PMID: 24531756

Haase, H., & Rink, L. (2014). Zinc signals and immune function. *BioFactors (Oxford, England), 40*(1), 27–40. DOI: 10.1002/biof.1114 PMID: 23804522

Hall, A. G., & King, J. C. (2022). Zinc fortification: Current trends and strategies. *Nutrients, 14*(19), 3895. DOI: 10.3390/nu14193895 PMID: 36235548

Hambidge, K. M. (1989). Mild zinc deficiency in children. In Mills, C. F. (Ed.), *Zinc in Human Biology* (pp. 285–295). Springer-Verlag. DOI: 10.1007/978-1-4471-3879-2_18

Hambidge, K. M. (1992). Zinc and diarrhea. *Acta Paediatrica (Oslo, Norway), 381*(s383), 82–86. DOI: 10.1111/j.1651-2227.1992.tb12377.x PMID: 1421947

Hambidge, K. M. (2000). Human zinc deficiency. *The Journal of Nutrition, 130*(5), S1344–S1349. DOI: 10.1093/jn/130.5.1344S PMID: 10801941

Hambidge, K. M. (2010). Micronutrient bioavailability: Dietary Reference Intakes and a future perspective. *The American Journal of Clinical Nutrition, 91*(5), 1430S–1432S. DOI: 10.3945/ajcn.2010.28674B PMID: 20200261

Hambidge, K. M., & Krebs, N. F. (2007). Zinc Deficiency: A Special Challenge1. *The Journal of Nutrition, 137*(4), 1101–1105. DOI: 10.1093/jn/137.4.1101 PMID: 17374687

Hambidge, K. M., Miller, L. V., Westcott, J. E., Sheng, X., & Krebs, N. F. (2010). Zinc bioavailability and homeostasis. *The American Journal of Clinical Nutrition, 91*(5), 1478S–1483S. DOI: 10.3945/ajcn.2010.28674I PMID: 20200254

Hambidge, K. M., & Walravens, P. A. (1982). Disorders of mineral metabolism. *Clinics in Gastroenterology*, *11*(1), 87–117. DOI: 10.1016/S0300-5089(21)00496-X PMID: 6277535

Hambidge, M., Cousins, R. J., & Costello, R. B. (2000). Introduction. *The Journal of Nutrition*, *130*(5), 1341S–1343S. DOI: 10.1093/jn/130.5.1341S PMID: 10801940

Han, S. M., Devaraj, S., Derraik, J. G., Vickers, M. H., Huang, F., Dubascoux, S., Godfrey, K. M., Chan, S.-Y., Pang, W. W., Thakkar, S. K., & Cutfield, W. S. (2023). A nutritional supplement containing zinc during preconception and pregnancy increases human milk zinc concentrations. *Frontiers in Nutrition*, *9*, 1034828. DOI: 10.3389/fnut.2022.1034828 PMID: 36704795

Hara, T., Takeda, T. A., Takagishi, T., Fukue, K., Kambe, T., & Fukada, T. (2017). Physiological roles of zinc transporters: Molecular and genetic importance in zinc homeostasis. *The Journal of Physiological Sciences; JPS*, *67*(2), 283–301.

Hara, T., Yoshigai, E., Ohashi, T., & Fukada, T. (2023). Zinc in cardiovascular functions and diseases: Epidemiology and molecular mechanisms for therapeutic development. *International Journal of Molecular Sciences*, *24*(8), 7152. DOI: 10.3390/ijms24087152 PMID: 37108314

Harrington, S. A., Connorton, J. M., Nyangoma, N. I., McNelly, R., Morgan, Y. M., Aslam, M. F., Sharp, P. A., Johnson, A. A. T., Uauy, C., & Balk, J. (2023). A two-gene strategy increases iron and zinc concentrations in wheat flour, improving mineral bioaccessibility. *Plant Physiology*, *191*(1), 528–541. DOI: 10.1093/plphys/kiac499 PMID: 36308454

Hassan, A., Sada, K.-K., Ketheeswaran, S., Dubey, A. K., & Bhat, M. S. (2020). Role of Zinc in Mucosal Health and Disease: A Review of Physiological, Biochemical, and Molecular Processes. *Cureus*. Advance online publication. DOI: 10.7759/cureus.8197 PMID: 32572355

Hatch-McChesney, A., & Smith, T. J. (2023). Nutrition, immune function, and infectious disease in military personnel: A narrative review. *Nutrients*, *15*(23), 4999. DOI: 10.3390/nu15234999 PMID: 38068857

Hemilä, H. (2017). Zinc lozenges and the common cold: A meta-analysis comparing zinc acetate and zinc gluconate, and the role of zinc dosage. *JRSM Open*, *8*(5), 205427041769429. DOI: 10.1177/2054270417694291 PMID: 28515951

Hemilä, H., & Chalker, E. (2015). The effectiveness of high dose zinc acetate lozenges on various common cold symptoms: A meta-analysis. *BMC Family Practice*, *16*(1), 24. DOI: 10.1186/s12875-015-0237-6 PMID: 25888289

Henkin, R. I. (1984). Zinc in taste function: A critical review. *Biological Trace Element Research, 6*(3), 263–280. DOI: 10.1007/BF02917511 PMID: 24264025

Hennigar, S. R., Lieberman, H. R., Fulgoni, V. L.III, & McClung, J. P. (2018). Serum zinc concentrations in the US population are related to sex, age, and time of blood draw but not dietary or supplemental zinc. *The Journal of Nutrition, 148*(8), 1341–1351. DOI: 10.1093/jn/nxy105 PMID: 29947812

Hess, S. Y., & Brown, K. H. (2009). Impact of zinc fortification on zinc nutrition. *Food and Nutrition Bulletin, 30*(1, suppl1), S79–S107. DOI: 10.1177/15648265090301S106 PMID: 19472603

Hess, S. Y., McLain, A. C., Lescinsky, H., Brown, K. H., Afshin, A., Atkin, R., & Osendarp, S. J. (2022). Basis for changes in the disease burden estimates related to vitamin A and zinc deficiencies in the 2017 and 2019 Global Burden of Disease Studies. *Public Health Nutrition, 25*(8), 2225–2231. DOI: 10.1017/S1368980021004821 PMID: 34889182

Heyland, D. K., Jones, N., Cvijanovich, N. Z., & Wong, H. (2008). Zinc Supplementation in Critically Ill Patients: A Key Pharmaconutrient? *JPEN. Journal of Parenteral and Enteral Nutrition, 32*(5), 509–519. DOI: 10.1177/0148607108322402 PMID: 18669902

Himoto, T., & Masaki, T. (2018). Associations between zinc deficiency and metabolic abnormalities in patients with chronic liver disease. *Nutrients, 10*(1), 88. DOI: 10.3390/nu10010088 PMID: 29342898

Hina, A., Abbasi, A., Imtiaz, S., Ul Haq, I., Ul Hassan, A., & Chaudhry, A. (2023). General Aspects of Genetic Improvement (Traditional and Transgenic Methods) Aiming to Food Biofortification. In *Legumes Biofortification* (pp. 73–109). Springer International Publishing., DOI: 10.1007/978-3-031-33957-8_4

Hobbs, R. P., & Bernstein, P. S. (2014). Nutrient supplementation for age-related macular degeneration, cataract, and dry eye. *Journal of Ophthalmic & Vision Research, 9*(4), 487. DOI: 10.4103/2008-322X.150829 PMID: 25709776

Hoffman, H. N.II, Phyliky, R. L., & Fleming, C. R. (1988). Zinc-induced copper deficiency. *Gastroenterology, 94*(2), 508–512. DOI: 10.1016/0016-5085(88)90445-3 PMID: 3335323

Hoque, M., Emon, K., Malo, P. C., Hossain, M. H., Tannu, S. I., & Roshed, M. M. (2023). Comprehensive guide to vitamin and mineral sources with their requirements. *Indiana Journal of Agriculture and Life Sciences, 3*(6), 23–31. DOI: 10.5281/zenodo.10284736

Hotz, C., & Brown, K. H. (2004). Assessment of the risk of zinc deficiency in populations and options for its control.

Hotz, C., & Brown, K. H. (2004). *Assessment of the risk of zinc deficiency in populations and options for its control.* https://citeseerx.ist.psu.edu/document?repid=rep1&type=pdf&doi=4fffa0f903be10224b0651fed1d27bb144feb1ac

Hotz, C. (2009). The Potential to Improve Zinc Status through Biofortification of Staple Food Crops with Zinc. *Food and Nutrition Bulletin, 30*(1, suppl1), S172–S178. DOI: 10.1177/15648265090301S109 PMID: 19472606

Hotz, C., & Gibson, R. S. (2007). Traditional Food-Processing and Preparation Practices to Enhance the Bioavailability of Micronutrients in Plant-Based Diets1. *The Journal of Nutrition, 137*(4), 1097–1100. DOI: 10.1093/jn/137.4.1097 PMID: 17374686

Huang, L., Teng, T., Zhao, J., Bian, B., Yao, W., Yu, X., Wang, Z., Xu, Z., & Sun, Y. (2018). The relationship between serum zinc levels, cardiac markers and the risk of acute myocardial infarction by zinc quartiles. *Heart Lung and Circulation, 27*(1), 66–72. DOI: 10.1016/j.hlc.2017.01.022 PMID: 28408092

Huang, S., Sasaki, A., Yamaji, N., Okada, H., Mitani-Ueno, N., & Ma, J. F. (2020). The ZIP transporter family member OsZIP9 contributes to root zinc uptake in rice under zinc-limited conditions. *Plant Physiology, 183*(3), 1224–1234. DOI: 10.1104/pp.20.00125 PMID: 32371522

Hussain, A., Jiang, W., Wang, X., Shahid, S., Saba, N., Ahmad, M., Dar, A., Masood, S. U., Imran, M., & Mustafa, A. (2022). Mechanistic Impact of Zinc Deficiency in Human Development. *Frontiers in Nutrition, 9*, 717064. DOI: 10.3389/fnut.2022.717064 PMID: 35356730

Ibrahim, S., Saleem, B., Rehman, N., Zafar, S. A., Naeem, M. K., & Khan, M. R. (2022). CRISPR/Cas9 mediated disruption of Inositol Pentakisphosphate 2-Kinase 1 (TaIPK1) reduces phytic acid and improves iron and zinc accumulation in wheat grains. *Journal of Advanced Research, 37*, 33–41. DOI: 10.1016/j.jare.2021.07.006 PMID: 35499048

Iida, D., Shigemura, T., Yamamoto, Y., & Murata, Y. (2023). *Prevalence and Predictive Factors of Zinc Deficiency in Orthopaedic Inpatients.* Medicine and Pharmacology. DOI: 10.20944/preprints202312.0416.v1

Imdad, A., Rogner, J., Sherwani, R. N., Sidhu, J., Regan, A., Haykal, M. R., Tsistinas, O., Smith, A., Chan, X. H. S., Mayo-Wilson, E., & Bhutta, Z. A. (2023). Zinc supplementation for preventing mortality, morbidity, and growth failure in children aged 6 months to 12 years. *Cochrane Database of Systematic Reviews, 2023*(3). DOI: 10.1002/14651858.CD009384.pub3

Inabangan-Asilo, M. A., Swamy, B. P. M., Amparado, A. F., Descalsota-Empleo, G. I., Arocena, E. C., & Reinke, R. (2019). Stability and G×E analysis of zinc-biofortified rice genotypes evaluated in diverse environments. *Euphytica, 215*(3), 1–7. DOI: 10.1007/s10681-019-2384-7

Institute of Medicine. (2001). *Dietary Reference Intakes for Vitamin A, Vitamin K, Arsenic, Boron, Chromium, Copper, Iodine, Iron, Manganese, Molybdenum, Nickel, Silicon, Vanadium, and Zinc*. The National Academies Press., DOI: 10.17226/10026

Islam, M. M., Black, R. E., Krebs, N. F., Westcott, J., Long, J., Islam, K. M., Peerson, J. M., Sthity, R. A., Khandaker, A. M., Hasan, M., El Arifeen, S., Ahmed, T., King, J. C., & McDonald, C. M. (2022). Different doses, forms, and frequencies of zinc supplementation for the prevention of diarrhea and promotion of linear growth among young Bangladeshi children: A six-arm, randomized, community-based efficacy trial. *The Journal of Nutrition, 152*(5), 1306–1315. DOI: 10.1093/jn/nxab439 PMID: 35015856

Islam, M. M., McDonald, C. M., Krebs, N. F., Westcott, J., Rahman, A. E., El Arifeen, S., Ahmed, T., King, J. C., & Black, R. E. (2018). Study protocol for a randomized, double-blind, community-based efficacy trial of various doses of zinc in micronutrient powders or tablets in young Bangladeshi children. *Nutrients, 10*(2), 132. DOI: 10.3390/nu10020132 PMID: 30720778

Itsumura, N., Inamo, Y., Okazaki, F., Teranishi, F., Narita, H., Kambe, T., & Kodama, H. (2013). Compound heterozygous mutations in SLC30A2/ZnT2 results in low milk zinc concentration. A novel mechanism for zinc deficiency in a breast fed infant. *PLoS One, 8*(5), e64045. DOI: 10.1371/journal.pone.0064045 PMID: 23741301

Jankowska, M., Rutkowski, B., & Dębska-Ślizień, A. (2017). Vitamins and microelement bioavailability in different stages of chronic kidney disease. *Nutrients, 9*(3), 282. DOI: 10.3390/nu9030282 PMID: 28294976

Jin, D., Wei, X., He, Y., Zhong, L., Lu, H., Lan, J., Wei, Y., Liu, Z., & Liu, H. (2024). The nutritional roles of zinc for immune system and COVID-19 patients. *Frontiers in Nutrition, 11*, 1385591. DOI: 10.3389/fnut.2024.1385591 PMID: 38706559

Jindal, A. (2023). Zinc enrichment strategies in legumes and cereals: Assessing current advancements and future prospects. *The Pharma Innovation Journal, 12*(8), 935–944.

Jones, P. W., & Williams, D. R. (2004). The use and role of zinc and its compounds in wound healing. *Metal Ions in Biological Systems*, *41*, 139–184. DOI: 10.1201/9780203913703.ch5 PMID: 15206116

Joo, Y. S., Kim, H. W., Lee, S., Nam, K. H., Yun, H.-R., Jhee, J. H., Han, S. H., Yoo, T.-H., Kang, S.-W., & Park, J. T. (2021). Dietary zinc intake and incident chronic kidney disease. *Clinical Nutrition (Edinburgh, Lothian)*, *40*(3), 1039–1045. DOI: 10.1016/j.clnu.2020.07.005 PMID: 32753349

Kabu, K., Yamasaki, S., Kamimura, D., Ito, Y., Hasegawa, A., Sato, E., Kitamura, H., Nishida, K., & Hirano, T. (2006). Zinc is required for Fc epsilon RI-mediated mast cell activation. *The Journal of Immunology : Official Journal of the American Association of Immunologists*, *177*(2), 1296–1305. DOI: 10.4049/jimmunol.177.2.1296 PMID: 16818790

Kahane, R., Hodgkin, T., Jaenicke, H., Hoogendoorn, C., Hermann, M., Keatinge, J. D. H., d'Arros Hughes, J., Padulosi, S., & Looney, N. (2013). Agrobiodiversity for food security, health and income. *Agronomy for Sustainable Development*, *33*, 671–693. DOI: 10.1007/s13593-013-0147-8

Kamalov, G., Holewinski, J. P., Bhattacharya, S. K., Ahokas, R. A., Sun, Y., Gerling, I. C., & Weber, K. T. (2009). Nutrient dyshomeostasis in congestive heart failure. *The American Journal of the Medical Sciences*, *338*(1), 28–33. DOI: 10.1097/MAJ.0b013e3181aaee63 PMID: 19593100

Kamaral, C., Neate, S. M., Gunasinghe, N., Milham, P. J., Paterson, D. J., Kopittke, P. M., & Seneweera, S. (2022). Genetic biofortification of wheat with zinc: Opportunities to fine-tune zinc uptake, transport and grain loading. *Physiologia Plantarum*, *174*(1), e13612. DOI: 10.1111/ppl.13612 PMID: 34970752

Kambe, T., Tsuji, T., Hashimoto, A., & Itsumura, N. (2015). The Physiological, Biochemical, and Molecular Roles of Zinc Transporters in Zinc Homeostasis and Metabolism. *Physiological Reviews*, *95*(3), 749–784. DOI: 10.1152/physrev.00035.2014 PMID: 26084690

Kapper, C., Oppelt, P., Ganhör, C., Gyunesh, A. A., Arbeithuber, B., Stelzl, P., & Rezk-Füreder, M. (2024). Minerals and the Menstrual Cycle: Impacts on Ovulation and Endometrial Health. *Nutrients*, *16*(7), 1008. DOI: 10.3390/nu16071008 PMID: 38613041

Karagulova, G., Yue, Y., Moreyra, A., Boutjdir, M., & Korichneva, I. (2007). Protective role of intracellular zinc in myocardial ischemia/reperfusion is associated with preservation of protein kinase C isoforms. *The Journal of Pharmacology and Experimental Therapeutics*, *321*(2), 517–525. DOI: 10.1124/jpet.107.119644 PMID: 17322024

Karimi, A., Bagheri, S., Nematy, M., & Saeidi, M. (2012). Zinc deficiency in pregnancy and fetal-neonatal outcomes and impact of the supplements on pregnancy outcomes. *Iranian Journal of Neonatology IJN*, *3*(2), 77–83.

Katayama, K., Kawaguchi, T., Shiraishi, K., Ito, T., Suzuki, K., Koreeda, C., Ohtake, T., Iwasa, M., Tokumoto, Y., Endo, R., Kawamura, N., Shiraki, M., Hanai, T., Habu, D., Tsuruta, S., Sakai, H., Miwa, Y., Kawada, N., Kato, A., & Suzuki, K. (2018). The prevalence and implication of zinc deficiency in patients with chronic liver disease. *Journal of Clinical Medicine Research*, *10*(5), 437–444. DOI: 10.14740/jocmr3374w PMID: 29581807

Katimba, H. A., Wang, R., Cheng, C., Zhang, Y., Lu, W., & Ma, Y. (2024). Zinc Absorption & Homeostasis in the Human Body: A General Overview. *Food Reviews International*, *40*(2), 715–739. DOI: 10.1080/87559129.2023.2195188

Kaur, K., Gupta, R., Saraf, S. A., & Saraf, S. K. (2014). Zinc: The Metal of Life. *Comprehensive Reviews in Food Science and Food Safety*, *13*(4), 358–376. DOI: 10.1111/1541-4337.12067 PMID: 33412710

Kay, R. G. (1975). Tasman-Jones C. Acute zinc deficiency in man during intravenous alimentation. *ANZ Journal of Surgery*, *45*, 325–330. PMID: 813623

Kelishadi, R., Alikhassy, H., & Amiri, M. (2002). Zinc and copper status in children with high family risk of premature cardiovascular disease. *Annals of Saudi Medicine*, *22*(5-6), 291–294. DOI: 10.5144/0256-4947.2002.291 PMID: 17146244

Kemp, J. F., Hambidge, K. M., Westcott, J. L., Ali, S. A., Saleem, S., Garcés, A., Figueroa, L., Somannavar, M. S., Goudar, S. S., Long, J. M., Hendricks, A. E., Krebs, N. F., Dhaded, S. M., Vernekar, S. S., Herekar, V. R., Yogeshkumar, S., McClure, E. M., Das, A., Thorsten, V. R., & Koso-Thomas, M. W. (2024). Zinc supplementation initiated prior to or during pregnancy modestly impacted maternal status and high prevalence of hypozincemia in pregnancy and lactation: The Women First Preconception Maternal Nutrition Trial. *The Journal of Nutrition*, *154*(6), 1917–1926. Advance online publication. DOI: 10.1016/j.tjnut.2024.04.018 PMID: 38621624

Kewcharoenwong, C., Schuster, G. U., Wessells, K. R., Hinnouho, G.-M., Barffour, M. A., Kounnavong, S., Brown, K. H., Hess, S. Y., Samer, W., Tussakhon, I., Peerson, J. M., Lertmemongkolchai, G., & Stephensen, C. B. (2020). Daily preventive zinc supplementation decreases lymphocyte and eosinophil concentrations in rural Laotian children from communities with a high prevalence of zinc deficiency: Results of a randomized controlled trial. *The Journal of Nutrition*, *150*(8), 2204–2213. DOI: 10.1093/jn/nxaa037 PMID: 32119742

Khadamy, J. (n.d.). *Nutrients for Eye Health and Disease Management*. Retrieved May 25, 2024, from https://www.researchgate.net/profile/Joobin-Khadamy/publication/376582120_Nutrients_for_Eye_Health_and_Disease_Management/links/657df780aff8b16813ad8fda/Nutrients-for-Eye-Health-and-Disease-Management.pdf

Khalid, M. S., Aljohani, M. M., Alomrani, N. A., Oyouni, A. A. A., Alzahrani, O., & Ahmad, M. A.. (2020). COVID-19 and immune function—"A significant" zinc. *Oriental Journal of Chemistry*, *36*(6), 1026. DOI: 10.13005/ojc/360604

Khan, S. T., Malik, A., Alwarthan, A., & Shaik, M. R. (2022). The enormity of the zinc deficiency problem and available solutions; an overview. *Arabian Journal of Chemistry*, *15*(3), 103668. DOI: 10.1016/j.arabjc.2021.103668

Khayat, S., Fanaei, H., & Ghanbarzehi, A. (2017). Minerals in pregnancy and lactation: A review article. *Journal of Clinical and Diagnostic Research : JCDR*, *11*(9), QE01. DOI: 10.7860/JCDR/2017/28485.10626 PMID: 29207789

Khoo, H. E., Ng, H. S., Yap, W.-S., Goh, H. J. H., & Yim, H. S. (2019). Nutrients for prevention of macular degeneration and eye-related diseases. *Antioxidants*, *8*(4), 85. DOI: 10.3390/antiox8040085 PMID: 30986936

Kido, T., Suka, M., & Yanagisawa, H. (2022). Effectiveness of interleukin-4 administration or zinc supplementation in improving zinc deficiency–associated thymic atrophy and fatty degeneration and in normalizing T cell maturation process. *Immunology*, *165*(4), 445–459. DOI: 10.1111/imm.13452 PMID: 35138640

Kil, M. S., Kim, C. W., & Kim, S. S. (2013). Analysis of serum zinc and copper concentration in hair loss. *Annals of Dermatology*, *25*(4), 405–409. DOI: 10.5021/ad.2013.25.4.405 PMID: 24371385

Kim, B., & Lee, W.-W. (2021). Regulatory Role of Zinc in Immune Cell Signaling. *Molecules and Cells*, *44*(5), 335–341. DOI: 10.14348/molcells.2021.0061 PMID: 33986184

King, J. C. (2000). Physiology of pregnancy and nutrient metabolism. *The American Journal of Clinical Nutrition*, *71*(5), 1218S–1225S. DOI: 10.1093/ajcn/71.5.1218s PMID: 10799394

King, J. C. (2011). Zinc: An essential but elusive nutrient. *The American Journal of Clinical Nutrition*, *94*(2), 679S–684S. DOI: 10.3945/ajcn.110.005744 PMID: 21715515

King, J. C., Brown, K. H., Gibson, R. S., Krebs, N. F., Lowe, N. M., Siekmann, J. H., & Raiten, D. J. (2016). Biomarkers of Nutrition for Development (BOND)—Zinc review. *The Journal of Nutrition*, *146*(4), 858S–885S. DOI: 10.3945/jn.115.220079 PMID: 26962190

King, J. C., Shames, D. M., & Woodhouse, L. R. (2000). Zinc Homeostasis in Humans. *The Journal of Nutrition*, *130*(5), 1360S–1366S. DOI: 10.1093/jn/130.5.1360S PMID: 10801944

Kiouri, D. P., Tsoupra, E., Peana, M., Perlepes, S. P., Stefanidou, M. E., & Chasapis, C. T. (2023). Multifunctional role of zinc in human health: An update. *EXCLI Journal*, *22*, 809. PMID: 37780941

Kiran, A., Wakeel, A., Mahmood, K., Mubaraka, R., Hafsa, , & Haefele, S. M. (2022). Biofortification of Staple Crops to Alleviate Human Malnutrition: Contributions and Potential in Developing Countries. *Agronomy (Basel)*, *12*(2), 452. DOI: 10.3390/agronomy12020452

Kloubert, V., Wessels, I., Wolf, J., Blaabjerg, K., Janssens, V., Hapala, J., Wagner, W., & Rink, L. (2021). Zinc deficiency leads to reduced interleukin-2 production by active gene silencing due to enhanced CREMα expression in T cells. *Clinical Nutrition (Edinburgh, Lothian)*, *40*(5), 3263–3278. DOI: 10.1016/j.clnu.2020.10.052 PMID: 33183881

Klug, A. (1999). Zinc finger peptides for the regulation of gene expression. *Journal of Molecular Biology*, *293*(2), 215–218. DOI: 10.1006/jmbi.1999.3007 PMID: 10529348

Knez, M., & Stangoulis, J. C. (2023). Dietary Zn deficiency, the current situation and potential solutions. *Nutrition Research Reviews*, *36*(2), 199–215. DOI: 10.1017/S0954422421000342 PMID: 37062532

Kohn, S., Kohn, D., & Schiller, D. (2000). Effect of zinc supplementation on epidermal Langerhans'cells of elderly patients with decubital ulcers. *The Journal of Dermatology*, *27*(4), 2558–2563. DOI: 10.1111/j.1346-8138.2000.tb02161.x PMID: 10824490

Kondaiah, P., Yaduvanshi, P. S., Sharp, P. A., & Pullakhandam, R. (2019). Iron and zinc homeostasis and interactions: Does enteric zinc excretion cross-talk with intestinal iron absorption? *Nutrients, 11*(8), 1885. DOI: 10.3390/nu11081885 PMID: 31412634

Koop, A. H., Mousa, O. Y., Pham, L. E., Corral-Hurtado, J. E., Pungpapong, S., & Keaveny, A. P. (2018). An argument for vitamin D, A, and zinc monitoring in cirrhosis. *Annals of Hepatology, 17*(6), 920–932. DOI: 10.5604/01.3001.0012.7192 PMID: 30600288

Korichneva, I. (2006). Zinc dynamics in the myocardial redox signaling network. *Antioxidants & Redox Signaling, 8*(9-10), 1707–1721. DOI: 10.1089/ars.2006.8.1707 PMID: 16987023

Kotnis, A., Bhatt, G. C., Joshi, D., Shukla, A. K., Gupta, P., Shah, D., Choudhary, B., Patil, R., Dubey, S. K., Shukla, M., Joshi, A., & Pakhare, A. P. (2022). Assessment of zinc inadequacy among tribal adolescent population of central India-A cross-sectional study. *The Indian Journal of Medical Research, 156*(2), 339–347. DOI: 10.4103/ijmr.ijmr_3130_21 PMID: 36629194

Kottala, S. Y., & Sahu, A. K. (2023). Evaluating ergonomics and financial distress in manufacturing organization behavior: Resiliency framework from operations and strategic management. *The Learning Organization*. Advance online publication. DOI: 10.1108/TLO-03-2023-0041

Krebs, N. F. (1998). Zinc supplementation during lactation. *The American Journal of Clinical Nutrition, 68*(2, SUPPL.), 509S–512S. Advance online publication. DOI: 10.1093/ajcn/68.2.509S PMID: 9701169

Krebs, N. F. (2000). Overview of zinc absorption and excretion in the human gastrointestinal tract. *The Journal of Nutrition, 130*(5), 1374S–1377S. DOI: 10.1093/jn/130.5.1374S PMID: 10801946

Krebs, N. F. (2013). Update on Zinc Deficiency and Excess in Clinical Pediatric Practice. *Annals of Nutrition & Metabolism, 62*(Suppl. 1), 19–29. DOI: 10.1159/000348261 PMID: 23689110

Kumar, A., Kerketta, A., Dewali, S., Sharma, N., Kumari Panda, A., & Singh Bisht, S. (2023). Tackling Hidden Hunger: Understanding Micronutrient Deficiency and Effective Mitigation Strategies. In *Emerging Solutions in Sustainable Food and Nutrition Security* (pp. 305–319). Springer International Publishing., DOI: 10.1007/978-3-031-40908-0_12

Kumari, D., Garg, S., & Bhawrani, P. (2022). Zinc homeostasis in immunity and its association with preterm births. *Scandinavian Journal of Immunology*, *95*(4), e13142. DOI: 10.1111/sji.13142 PMID: 35007353

Kumari, D., Nair, N., & Bedwal, R. (2024). Effects of dietary zinc deficiency and supplementation on prepubertal rat testes: Sulfhydryl and antioxidant status. *Indian Journal of Clinical Biochemistry : IJCB*, *39*(4), 539–547. DOI: 10.1007/s12291-023-01167-8 PMID: 39346712

Kumar, N., Krishnani, K. K., & Singh, N. P. (2018). Effect of dietary zinc-nanoparticles on growth performance, anti-oxidative and immunological status of fish reared under multiple stressors. *Biological Trace Element Research*, *186*(1), 267–278. DOI: 10.1007/s12011-018-1285-2 PMID: 29524193

Kumssa, D. B., Joy, E. J. M., Ander, E. L., Watts, M. J., Young, S. D., Walker, S., & Broadley, M. R. (2015). Dietary calcium and zinc deficiency risks are decreasing but remain prevalent. *Scientific Reports*, *5*(1), 10974. DOI: 10.1038/srep10974 PMID: 26098577

Kvamme, J.-M., Grønli, O., Jacobsen, B. K., & Florholmen, J. (2015). Risk of malnutrition and zinc deficiency in community-living elderly men and women: The Tromsø Study. *Public Health Nutrition*, *18*(11), 1907–1913. DOI: 10.1017/S1368980014002420 PMID: 25373445

Ladipo, O. A. (2000). Nutrition in pregnancy: Mineral and vitamin supplements. *The American Journal of Clinical Nutrition*, *72*(1), 280S–290S. DOI: 10.1093/ajcn/72.1.280S PMID: 10871594

Laity, J. H., Lee, B. M., & Wright, P. E. (2001). Zinc finger proteins: New insights into structural and functional diversity. *Current Opinion in Structural Biology*, *11*(1), 39–46. DOI: 10.1016/S0959-440X(00)00167-6 PMID: 11179890

Lakey-Beitia, J., Burillo, A. M., La Penna, G., Hegde, M. L., & Rao, K. (2021). Polyphenols as potential metal chelation compounds against Alzheimer's disease. *Journal of Alzheimer's Disease*, *82*(s1), S335–S357. DOI: 10.3233/JAD-200185 PMID: 32568200

Lakshmi, V., & Bandi, K. (2024). Zinc Deficiency. In Nayak, A., & Misra, S. (Eds.), *Advances in Medical Diagnosis, Treatment, and Care* (pp. 248–263). IGI Global., DOI: 10.4018/979-8-3693-2947-4.ch014

Lamberti, L. M., Walker, C. L. F., & Black, R. E. (2016). Zinc deficiency in childhood and pregnancy: Evidence for intervention effects and program responses, Hidden hunger. *Karger Publishers, 115*, 125–133.

Lamberti, L. M., Fischer Walker, C. L., Chan, K. Y., Jian, W.-Y., & Black, R. E. (2013). Oral zinc supplementation for the treatment of acute diarrhea in children: A systematic review and meta-analysis. *Nutrients*, *5*(11), 4715–4740. DOI: 10.3390/nu5114715 PMID: 24284615

Lansdown, A. B. G. (1996). Zinc in the healing wound. *Lancet*, *347*(9003), 706–707. DOI: 10.1016/S0140-6736(96)90072-0 PMID: 8601997

Larson, C. P., Koehlmoos, T. P., Sack, D. A., & Team, S. U. (2012). Scaling up zinc treatment of childhood diarrhoea in Bangladesh: Theoretical and practical considerations guiding the SUZY Project. *Health Policy and Planning*, *27*(2), 102–114. DOI: 10.1093/heapol/czr015 PMID: 21343236

Larson-Meyer, D. E., Woolf, K., & Burke, L. (2018). Assessment of nutrient status in athletes and the need for supplementation. *International Journal of Sport Nutrition and Exercise Metabolism*, *28*(2), 139–158. DOI: 10.1123/ijsnem.2017-0338 PMID: 29252049

Lassi, Z. S., Kurji, J., de Oliveira, C. S., Moin, A., & Bhutta, Z. A. (2020). Zinc supplementation for the promotion of growth and prevention of infections in infants less than six months of age. *Cochrane Database of Systematic Reviews*, *2020*(4). Advance online publication. DOI: 10.1002/14651858.CD010205.pub2 PMID: 32266964

Lazarczyk, M., Pons, C., Mendoza, J. A., Cassonnet, P., Jacob, Y., & Favre, M. (2008). Regulation of cellular zinc balance as a potential mechanism of EVER- mediated protection against pathogenesis by cutaneous oncogenic human papillomaviruses. *The Journal of Experimental Medicine*, *205*(1), 35–42. DOI: 10.1084/jem.20071311 PMID: 18158319

Lee, H. H., Prasad, A. S., Brewer, G. J., & Owyang, C. (1989). Zinc absorption in human small intestine. *The American Journal of Physiology*, *256*, G87–G91. PMID: 2912154

Lee, J., Tucker, R. M., Tan, S. Y., Running, C. A., Jones, J. B., & Mattes, R. D. (2015). Nutritional Implications of Taste and Smell Dysfunction. In Doty, R. L. (Ed.), *Handbook of Olfaction and Gustation* (1st ed., pp. 829–864). Wiley., DOI: 10.1002/9781118971758.ch37

Lee, S. R. (2018). Critical Role of Zinc as Either an Antioxidant or a Prooxidant in Cellular Systems. *Oxidative Medicine and Cellular Longevity*, *2018*(1), 1–11. DOI: 10.1155/2018/9156285 PMID: 29743987

Lei, G. J., Yamaji, N., & Ma, J. F. (2021). Two metallothionein genes highly expressed in rice nodes are involved in distribution of Zn to the grain. *The New Phytologist*, *229*(2), 1007–1020. DOI: 10.1111/nph.16860 PMID: 32772382

Li, Z., Liu, Y., Wei, R., Yong, V. W., & Xue, M. (2023). The Important Role of Zinc in Neurological Diseases. In *Biomolecules* (Vol. 13, Issue 1). MDPI. DOI: 10.3390/biom13010028

Lichten, L. A., & Cousins, R. J. (2009). Mammalian Zinc Transporters: Nutritional and Physiologic Regulation. *Annual Review of Nutrition*, *29*(1), 153–176. DOI: 10.1146/annurev-nutr-033009-083312 PMID: 19400752

Li, J., Cao, D., Huang, Y., Chen, B., Chen, Z., Wang, R., Dong, Q., Wei, Q., & Liu, L. (2022). Zinc intakes and health outcomes: An umbrella review. *Frontiers in Nutrition*, *9*, 798078. DOI: 10.3389/fnut.2022.798078 PMID: 35211497

Li, L., He, Y., Song, K., Xie, F., Li, H., & Sun, F. (2021). Derivation of water quality criteria of zinc to protect aquatic life in Taihu Lake and the associated risk assessment. *Journal of Environmental Management*, *296*, 113175. DOI: 10.1016/j.jenvman.2021.113175 PMID: 34243093

Lindenmayer, G. W., Stoltzfus, R. J., & Prendergast, A. J. (2014). Interactions between Zinc Deficiency and Environmental Enteropathy in Developing Countries. *Advances in Nutrition*, *5*(1), 1–6. DOI: 10.3945/an.113.004838 PMID: 24425714

Lin, P.-H., Sermersheim, M., Li, H., Lee, P. H. U., Steinberg, S. M., & Ma, J. (2017). Zinc in Wound Healing Modulation. *Nutrients*, *10*(1), 16. DOI: 10.3390/nu10010016 PMID: 29295546

Liu, E., Pimpin, L., Shulkin, M., Kranz, S., Duggan, C. P., Mozaffarian, D., & Fawzi, W. (2018). Effect of zinc supplementation on growth outcomes in children under 5 years of age. *Nutrients*, *10*(3), 377. DOI: 10.3390/nu10030377 PMID: 29558383

Liu, H. Y., Gale, J. R., Reynolds, I. J., Weiss, J. H., & Aizenman, E. (2021). The multifaceted roles of zinc in neuronal mitochondrial dysfunction. *Biomedicines*, *9*(5), 489. DOI: 10.3390/biomedicines9050489 PMID: 33946782

Liu, Y., Chen, S., Zühlke, L., Black, G. C., Choy, M., Li, N., & Keavney, B. D. (2019). Global birth prevalence of congenital heart defects 1970–2017: Updated systematic review and meta-analysis of 260 studies. *International Journal of Epidemiology*, *48*(2), 455–463. DOI: 10.1093/ije/dyz009 PMID: 30783674

Livingstone, C. (2015). Zinc: Physiology, Deficiency, and Parenteral Nutrition. *Nutrition in Clinical Practice*, *30*(3), 371–382. DOI: 10.1177/0884533615570376 PMID: 25681484

Li, X., Yadav, R., & Siddique, K. H. (2020). Neglected and underutilized crop species: The key to improving dietary diversity and fighting hunger and malnutrition in Asia and the Pacific. *Frontiers in Nutrition*, *7*, 593711. DOI: 10.3389/fnut.2020.593711 PMID: 33330593

Lockyer, S., White, A., & Buttriss, J. L. (2018). Biofortified crops for tackling micronutrient deficiencies – what impact are these having in developing countries and could they be of relevance within Europe? *Nutrition Bulletin*, *43*(4), 319–357. DOI: 10.1111/nbu.12347

Loechl, C. U., Datta-Mitra, A., Fenlason, L., Green, R., Hackl, L., Itzkowitz, L., Koso-Thomas, M., Moorthy, D., Owino, V. O., Pachón, H., Stoffel, N., Zimmerman, M. B., & Raiten, D. J. (2023). Approaches to address the anemia challenge. *The Journal of Nutrition*, *153*, S42–S59. DOI: 10.1016/j.tjnut.2023.07.017 PMID: 37714779

Lönnerdal, B. (2000). Dietary factors influencing zinc absorption. *The Journal of Nutrition*, *130*(5, SUPPL.), 1378S–1383S. Advance online publication. DOI: 10.1093/jn/130.5.1378S PMID: 10801947

Lönnerdal, B. (2003). Genetically modified plants for improved trace element nutrition. *The Journal of Nutrition*, *133*(5), 1490S–S1493. DOI: 10.1093/jn/133.5.1490S PMID: 12730450

Lopes-Pires, M. E., Ahmed, N. S., Vara, D., Gibbins, J. M., Pula, G., & Pugh, N. (2021). Zinc regulates reactive oxygen species generation in platelets. *Platelets*, *32*(3), 368–377. DOI: 10.1080/09537104.2020.1742311 PMID: 32248725

Lotfi, M., Venkatesh Mannar, M. G., Merx, R. J., & Naber-van den Heuvel, P. (1996). *Micronutrient fortification of foods: Current practices, research, and opportunities*. IDRC, Micronutrient Initiative., https://idl-bnc-idrc.dspacedirect.org/bitstream/handle/10625/14002/104386.pdf?sequence=1

Lovat, L. B. (1996). Age related changes in gut physiology and nutritional status. *Gut*, *38*(3), 306–309. DOI: 10.1136/gut.38.3.306 PMID: 8675079

Lowe, N. M., Hall, A. G., Broadley, M. R., Foley, J., Boy, E., & Bhutta, Z. A. (2024). Preventing and Controlling Zinc Deficiency Across the Life Course: A Call to Action. *Advances in Nutrition*, *15*(3), 100181. DOI: 10.1016/j.advnut.2024.100181 PMID: 38280724

Luan, R., Ding, D., Xue, Q., Li, H., Wang, Y., & Yang, J. (2023). Protective role of zinc in the pathogenesis of respiratory diseases. *European Journal of Clinical Nutrition*, *77*(4), 427–435. DOI: 10.1038/s41430-022-01191-6 PMID: 35982216

Ludwig, Y., Dueñas, C.Jr, Arcillas, E., Macalalad-Cabral, R. J., Kohli, A., Reinke, R., & Slamet-Loedin, I. H. (2024). CRISPR-mediated promoter editing of a cis-regulatory element of OsNAS2 increases Zn uptake/translocation and plant yield in rice. *Frontiers in Genome Editing*, *5*, 1308228. DOI: 10.3389/fgeed.2023.1308228 PMID: 38322756

Lu, J., Zhang, H., Cao, W., Jiang, S., Fang, H., Yu, D., & Yang, L. (2023). Study on the Zinc Nutritional Status and Risk Factors of Chinese 6–18-Year-Old Children. *Nutrients*, *15*(7), 1685. DOI: 10.3390/nu15071685 PMID: 37049525

MacDonald, R. S. (2000). The Role of Zinc in Growth and Cell Proliferation. *The Journal of Nutrition*, *130*(5), 1500S–1508S. DOI: 10.1093/jn/130.5.1500S PMID: 10801966

Ma, G., Jin, Y., Li, Y., Zhai, F., Kok, F. J., Jacobsen, E., & Yang, X. (2008). Iron and zinc deficiencies in China: What is a feasible and cost-effective strategy? *Public Health Nutrition*, *11*(6), 632–638. DOI: 10.1017/S1368980007001085 PMID: 17894916

Maggini, S., Maldonado, P., Cardim, P., Fernandez Newball, C., & Sota Latino, E. (2017). Vitamins C, D and zinc: Synergistic roles in immune function and infections. *Vitam Miner*, *6*(167), 2376–1318. DOI: 10.4172/2376-1318.1000167

Maggini, S., Pierre, A., & Calder, P. (2018). Immune Function and Micronutrient Requirements Change over the Life Course. *Nutrients*, *10*(10), 1531. DOI: 10.3390/nu10101531 PMID: 30336639

Malavolta, M., Costarelli, L., Giacconi, R., Basso, A., Piacenza, F., Pierpaoli, E., Provinciali, M., Ogo, O. A., & Ford, D. (2017). Changes in Zn homeostasis during long term culture of primary endothelial cells and effects of Zn on endothelial cell senescence. *Experimental Gerontology*, *99*, 35–45. DOI: 10.1016/j.exger.2017.09.006 PMID: 28918363

Manford, M. (2017). Recent advances in epilepsy. *Journal of Neurology*, *264*(8), 1811–1824. DOI: 10.1007/s00415-017-8394-2 PMID: 28120042

Manzeke-Kangara, M. G., Joy, E. J. M., Mtambanengwe, F., Chopera, P., Watts, M. J., Broadley, M. R., & Mapfumo, P. (2021). Good soil management can reduce dietary zinc deficiency in Zimbabwe. *CABI Agriculture and Bioscience*, *2*(1), 36. DOI: 10.1186/s43170-021-00057-4

Manzoor, M. F., Ali, A., Ain, H. B. U., Kausar, S., Khalil, A. A., Aadil, R. M., & Zeng, X.-A. (2024). Bioaccessibility mechanisms, fortification strategies, processing impact on bioavailability, and therapeutic potentials of minerals in cereals. *Future Foods : a Dedicated Journal for Sustainability in Food Science*, *10*, 100425. DOI: 10.1016/j.fufo.2024.100425

Mao, C., Shen, Z., Long, D., Liu, M., Xu, X., Gao, X., Lin, Y., & Wang, X. (2024). Epidemiological study of paediatric nutritional deficiencies: An analysis from the global burden of disease study 2019. *Nutrition Journal*, *23*(1), 44. DOI: 10.1186/s12937-024-00945-1 PMID: 38637763

Maret, W. (2001). Zinc biochemistry, physiology, and homeostasis: Recent insights and current trends. *Biometals*, *14*(3/4), 187–190. DOI: 10.1023/A:1012945110820

Maret, W., & Sandstead, H. H. (2006). Zinc requirements and the risks and benefits of zinc supplementation. *Journal of Trace Elements in Medicine and Biology*, *20*(1), 3–18. DOI: 10.1016/j.jtemb.2006.01.006 PMID: 16632171

Marger, L., Schubert, C., & Bertrand, D. (2014). Zinc: An underappreciated modulatory factor of brain function. *Biochemical Pharmacology*, *91*(4), 426–435. DOI: 10.1016/j.bcp.2014.08.002 PMID: 25130547

Mariotti, F. (2023). Nutritional and health benefits and risks of plant-based substitute foods. *Proceedings of the Nutrition Society*, 1-14.DOI: 10.1017/S0029665123004767

Ma, Y., Wen, Y., Wang, C., Wu, Z., Yuan, X., Xiong, Y., Chen, K., He, L., Zhang, Y., Wang, Z., Li, L., Yang, Z., Sun, Y., Chen, Z., & Ma, J. (2023). ZIP genes are involved in the retransfer of zinc ions during the senescence of zinc-deficient rice leaves. *International Journal of Molecular Sciences*, *24*(18), 13989. DOI: 10.3390/ijms241813989 PMID: 37762290

Mayo-Wilson, E., Junior, J. A., Imdad, A., Dean, S., Chan, X. H., Chan, E. S., Jaswal, A., & Bhutta, Z. A. (2014). Zinc supplementation for preventing mortality, morbidity, and growth failure in children aged 6 months to 12 years of age. *Cochrane Database of Systematic Reviews*, *2014*(5), CD009384. DOI: 10.1002/14651858.CD009384.pub2 PMID: 24826920

Maywald, M., & Rink, L. (2022). Zinc in human health and infectious diseases. *Biomolecules*, *12*(12), 1748. DOI: 10.3390/biom12121748 PMID: 36551176

McClements, I. F., & McClements, D. J. (2023). Designing healthier plant-based foods: Fortification, digestion, and bioavailability. *Food Research International*, *169*, 112853. DOI: 10.1016/j.foodres.2023.112853 PMID: 37254427

McCusker, M. M., Durrani, K., Payette, M. J., & Suchecki, J. (2016). An eye on nutrition: The role of vitamins, essential fatty acids, and antioxidants in age-related macular degeneration, dry eye syndrome, and cataract. *Clinics in Dermatology*, *34*(2), 276–285. DOI: 10.1016/j.clindermatol.2015.11.009 PMID: 26903189

McDonald, C. M., Suchdev, P. S., Krebs, N. F., Hess, S. Y., Wessells, K. R., Ismaily, S., Rahman, S., Wieringa, F. T., Williams, A. M., Brown, K. H., & King, J. C. (2020). Adjusting plasma or serum zinc concentrations for inflammation: Biomarkers Reflecting Inflammation and Nutritional Determinants of Anemia (BRINDA) project. *The American Journal of Clinical Nutrition*, *111*(4), 927–937. DOI: 10.1093/ajcn/nqz304 PMID: 32266402

Mehata, S., Tamang, M. K., Parajuli, K. R., Rayamajhee, B., Yadav, U. N., Mehta, R. K., & Singh, D. R. (2021). Serum zinc status is a matter of concern among children and non-pregnant women in a nationwide survey of Nepal. *Scientific Reports*, *11*(1), 14904. DOI: 10.1038/s41598-021-94344-9 PMID: 34290324

Mentella, M. C., Scaldaferri, F., Pizzoferrato, M., Gasbarrini, A., & Miggiano, G. A. D. (2020). Nutrition, IBD and gut microbiota: A review. *Nutrients*, *12*(4), 944. DOI: 10.3390/nu12040944 PMID: 32235316

Mertens, A., Benjamin-Chung, J., Colford, J. M.Jr, Coyle, J., Van der Laan, M. J., Hubbard, A. E., & Arnold, B. F. (2023). Causes and consequences of child growth faltering in low-resource settings. *Nature*, *621*(7979), 568–576. DOI: 10.1038/s41586-023-06501-x PMID: 37704722

Mezzaroba, L., Alfieri, D. F., Simão, A. N. C., & Reiche, E. M. V. (2019). The role of zinc, copper, manganese and iron in neurodegenerative diseases. *Neurotoxicology*, *74*, 230–241. DOI: 10.1016/j.neuro.2019.07.007 PMID: 31377220

Mirnamniha, M., Faroughi, F., Tahmasbpour, E., Ebrahimi, P., & Beigi Harchegani, A. (2019). An overview on role of some trace elements in human reproductive health, sperm function and fertilization process. *Reviews on Environmental Health*, *34*(4), 339–348. DOI: 10.1515/reveh-2019-0008 PMID: 31203261

Mocchegiani, E., Romeo, J., Malavolta, M., Costarelli, L., Giacconi, R., Diaz, L.-E., & Marcos, A. (2013). Zinc: Dietary intake and impact of supplementation on immune function in elderly. *Age (Dordrecht, Netherlands)*, *35*(3), 839–860. DOI: 10.1007/s11357-011-9377-3 PMID: 22222917

Mohammadi, H., Talebi, S., Ghavami, A., Rafiei, M., Sharifi, S., Faghihimani, Z., Ranjbar, G., Miraghajani, M., & Askari, G. (2021). Effects of zinc supplementation on inflammatory biomarkers and oxidative stress in adults: A systematic review and meta-analysis of randomized controlled trials. *Journal of Trace Elements in Medicine and Biology*, *68*, 126857. DOI: 10.1016/j.jtemb.2021.126857 PMID: 34560424

Mohammad, M. K., Zhou, Z., Cave, M., Barve, A., & McClain, C. J. (2012). Zinc and Liver Disease. *Nutrition in Clinical Practice*, *27*(1), 8–20. DOI: 10.1177/0884533611433534 PMID: 22307488

Mohanan, S., Gupta, D., Chandrashekhar, L., Thappa, D. M., & Rajesh, N. G. (2012). Acquired zinc deficiency in an adult female. *Indian Journal of Dermatology*, *57*(6), 492–494. DOI: 10.4103/0019-5154.103073 PMID: 23248371

MoHFW. UNICEF. (2019). *Comprehensive National Nutrition Survey 2016–2018* [Comprehensive National Nutrition Survey (CNNS)]. Ministry of Health and Family Welfare (MoHFW), Government of India, UNICEF and Population Council. https://www.unicef.org/india/media/2646/file/CNNS-report.pdf

Mohn, E., Kern, H., Saltzman, E., Mitmesser, S., & McKay, D. (2018). Evidence of Drug–Nutrient Interactions with Chronic Use of Commonly Prescribed Medications: An Update. *Pharmaceutics*, *10*(1), 36. DOI: 10.3390/pharmaceutics10010036 PMID: 29558445

Molenda, M., & Kolmas, J. (2023). The Role of Zinc in Bone Tissue Health and Regeneration—A Review. *Biological Trace Element Research*, *201*(12), 5640–5651. DOI: 10.1007/s12011-023-03631-1 PMID: 37002364

Montoro-Huguet, M. A., Belloc, B., & Domínguez-Cajal, M. (2021). Small and Large Intestine (I): Malabsorption of Nutrients. *Nutrients*, *13*(4), 1254. DOI: 10.3390/nu13041254 PMID: 33920345

Morel, L. N., Schaefer, S. M., & Hivnor, C. M. (2018). Nutritional diseases. In Bolognia, J. L., Schaffer, J. V., & Cerroni, L. (Eds.), *Dermatology* (4th ed., p. 804). Elsevier.

Morgan, C. I., Ledford, J. R., Zhou, P., & Page, K. (2011). Zinc supplementation alters airway inflammation and airway hyperresponsiveness to a common allergen. *Journal of Inflammation (London, England)*, *8*(1), 36. DOI: 10.1186/1476-9255-8-36 PMID: 22151973

Moser-Veillon, P. B. (1990). Zinc: Consumption patterns and dietary recommendations. *Journal of the American Dietetic Association*, *90*(8), 1089–1094. DOI: 10.1016/S0002-8223(21)01706-5 PMID: 2166098

Mossad, S. B., Macknin, M. L., Mendendorp, S. V., & Mason, P. (1996). Zinc Gluconate Lozenges for Treating the Common Cold: A Randomized, Double-Blind, Placebo-Controlled Study. *Annals of Internal Medicine*, *125*(2), 81–88. DOI: 10.7326/0003-4819-125-2-199607150-00001 PMID: 8678384

Mozaffar, B., Ardavani, A., Muzafar, H., & Idris, I. (2023). The Effectiveness of Zinc Supplementation in Taste Disorder Treatment: A Systematic Review and Meta-Analysis of Randomized Controlled Trials. *Journal of Nutrition and Metabolism*, *2023*, 1–13. DOI: 10.1155/2023/6711071 PMID: 36937245

Muddasani, S., Lin, G., Hooper, J., & Sloan, S. B. (2021). Nutrition and nail disease. *Clinics in Dermatology*, *39*(5), 819–828. DOI: 10.1016/j.clindermatol.2021.05.009 PMID: 34785009

Mukhopadhyay, S., Mukherjee, S., Hashim, M. A., Sahu, J. N., Martinez-Villegas, N., & Gupta, B. S. (2018). Zinc removal from soil by washing with saponin obtained from *Sapindus mukorossi.Journal of Environmental Analytical Chemistry*, *5*(4). Advance online publication. DOI: 10.4172/2380-2391.1000249

Muller, O., Becher, H., van Zweeden, A. B., Ye, Y., Diallo, D. A., Konate, A. T., Gbangou, A., Kouyate, B., & Garenne, M. (2001). Effect of zinc supplementation on malaria and other causes of morbidity in west African children: Randomised double blind placebo-controlled trial. *British Medical Journal*, *322*(7302), 1567–1574. DOI: 10.1136/bmj.322.7302.1567 PMID: 11431296

Munshi, A., Babu, S., Kaul, S., Shafi, G., Rajeshwar, K., Alladi, S., & Jyothy, A. (2010). Depletion of serum zinc in ischemic stroke patients. *Methods and Findings in Experimental and Clinical Pharmacology*, *32*(6), 433–436. DOI: 10.1358/mf.2010.32.6.1487084 PMID: 20852753

Murray, R. M., Davis, A. L., Shepler, L. J., Moore-Merrell, L., Troup, W. J., Allen, J. A., & Taylor, J. A. (2020). A Systematic Review of Workplace Violence Against Emergency Medical Services Responders. *New Solutions*, *29*(4), 487–503. DOI: 10.1177/1048291119893388 PMID: 31841060

Muthukumar, J., Selvasekaran, P., Lokanadham, M., & Chidambaram, R. (2020). Food and food products associated with food allergy and food intolerance – An overview. *Food Research International*, *138*, 109780. DOI: 10.1016/j.foodres.2020.109780 PMID: 33288166

Mwangi, M. N., Oonincx, D. G., Stouten, T., Veenenbos, M., Melse-Boonstra, A., Dicke, M., & Van Loon, J. J. (2018). Insects as sources of iron and zinc in human nutrition. *Nutrition Research Reviews*, *31*(2), 248–255. DOI: 10.1017/S0954422418000094 PMID: 30033906

Myers, S. S., Wessells, K. R., Kloog, I., Zanobetti, A., & Schwartz, J. (2015). Effect of increased concentrations of atmospheric carbon dioxide on the global threat of zinc deficiency: A modelling study. *The Lancet. Global Health*, *3*(10), e639–e645. DOI: 10.1016/S2214-109X(15)00093-5 PMID: 26189102

Naem, N. E., El-Sayed, N. M., Nossier, S. A., & Zeid, A. A. A. (2014). Zinc status and dietary intake of pregnant women, Alexandria, Egypt. *The Journal of the Egyptian Public Health Association*, *89*(1), 35–41. DOI: 10.1097/01.EPX.0000443987.44261.9b PMID: 24717399

Naik, B., Kumar, V., Rizwanuddin, S., Mishra, S., Kumar, V., Saris, P. E. J., Khanduri, N., Kumar, A., Pandey, P., Gupta, A. K., Khan, J. M., & Rustagi, S. (2024). Biofortification as a solution for addressing nutrient deficiencies and malnutrition. *Heliyon*, *10*(9), e30595. DOI: 10.1016/j.heliyon.2024.e30595 PMID: 38726166

Nair, M. K., Augustine, L. F., & Konapur, A. (2016). Food-Based Interventions to Modify Diet Quality and Diversity to Address Multiple Micronutrient Deficiency. *Frontiers in Public Health*, *3*. Advance online publication. DOI: 10.3389/fpubh.2015.00277 PMID: 26779472

Nalyotov, A. V., Matsynin, A. N., & Matsynina, M. A. (2022). Zinc Availability is an Important Indicator of Human Health. *Health. Food Biotechnology*, *4*(3), 12–18.

Nasiadek, M., Stragierowicz, J., Klimczak, M., & Kilanowicz, A. (2020). The role of zinc in selected female reproductive system disorders. *Nutrients*, *12*(8), 2464. DOI: 10.3390/nu12082464 PMID: 32824334

National Institutes of Health. (2022, January 3). *Zinc: Fact Sheet for Health Professionals*. Office of Dietary Supplements. https://ods.od.nih.gov/factsheets/Zinc-HealthProfessional

Nestel, P., Bouis, H. E., Meenakshi, J. V., & Pfeiffer, W. (2006). Biofortification of staple food crops. *The Journal of Nutrition*, *136*(4), 1064–1067. DOI: 10.1093/jn/136.4.1064 PMID: 16549478

Neufingerl, N., & Eilander, A. (2021). Nutrient intake and status in adults consuming plant-based diets compared to meat-eaters: A systematic review. *Nutrients*, *14*(1), 29. DOI: 10.3390/nu14010029 PMID: 35010904

Nissar, J., Ahad, T., Naik, H. R., & Hussain, S. Z. (2017). A review phytic acid: As antinutrient or nutraceutical. *Journal of Pharmacognosy and Phytochemistry*, *6*(6), 1554–1560.

Nissar, J., Ahad, T., Naik, H., & Hussain, S. (2017). A review: Phytic acid—As antinutrient or nutraceutical. *Journal of Pharmacognosy and Phytochemistry, 6*(6), 1554–1560.

Nolla, N. P., Sop, M. M. K., Mananga, M. J., & Gouado, I. (2021). Nutrition Education of Mothers and Zinc Supplementation among Children in the Rural Community, Cameroon. *European Journal of Nutrition & Food Safety, 13*(1), 59–69. DOI: 10.9734/ejnfs/2021/v13i130348

Norman, K., Haß, U., & Pirlich, M. (2021). Malnutrition in Older Adults—Recent Advances and Remaining Challenges. *Nutrients, 13*(8), 2764. DOI: 10.3390/nu13082764 PMID: 34444924

Noulas, C., Tziouvalekas, M., & Karyotis, T. (2018). Zinc in soils, water and food crops. *Journal of Trace Elements in Medicine and Biology, 49*, 252–260. DOI: 10.1016/j.jtemb.2018.02.009 PMID: 29472130

Nriagu, J. (2007). Zinc toxicity in humans. *School of Public Health, University of Michigan*, 1–7.

O'dell, B. L., Burpo, C. E., & Savage, J. E. (1972). Evaluation of zinc availability in foodstuffs of plant and animal origin. *The Journal of Nutrition, 102*(5), 653–660. DOI: 10.1093/jn/102.5.653 PMID: 5063219

Obeagu, E. I., Ubosi, N. I., & Uzoma, G. (2023). Antioxidant Supplementation in Pregnancy: Effects on Maternal and Infant Health. *Int. J. Adv. Multidiscip. Res, 10*(11), 60–70.

Ogawa, Y., Kawamura, T., & Shimada, S. (2016). Zinc and skin biology. *Archives of Biochemistry and Biophysics, 611*, 113–119. DOI: 10.1016/j.abb.2016.06.003 PMID: 27288087

Ogawa, Y., Kinoshita, M., Shimada, S., & Kawamura, T. (2018). Zinc and skin disorders. *Nutrients, 10*(2), 199. DOI: 10.3390/nu10020199 PMID: 29439479

Ohanenye, I. C., Emenike, C. U., Mensi, A., Medina-Godoy, S., Jin, J., Ahmed, T., Sun, X., & Udenigwe, C. C. (2021). Food fortification technologies: Influence on iron, zinc and vitamin A bioavailability and potential implications on micronutrient deficiency in sub-Saharan Africa. *Scientific African, 11*, e00667. DOI: 10.1016/j.sciaf.2020.e00667

Oh, C., Keats, E., & Bhutta, Z. (2020). Vitamin and Mineral Supplementation During Pregnancy on Maternal, Birth, Child Health and Development Outcomes in Low- and Middle-Income Countries: A Systematic Review and Meta-Analysis. *Nutrients, 12*(2), 491. DOI: 10.3390/nu12020491 PMID: 32075071

Orth, G. (2008). Host defenses against human papillomaviruses: Lessons from epidermodysplasia verruciformis. *Current Topics in Microbiology and Immunology*, *321*, 59–83. DOI: 10.1007/978-3-540-75203-5_3 PMID: 18727487

Osmani, S., Smidt, A. C., Phan, C. M., & Johnson, D. W. (2021). Acquired acrodermatitis enteropathica from a ketogenic diet. *JAAD Case Reports*, *9*, 75–77. DOI: 10.1016/j.jdcr.2021.01.016 PMID: 33665283

Osredkar, J., & Sustar, N. (2011). Copper and zinc, biological role and significance of copper/zinc imbalance. *J Clinic Toxicol s, 3*(2161), 0495.

Oteiza, P. I., & Mackenzie, G. G. (2005). Zinc, oxidant-triggered cell signaling, and human health. *Molecular Aspects of Medicine*, *26*(4–5), 245–255. DOI: 10.1016/j.mam.2005.07.012 PMID: 16115673

Outten, C. E., & O'Halloran, T. V. (2001). Femtomolar Sensitivity of Metalloregulatory Proteins Controlling Zinc Homeostasis. *Science*, *292*(5526), 2488–2492. DOI: 10.1126/science.1060331 PMID: 11397910

Oz, A. T., & Kafkas, E. (2017). Phytochemicals in fruits and vegetables. In Waisundara, V. (Ed.), *Superfood and functional food* (pp. 175–184). IntechOpen.

Ozturk, H., Niazi, P., Mansoor, M., Monib, A. W., Alikhail, M., & Azizi, A. (2023). The function of zinc in animal, plant, and human nutrition. *Journal for Research in Applied Sciences and Biotechnology*, *2*(2), 35–43. DOI: 10.55544/jrasb.2.2.6

Pachón, H., Reynolds, B., Duong, M., Tsang, B. L., Childs, L., Luthringer, C. L., Kang, Y., Vasta, F. C., & Codling, K. (2021). The potential contribution of fortified maize flour, oil, rice, salt, and wheat flour to estimated average requirements and tolerable upper intake levels for 15 nutrients in 153 countries. *Nutrients*, *13*(2), 579. DOI: 10.3390/nu13020579 PMID: 33572488

Pajarillo, E. A. B., Lee, E., & Kang, D. K. (2021). Trace metals and animal health: Interplay of the gut microbiota with iron, manganese, zinc, and copper. *Animal Nutrition*, *7*(3), 750–761. DOI: 10.1016/j.aninu.2021.03.005 PMID: 34466679

Palacios, A. M., Hurley, K. M., De-Ponce, S., Alfonso, V., Tilton, N., Lambden, K. B., Reinhart, G. A., Freeland-Graves, J. H., Villanueva, L. M., & Black, M. M. (2020). Zinc deficiency associated with anaemia among young children in rural Guatemala. *Maternal and Child Nutrition*, *16*(1), e12885. DOI: 10.1111/mcn.12885 PMID: 31595712

Palmer, A. C., Bedsaul-Fryer, J. R., & Stephensen, C. B. (2024). Interactions of Nutrition and Infection: The Role of Micronutrient Deficiencies in the Immune Response to Pathogens and Implications for Child Health. *Annual Review of Nutrition*, *44*(1), 99–124. Advance online publication. DOI: 10.1146/annurev-nutr-062122-014910 PMID: 38724105

Palmiter, R. D., & Huang, L. (2004). Efflux and compartmentalization of zinc by members of the SLC30 family of solute carriers. *Pflügers Archiv*, *447*(5), 744–751. DOI: 10.1007/s00424-003-1070-7 PMID: 12748859

Panchariya, L., Khan, W. A., Kuila, S., Sonkar, K., Sahoo, S., Ghoshal, A., Kumar, A., Verma, D. K., Hasan, A., Khan, M. A., Jain, N., Mohapatra, A. K., Das, S., Thakur, J. K., Maiti, S., Nanda, R. K., Halder, R., Sunil, S., & Arockiasamy, A. (2021). $Zinc^{2+}$ ion inhibits SARS-CoV-2 main protease and viral replication in vitro. *Chemical Communications (Cambridge)*, *57*(78), 10083–10086. DOI: 10.1039/D1CC03563K PMID: 34514483

Parca, F., Koca, Y. O., & Unay, A. (2018). Nutritional and antinutritional factors of some pulses seed and their effects on human health. *International Journal of Secondary Metabolite*, *5*(4), 331–342. DOI: 10.21448/ijsm.488651

Parham, M., Amini, M., Aminorroaya, A., & Heidarian, E. (2008). Effect of zinc supplementation on microalbuminuria in patients with type 2 diabetes: A double blind, randomized, placebo-controlled, cross-over trial. *The Review of Diabetic Studies; RDS*, *5*(2), 102–109. DOI: 10.1900/RDS.2008.5.102 PMID: 18795212

Patil, R., Sontakke, T., Biradar, A., & Nalage, D. (2023). Zinc: An essential trace element for human health and beyond. *Food Health*, *5*(3), 13. DOI: 10.53388/FH2023013

Pellinen, T., Päivärinta, E., Isotalo, J., Lehtovirta, M., Itkonen, S. T., Korkalo, L., & Pajari, A. M. (2022). Replacing dietary animal-source proteins with plant-source proteins changes dietary intake and status of vitamins and minerals in healthy adults: A 12-week randomized controlled trial. *European Journal of Nutrition*, •••, 1–14. PMID: 34837522

Penny, M. E. (2013). Zinc Supplementation in Public Health. *Annals of Nutrition & Metabolism*, *62*(Suppl. 1), 31–42. DOI: 10.1159/000348263 PMID: 23689111

Pérez-Escamilla, R., & Engmann, C. (2019). Integrating nutrition services into health care systems platforms: Where are we and where do we go from here. *Maternal and Child Nutrition*, *15*(S1), e12743. DOI: 10.1111/mcn.12743 PMID: 30748115

Pereznieto, P., & Taylor, G. (2014). A review of approaches and methods to measure economic empowerment of women and girls. *Gender and Development*, *22*(2), 233–251. DOI: 10.1080/13552074.2014.920976

Petrilli, M. A., Kranz, T. M., Kleinhaus, K., Joe, P., Getz, M., Johnson, P., Chao, M. V., & Malaspina, D. (2017). The emerging role for zinc in depression and psychosis. *Frontiers in Pharmacology*, *8*, 414. DOI: 10.3389/fphar.2017.00414 PMID: 28713269

Philipo, M., Ndakidemi, P. A., & Mbega, E. R. (2021). Importance of common bean genetic zinc biofortification in alleviating human zinc deficiency in sub-Saharan Africa. *Cogent Food & Agriculture*, *7*(1), 1907954. DOI: 10.1080/23311932.2021.1907954

Picolo, M., Barros, I., Joyeux, M., Gottwalt, A., Possolo, E., Sigauque, B., & Kavle, J. A. (2019). Rethinking integrated nutrition-health strategies to address micronutrient deficiencies in children under five in Mozambique. *Maternal and Child Nutrition*, *15*(S1), e12721. DOI: 10.1111/mcn.12721 PMID: 30748114

Pinzón-Rondón, Á. M., Hoyos-Martínez, A., Parra-Correa, D., Pedraza-Flechas, A. M., & Ruiz-Sternberg, Á. M. (2019). Association of nutritional support programs with zinc deficiency in Colombian children: A cross-sectional study. *BMC Nutrition*, *5*(1), 42. DOI: 10.1186/s40795-019-0305-8 PMID: 32153955

Płaczek, A., Machaj, D., Białas, F., Cyboran, K., & Kuc, M. (2022). Consequences of zinc deficiency in selected diseases—Literature review. *Journal of Education, Health and Sport*, *12*(7), 775–779. DOI: 10.12775/JEHS.2022.12.07.076

Plum, L. M., Rink, L., & Haase, H. (2010). The essential toxin: Impact of zinc on human health. *International Journal of Environmental Research and Public Health*, *7*(4), 1342–1365. DOI: 10.3390/ijerph7041342 PMID: 20617034

Pompano, L. M., & Boy, E. (2021). Effects of dose and duration of zinc interventions on risk factors for Type 2 Diabetes and cardiovascular disease: A systematic review and meta-analysis. *Advances in Nutrition*, *12*(1), 141–160. DOI: 10.1093/advances/nmaa087 PMID: 32722790

Poudel, P., Di Gioia, F., Lambert, J. D., & Connolly, E. L. (2023). Zinc biofortification through seed nutri-priming using alternative zinc sources and concentration levels in pea and sunflower microgreens. *Frontiers in Plant Science*, *14*, 1177844. DOI: 10.3389/fpls.2023.1177844 PMID: 37139105

Powell, J. J., Jugdaohsingh, R., & Thompson, R. P. H. (1999). The regulation of mineral absorption in the gastrointestinal tract. *The Proceedings of the Nutrition Society*, *58*(1), 147–153. DOI: 10.1079/PNS19990020 PMID: 10343352

Praharaj, S., Skalicky, M., Maitra, S., Bhadra, P., Shankar, T., Brestic, M., Hejnak, V., Vachova, P., & Hossain, A. (2021). Zinc biofortification in food crops could alleviate the zinc malnutrition in human health. *Molecules (Basel, Switzerland)*, *26*(12), 3509. DOI: 10.3390/molecules26123509 PMID: 34207649

Prakash, A., Bharti, K., & Majeed, A. B. A. (2015). Zinc: Indications in brain disorders. *Fundamental & Clinical Pharmacology*, *29*(2), 131–149. DOI: 10.1111/fcp.12110 PMID: 25659970

Prasad, A. S. (1988). Zinc in growth and development and spectrum of human zinc deficiency. *Journal of the American College of Nutrition*, *7*(5), 377–384. DOI: 10.1080/07315724.1988.10720255 PMID: 3053862

Prasad, A. S. (1996). Zinc deficiency in women, infants and children. *Journal of the American College of Nutrition*, *15*(2), 113–120. DOI: 10.1080/07315724.1996.10718575 PMID: 8778139

Prasad, A. S. (1998). Zinc in human health: An update. *The Journal of Trace Elements in Experimental Medicine*, *11*(2–3), 63–87. DOI: 10.1002/(SICI)1520-670X(1998)11:2/3<63::AID-JTRA2>3.0.CO;2-5

Prasad, A. S. (2004). Zinc deficiency: Its characterization and treatment. *Metal Ions in Biological Systems*, *41*, 103–138. PMID: 15206115

Prasad, A. S. (2008). Zinc in Human Health: Effect of Zinc on Immune Cells. *Molecular Medicine (Cambridge, Mass.)*, *14*(5–6), 353–357. DOI: 10.2119/2008-00033.Prasad PMID: 18385818

Prasad, A. S. (2009). Zinc: Role in immunity, oxidative stress and chronic inflammation. *Current Opinion in Clinical Nutrition and Metabolic Care*, *12*(6), 646–652. DOI: 10.1097/MCO.0b013e3283312956 PMID: 19710611

Prasad, A. S. (2013). Discovery of Human Zinc Deficiency: Its Impact on Human Health and Disease. *Advances in Nutrition*, *4*(2), 176–190. DOI: 10.3945/an.112.003210 PMID: 23493534

Prasad, A. S. (2020). Lessons learned from experimental human model of zinc deficiency. *Journal of Immunology Research*, *2020*, 1–12. Advance online publication. DOI: 10.1155/2020/9207279 PMID: 32411807

Prasad, S., & Lall, R. (2022). Zinc-curcumin based complexes in health and diseases: An approach in chemopreventive and therapeutic improvement. *Journal of Trace Elements in Medicine and Biology*, *73*, 127023. DOI: 10.1016/j.jtemb.2022.127023 PMID: 35780653

Prashanth, G. P., & Hegde, D. G. (2023). Zinc Prophylaxis to Reduce Mortality and Morbidity in Under-5 Children: Clinical and Global Health Points of View. Global Pediatric Health, 10, 2333794X231156043. https://doi.org/DOI: 10.1177/2333794X23115604

Pujiastuti, I. T., Deliana, M., Mutiara, E., & Lubis, M. (2018). Effect of zinc supplementation on linear growth velocity of children with short stature. In *Stem Cell Oncology* (pp. 321–324). CRC Press. DOI: 10.1201/9781351190152-68

Pullakhandam, R., Agrawal, P. K., Peter, R., Ghosh, S., Reddy, G. B., Kulkarni, B., Thomas, T., Kurpad, A. V., Sachdev, H. S., Porwal, A., Khan, N., Ramesh, S., Acharya, R., Sarna, A., Kapil, U., Rajkumar, H., De Wagt, A., Deb, S., & Johnston, R. (2021). Prevalence of low serum zinc concentrations in Indian children and adolescents: Findings from the Comprehensive National Nutrition Survey 2016–18. *The American Journal of Clinical Nutrition*, *114*(2), 638–648. DOI: 10.1093/ajcn/nqab066 PMID: 33831945

Qi, S., He, J., Zheng, H., Chen, C., Jiang, H., & Lan, S. (2020). Zinc Supplementation Increased Bone Mineral Density, Improves Bone Histomorphology, and Prevents Bone Loss in Diabetic Rat. *Biological Trace Element Research*, *194*(2), 493–501. DOI: 10.1007/s12011-019-01810-7 PMID: 31363990

Quamme, S. H., & Iversen, P. O. (2022). Prevalence of child stunting in Sub-Saharan Africa and its risk factors. *Clinical Nutrition Open Science*, *42*, 49–61. DOI: 10.1016/j.nutos.2022.01.009

Rai, D., Chaudhary, C., Khatak, A., & Banyal, S. (2024). A Sustainable Approach to Combat Micronutrient Deficiencies and Ensure Global Food Security through Biofortification. *European Journal of Nutrition & Food Safety*, *16*(4), 15–30. DOI: 10.9734/ejnfs/2024/v16i41404

Rajput, R. (2018). A scientific hypothesis on the role of nutritional supplements for effective management of hair loss and promoting hair regrowth. *Journal of Nutritional Health & Food Science*, *6*(3), 1–11. DOI: 10.15226/jnhfs.2018.001132

Rawat, M., Varshney, A., Rai, M., Chikara, A., Pohty, A. L., Joshi, A., Binjola, A., Singh, C. P., Rawat, K., Rather, M. A., & Gupta, A. K. (2023). A comprehensive review on nutraceutical potential of underutilized cereals and cereal-based products. *Journal of Agriculture and Food Research*, *12*, 100619. DOI: 10.1016/j.jafr.2023.100619

Read, S. A., Obeid, S., Ahlenstiel, C., & Ahlenstiel, G. (2019). The role of zinc in antiviral immunity. *Advances in Nutrition*, *10*(4), 696–710. DOI: 10.1093/advances/nmz013 PMID: 31305906

Rehman, A., Farooq, M., Ozturk, L., Asif, M., & Siddique, K. H. M. (2018). Zinc nutrition in wheat-based cropping systems. *Plant and Soil*, *422*(1–2), 283–315. DOI: 10.1007/s11104-017-3507-3

Rehman, A., Farooq, M., Ullah, A., Nadeem, F., Im, S. Y., Park, S. K., & Lee, D.-J. (2020). Agronomic Biofortification of Zinc in Pakistan: Status, Benefits, and Constraints. *Frontiers in Sustainable Food Systems*, *4*, 591722. DOI: 10.3389/fsufs.2020.591722

Reynolds, D. (2018). *Skin Conditions: From Acne to Eczema*. Greenhaven Publishing LLC.

Rezazadegan, M., Shahdadian, F., Soheilipour, M., Tarrahi, M. J., & Amani, R. (2022). Zinc nutritional status, mood states and quality of life in diarrhea-predominant irritable bowel syndrome: A case–control study. *Scientific Reports*, *12*(1), 11002. DOI: 10.1038/s41598-022-15080-2 PMID: 35768522

Rinninella, E., Mele, M. C., Merendino, N., Cintoni, M., Anselmi, G., Caporossi, A., Gasbarrini, A., & Minnella, A. M. (2018). The role of diet, micronutrients and the gut microbiota in age-related macular degeneration: New perspectives from the gut–retina axis. *Nutrients*, *10*(11), 1677. DOI: 10.3390/nu10111677 PMID: 30400586

Rizwan, M., Abbas, A., Xu, H., Ahmed, U. I., Qing, P., He, P., Iqbal, M. A., & Shahzad, M. A. (2022). Role of nutrition information in acceptance and willingness to pay for biofortified cereal food: Implications for better health and sustainable diet. *Nutrients*, *14*(16), 3352. DOI: 10.3390/nu14163352 PMID: 36014858

Rodríguez-Carmona, Y., Denova-Gutiérrez, E., Sánchez-Uribe, E., Muñoz-Aguirre, P., Flores, M., & Salmerón, J. (2020). Zinc supplementation and fortification in Mexican children. *Food and Nutrition Bulletin*, *41*(1), 89–101. DOI: 10.1177/0379572119877757 PMID: 31955593

Roohani, N., Hurrell, R., Kelishadi, R., & Schulin, R. (2013). Zinc and its importance for human health: An integrative review. *Journal of Research in Medical Sciences : the Official Journal of Isfahan University of Medical Sciences*, *18*(2), 144. PMID: 23914218

Roohani, N., Hurrell, R., Kelishadi, R., & Schulin, R. (2013). Zinc and its importance in human health: An integrative review. *Journal of Research in Medical Sciences : the Official Journal of Isfahan University of Medical Sciences*, *18*(2), 144–157. PMID: 23914218

Roston, E. F., DeBuys, H. V., Madey, D. L., & Pinnell, S. R. (2002). Evidence supporting zinc as an important antioxidant for skin. *International Journal of Dermatology, 41*(9), 606–611. DOI: 10.1046/j.1365-4362.2002.01567.x PMID: 12358835

Rousseau, S., Kyomugasho, C., Celus, M., Hendrickx, M. E., & Grauwet, T. (2020). Barriers impairing mineral bioaccessibility and bioavailability in plant-based foods and the perspectives for food processing. *Critical Reviews in Food Science and Nutrition, 60*(5), 826–843. DOI: 10.1080/10408398.2018.1552243 PMID: 30632768

Rudolf, E., & Rudolf, K. (2017). Increases in Intracellular zinc enhance proliferative signalling as well as mitochondrial and lysosomal activity in human melanocytes. *Cellular Physiology and Biochemistry, 43*(1), 1–16. DOI: 10.1159/000480306 PMID: 28848213

Ruiz-Tagle, S. A., Figueira, M. M., Vial, V., Espinoza-Benavides, L., & Miteva, M. (2018). Micronutrients in hair loss. *Our Dermatology Online. Nasza Dermatologia Online, 9*(3), 320–328. https://www.odermatol.com/odermatology/20183/25.Micronutrients-Ruiz-TagleSA.pdf. DOI: 10.7241/ourd.20183.25

Rushton, D. H. (2002). Nutritional factors and hair loss. *Clinical and Experimental Dermatology, 27*(5), 396–404. DOI: 10.1046/j.1365-2230.2002.01076.x PMID: 12190640

Russell, R. M. (1992). Changes in gastrointestinal function attributed to aging. *The American Journal of Clinical Nutrition, 55*(6), 1203S–1207S. DOI: 10.1093/ajcn/55.6.1203S PMID: 1590257

Ryckman, T., Beal, T., Nordhagen, S., Murira, Z., & Torlesse, H. (2021). Affordability of nutritious foods for complementary feeding in South Asia. *Nutrition Reviews, 79*(Supplement_1), 52–68. DOI: 10.1093/nutrit/nuaa139 PMID: 33693914

Ryu, M. S. A. T. (2020). *Present Knowledge in Nutrition* (Bernadette P. Marriott, Diane F. Birt, Virginia A. Stalling, & Allison A. Yates, Eds.; 11th ed). Wiley-Blackwell.

Sadeghzadeh, B. (2013). A review of zinc nutrition and plant breeding. *Journal of Soil Science and Plant Nutrition, 13*(4), 905–927. DOI: 10.4067/S0718-95162013005000072

Salgueiro, M. J., Zubillaga, M. B., Lysionek, A. E., Caro, R. A., Weill, R., & Boccio, J. R. (2002). The role of zinc in the growth and development of children. *Nutrition (Burbank, Los Angeles County, Calif.), 18*(6), 510–519. DOI: 10.1016/S0899-9007(01)00812-7 PMID: 12044825

Sallé, A., Demarsy, D., Poirier, A. L., Lelièvre, B., Topart, P., Guilloteau, G., Bécouarn, G., & Rohmer, V. (2010). Zinc Deficiency: A Frequent and Underestimated Complication After Bariatric Surgery. *Obesity Surgery, 20*(12), 1660–1670. DOI: 10.1007/s11695-010-0237-5 PMID: 20706804

Sampson, D., Cely-Santos, M., Gemmill-Herren, B., Babin, N., Bernhart, A., Bezner Kerr, R., Blesh, J., Bowness, E., Feldman, M., Gonçalves, A. L., James, D., Kerssen, T., Klassen, S., Wezel, A., & Wittman, H. (2021). Food sovereignty and rights-based approaches strengthen food security and nutrition across the globe: A systematic review. *Frontiers in Sustainable Food Systems, 5*, 686492. DOI: 10.3389/fsufs.2021.686492

Samtiya, M., Aluko, R. E., & Dhewa, T. (2020). Plant food anti-nutritional factors and their reduction strategies: An overview. *Food Production, Processing and Nutrition, 2*(1), 6. DOI: 10.1186/s43014-020-0020-5

Sandstead, H. H., & Freeland-Graves, J. H. (2014). Dietary phytate, zinc and hidden zinc deficiency. *Journal of Trace Elements in Medicine and Biology, 28*(4), 414–417. DOI: 10.1016/j.jtemb.2014.08.011 PMID: 25439135

Sandström, B. (1997). Bioavailability of zinc. *European Journal of Clinical Nutrition, 51*(Suppl 1), S17–S19. PMID: 9023474

Sandström, B., Almgren, A., Kivistö, B., & Cederblad, Å. (1989). Effect of protein level and protein source on zinc absorption in humans. *The Journal of Nutrition, 119*(1), 48–53. DOI: 10.1093/jn/119.1.48 PMID: 2492337

Sandstrom, B., Davidsson, L., Cederblad, A., & Lönnerdal, B. (1985). Oral iron, dietary ligands and zinc absorption. *The Journal of Nutrition, 115*(3), 411–414. DOI: 10.1093/jn/115.3.411 PMID: 3973750

Sangeetha, V. J., Dutta, S., Moses, J. A., & Anandharamakrishnan, C. (2022). Zinc nutrition and human health: Overview and implications. *eFood, 3*(5), e17. DOI: 10.1002/efd2.17

Santos, C. A., Fonseca, J., Maria, T. M. L., Carolino, E., & Guerreiro, A. S. (2017). Serum zinc evolution in dysphagic patients that underwent endoscopic gastrostomy for long term enteral feeding. *Asia Pacific Journal of Clinical Nutrition, 26*(2). Advance online publication. DOI: 10.6133/apjcn.022016.03 PMID: 28244699

Santos, H. O., & Teixeira, F. J. (2019). Use of medicinal doses of zinc as a safe and efficient coadjutant in the treatment of male hypogonadism. *The Aging Male*. PMID: 30767598

Sanusi, K. O., Ibrahim, K. G., Abubakar, B., Malami, I., Bello, M. B., Imam, M. U., & Abubakar, M. B. (2021). Effect of maternal zinc deficiency on offspring health: The epigenetic impact. *Journal of Trace Elements in Medicine and Biology*, *65*, 126731. DOI: 10.1016/j.jtemb.2021.126731 PMID: 33610057

Saper, R. B., & Rash, R. (2009). Zinc: An essential micronutrient. *American Family Physician*, *79*(9), 768. PMID: 20141096

Sazawal, S., Black, R. E., Menon, V. P., Dinghra, P., Caulfield, L. E., Dhingra, U., & Bagati, A. (2001). Zinc supplementation in infants born small for gestational age reduces mortality: A prospective, randomized, controlled trial. *Pediatrics*, *108*(6), 1280–1286. DOI: 10.1542/peds.108.6.1280 PMID: 11731649

Scarpellini, E., Balsiger, L. M., Maurizi, V., Rinninella, E., Gasbarrini, A., Giostra, N., Santori, P., Abenavoli, L., & Rasetti, C. (2022). Zinc and gut microbiota in health and gastrointestinal disease under the COVID-19 suggestion. *BioFactors (Oxford, England)*, *48*(2), 294–306. DOI: 10.1002/biof.1829 PMID: 35218585

Schaefer, E., & Nock, D. (2019). The Impact of Preconceptional Multiple-Micronutrient Supplementation on Female Fertility. *Clinical Medicine Insights: Women's Health*, *12*, 1179562X1984386. DOI: 10.1177/1179562X19843868

Schmitt, S., Kury, S., Giraud, M., Dreno, B., Kharfi, M., & Bezieau, S. (2009). An update on mutations of the SLC39A4 gene in acrodermatitis enteropathica. *Human Mutation*, *30*(6), 926–933. DOI: 10.1002/humu.20988 PMID: 19370757

Scholmerich, J., Freudemann, A., Kottgen, E., Wietholtz, H., Steiert, B., Lohle, E., Haussinger, D., & Gerok, W. (1987). Bioavailability of zinc from zinc-histidine complexes. I. Comparison with zinc sulfate in healthy men. *The American Journal of Clinical Nutrition*, *45*(6), 1480–1486. DOI: 10.1093/ajcn/45.6.1480 PMID: 3591728

Schoofs, H., Schmit, J., & Rink, L. (2024). Zinc toxicity: Understanding the limits. *Molecules (Basel, Switzerland)*, *29*(13), 3130. DOI: 10.3390/molecules29133130 PMID: 38999082

Schwartz, J. R., Marsh, R. G., & Draelos, Z. D. (2005). Zinc and skin health: Overview of physiology and pharmacology. *Dermatologic Surgery*, *31*(7 Pt 2), 837–847. DOI: 10.1111/j.1524-4725.2005.31729 PMID: 16029676

Scrimgeour, A. G., Condlin, M. L., Otieno, L., & Bovill, M. E. (2011). Zinc Intervention Strategies: Costs and Health Benefits. In Gerald, J. K., Watson, R. R., & Preedy, V. R. (Eds.), *Nutrients, Dietary Supplements, and Nutriceuticals* (pp. 189–214). Humana Press., DOI: 10.1007/978-1-60761-308-4_13

Searle, T., Ali, F. R., & Al-Niaimi, F. (2022). Zinc in dermatology. *The Journal of Dermatological Treatment*, *33*(5), 2455–2458. DOI: 10.1080/09546634.2022.2062282 PMID: 35437093

Seifi, N., Bahari, H., Ghiasi Hafezi, S., Ghotbani, F., Afzalinia, A., Ferns, G. A., Farkhani, E. M., & Ghayour-mobarhan, M. (2024). Dietary mineral intakes predict Coronavirus-disease 2019 (COVID-19) incidence and hospitalization in older adults. *BMC Nutrition*, *10*(1), 1–8. DOI: 10.1186/s40795-024-00821-5 PMID: 38439106

Semba, R. D., Ramsing, R., Rahman, N., Kraemer, K., & Bloem, M. W. (2021). Legumes as a sustainable source of protein in human diets. Global Food Security, 28(June 2020), 100520. DOI: 10.1016/j.gfs.2021.100520

Serhan, H., Alma'aitah, H., Irshaidat, S., Ameer, M., Asghar, M., & Tahir, M. (2022). Ophthalmic manifestations of nutritional deficiencies: A mini review. *Journal of Family Medicine and Primary Care*, *11*(10), 5899–5901. DOI: 10.4103/jfmpc.jfmpc_790_22 PMID: 36618247

Seth, R., Corniola, R. S., Gower-Winter, S. D., Morgan, T. J.Jr, Bishop, B., & Levenson, C. W. (2015). Zinc deficiency induces apoptosis via mitochondrial p53- and caspase-dependent pathways in human neuronal precursor cells. *Journal of Trace Elements in Medicine and Biology*, *30*, 59–65. DOI: 10.1016/j.jtemb.2014.10.010 PMID: 25467851

Seven, M., Basaran, S. Y., Cengiz, M., Unal, S., & Yuksel, A. (2013). Deficiency of selenium and zinc as a causative factor for idiopathic intractable epilepsy. *Epilepsy Research*, *104*(1-2), 35–39. DOI: 10.1016/j.eplepsyres.2012.09.013 PMID: 23103062

Severe, M. (n.d.). *Zinc: Everything you need to know about this vital mineral*. Retrieved May 25, 2024, from https://blog.cytoplan.co.uk/zinc-all-about-this-vital-mineral/

Sevryugin, O., Kasvis, P., Vigano, M., & Vigano, A. (2021). Taste and smell disturbances in cancer patients: A scoping review of available treatments. *Supportive Care in Cancer*, *29*(1), 49–66. DOI: 10.1007/s00520-020-05609-4 PMID: 32734392

Shah, D., Sachdev, H. S., Gera, T., De-Regil, L. M., & Peña-Rosas, J. P. (2016). Fortification of staple foods with zinc for improving zinc status and other health outcomes in the general population. *Cochrane Database of Systematic Reviews*, *2016*(6). DOI: 10.1002/14651858.CD010697.pub2

Shah, D., & Sachdev, H. (2006). Zinc deficiency in pregnancy and fetal outcome. *Nutrition Reviews*, *64*(1), 15–30. DOI: 10.1111/j.1753-4887.2006.tb00169.x PMID: 16491666

Shah, D., & Sachdev, H. S. (2001). Effect of gestational zinc deficiency on pregnancy outcomes: Summary of observation studies and zinc supplementation trials. *British Journal of Nutrition*, *85*(S2), S101–S108. DOI: 10.1079/BJN2000301 PMID: 11509097

Shams Tabrez, K., & Malik, A. (2021). *Microbial biofertilizers and micronutrient availability: The role of zinc in agriculture and human health*. Springer Nature. https://books.google.com/books?hl=en&lr=&id=andTEAAAQBAJ&oi=fnd&pg=PR8&dq=In+regions+where+animal-based+foods+are+scarce+or+expensive,+promoting+alternative+zinc-rich+plant+foods+and+fortifying+staple+crops+becomes+particularly+important.&ots=oYNloCTN6o&sig=jbrZnyMkop_tKH5Y8kaMZfDrrTI

Shankar, A. H. (2020). Mineral deficiencies. In *Hunter's Tropical Medicine and Emerging Infectious Diseases* (pp. 1048–1054). Elsevier., DOI: 10.1016/B978-0-323-55512-8.00145-9

Shankar, A. H., Genton, B., Baisor, M., Paino, J., Tamja, S., Adiguma, T., Wu, L., Rare, L., Bannon, D., Tielsch, J. M., West, K. P., & Alpers, M. P. (2000). The influence of zinc supplementation on morbidity due to Plasmodium falciparum: Arandomized trial in preschool children in Papua New Guinea. *The American Journal of Tropical Medicine and Hygiene*, *62*(6), 663–669. DOI: 10.4269/ajtmh.2000.62.663 PMID: 11304051

Shankar, A. H., & Prasad, A. S. (1998). Zinc and immune function: The biological basis of altered resistance to infection. *The American Journal of Clinical Nutrition*, *68*(2), 447S–463S. DOI: 10.1093/ajcn/68.2.447S PMID: 9701160

Shao, T., Verma, H. K., Pande, B., Costanzo, V., Ye, W., Cai, Y., & Bhaskar, L. (2021). Physical activity and nutritional influence on immune function: An important strategy to improve immunity and health status. *Frontiers in Physiology*, *12*, 751374. DOI: 10.3389/fphys.2021.751374 PMID: 34690818

Shariatipour, N., & Heidari, B. (2020). Genetic-Based Biofortification of Staple Food Crops to Meet Zinc and Iron Deficiency-Related Challenges. In Aftab, T., & Hakeem, K. R. (Eds.), *Plant Micronutrients* (pp. 173–223). Springer International Publishing., DOI: 10.1007/978-3-030-49856-6_8

Shayganfard, M. (2022). Are Essential Trace Elements Effective in Modulation of Mental Disorders? Update and Perspectives. *Biological Trace Element Research*, *200*(3), 1032–1059. DOI: 10.1007/s12011-021-02733-y PMID: 33904124

Shelenga, T. V., Kerv, Y. A., Perchuk, I. N. E., Solovyeva, A., Khlestkina, E. K. G., Loskutov, I., & Konarev, A. V. (2021). The potential of small grains crops in enhancing biofortification breeding strategies for human health benefit. *Agronomy (Basel)*, *11*(7), 1420. DOI: 10.3390/agronomy11071420

Shikora, S. A., Kim, J. J., & Tarnoff, M. E. (2007). Nutrition and Gastrointestinal Complications of Bariatric Surgery. *Nutrition in Clinical Practice*, *22*(1), 29–40. DOI: 10.1177/011542650702200129 PMID: 17242452

Shkembi, B., & Huppertz, T. (2021). Influence of dairy products on bioavailability of zinc from other food products: A review of complementarity at a meal level. *Nutrients*, *13*(12), 4253. DOI: 10.3390/nu13124253 PMID: 34959808

Shubham, K., Anukiruthika, T., Dutta, S., Kashyap, A., Moses, J. A., & Anandharamakrishnan, C. (2020). Iron deficiency anemia: A comprehensive review on iron absorption, bioavailability and emerging food fortification approaches. *Trends in Food Science & Technology*, *99*, 58–75. DOI: 10.1016/j.tifs.2020.02.021

Shukla, A. K., Behera, S. K., Prakash, C., Tripathi, A., Patra, A. K., Dwivedi, B. S., Trivedi, V., Rao, Ch. S., Chaudhari, S. K., Das, S., & Singh, A. K. (2021). Deficiency of phyto-available sulphur, zinc, boron, iron, copper and manganese in soils of India. *Scientific Reports*, *11*(1), 19760. DOI: 10.1038/s41598-021-99040-2 PMID: 34611190

Siddiqui, F. J., Belayneh, G., & Bhutta, Z. A. (2021). Nutrition and diarrheal disease and enteric pathogens. *Nutrition and infectious diseases: Shifting the clinical paradigm*, 219-241..DOI: 10.1007/978-3-030-56913-6_8

Singh, A., Rajput, V. D., Pandey, D., Sharma, R., Ghazaryan, K., & Minkina, T. (2023). Nano Zinc-Enabled Strategies in Crops for Combatting Zinc Malnutrition in Human Health. *Frontiers in Bioscience (Landmark Edition)*, *28*(8), 158. DOI: 10.31083/j.fbl2808158 PMID: 37664935

Singh, C. K., Chhabra, G., Patel, A., Chang, H., & Ahmad, N. (2021). Dietary phytochemicals in zinc homeostasis: A strategy for prostate cancer management. *Nutrients*, *13*(6), 1867. DOI: 10.3390/nu13061867 PMID: 34070833

Singh, G., & Pal, V. (2024). Agronomic innovations for enhancement of zinc content in pulses: A review. *Indian Journal of Pulses Research*, *37*(1), 11–21. DOI: 10.59797/jfl.v37.i1.173

Singh, P., & Prasad, S. (2023). A review on iron, zinc and calcium biological significance and factors affecting their absorption and bioavailability. *Journal of Food Composition and Analysis*, *123*, 105529. DOI: 10.1016/j.jfca.2023.105529

Singh, S., Kaur, J., Ram, H., Singh, J., & Kaur, S. (2023). Agronomic bio-fortification of wheat (Triticum aestivum L.) to alleviate zinc deficiency in human being. *Reviews in Environmental Science and Biotechnology*, *22*(2), 505–526. DOI: 10.1007/s11157-023-09653-4 PMID: 37234132

Singh, U., Praharaj, C. S., Chaturvedi, S. K., & Bohra, A. (2016). Biofortification: Introduction, Approaches, Limitations, and Challenges. In Singh, U., Praharaj, C. S., Singh, S. S., & Singh, N. P. (Eds.), *Biofortification of Food Crops* (pp. 3–18). Springer India., DOI: 10.1007/978-81-322-2716-8_1

Siwela, M., Pillay, K., Govender, L., Lottering, S., Mudau, F. N., Modi, A. T., & Mabhaudhi, T. (2020). Biofortified crops for combating hidden hunger in South Africa: Availability, acceptability, micronutrient retention and bioavailability. *Foods*, *9*(6), 815. DOI: 10.3390/foods9060815 PMID: 32575819

Skalny, A. V., Aschner, M., Lei, X. G., Gritsenko, V. A., Santamaria, A., Alekseenko, S. I., Prakash, N. T., Chang, J.-S., Sizova, E. A., Chao, J. C., Aaseth, J., & Tinkov, A. A. (2021). Gut microbiota as a mediator of essential and toxic effects of zinc in the intestines and other tissues. *International Journal of Molecular Sciences*, *22*(23), 13074. DOI: 10.3390/ijms222313074 PMID: 34884881

Skalny, A. V., Aschner, M., & Tinkov, A. A. (2021). Zinc. In *Advances in Food and Nutrition Research* (Vol. 96, pp. 251–310). Elsevier., DOI: 10.1016/bs.afnr.2021.01.003

Skalny, A. V., Sotnikova, T. I., Korobeynikova, T. V., & Tinkov, A. A. (2023). Significance of zinc deficiency correction for practical medicine: A review. *Sechenov Medical Journal*, *13*(4), 4–17. DOI: 10.47093/2218-7332.2022.13.4.4-17

Skrajnowska, D., & Bobrowska-Korczak, B. (2019). Role of zinc in immune system and anti-cancer defense mechanisms. *Nutrients*, *11*(10), 2273. DOI: 10.3390/nu11102273 PMID: 31546724

Skrovanek, S., DiGuilio, K., Bailey, R., Huntington, W., Urbas, R., Mayilvaganan, B., Mercogliano, G., & Mullin, J. M. (2014). Zinc and gastrointestinal disease. *World Journal of Gastrointestinal Pathophysiology*, *5*(4), 496–513. DOI: 10.4291/wjgp.v5.i4.496 PMID: 25400994

Smith, L. H. (1991). *Clinical guide to the use of vitamin C*. SEANET Corporation–Internet Services for the Puget Sound Region. https://www.seanet.com/~alexs/ascorbate/198x/smith-lh-clinical_guide_1988.htm

Solomons, N. W. (2001). Dietary Sources of Zinc and Factors Affecting its Bioavailability. *Food and Nutrition Bulletin*, *22*(2), 138–154. DOI: 10.1177/156482650102200204

Sorokman, T., Sokolnyk, S., Popelyuk, A.-M., Makarova, O., Bezruk, T., & Moldovan, P. (2019). Zinc level in children with short stature. *Romanian Journal of Pediatrics*, *68*(4), 248–254. DOI: 10.37897/RJP.2019.4.4

Speich, M., Pineau, A., & Ballereau, F. (2001). Minerals, trace elements and related biological variables in athletes and during physical activity. *Clinica Chimica Acta*, *312*(1–2), 1–11. DOI: 10.1016/S0009-8981(01)00598-8 PMID: 11580904

Squitti, R., Pal, A., Picozza, M., Avan, A., Ventriglia, M., Rongioletti, M. C., & Hoogenraad, T. (2020). Zinc Therapy in early Alzheimer's disease: Safety and potential therapeutic efficacy. *Biomolecules*, *10*(8), 1164. DOI: 10.3390/biom10081164 PMID: 32784855

Stanaway, J. D., Afshin, A., Gakidou, E., Lim, S. S., Abate, D., Abate, K. H., Abbafati, C., Abbasi, N., Abbastabar, H., Abd-Allah, F., Abdela, J., Abdelalim, A., Abdollahpour, I., Abdulkader, R. S., Abebe, M., Abebe, Z., Abera, S. F., Abil, O. Z., Abraha, H. N., & Murray, C. J. L. (2018). Global, regional, and national comparative risk assessment of 84 behavioural, environmental and occupational, and metabolic risks or clusters of risks for 195 countries and territories, 1990–2017: A systematic analysis for the Global Burden of Disease Study 2017. *Lancet*, *392*(10159), 1923–1994. DOI: 10.1016/S0140-6736(18)32225-6 PMID: 30496105

Stefanidou, M., Maravelias, C., Dona, A., & Spiliopoulou, C. (2006). Zinc: A multipurpose trace element. *Archives of Toxicology*, *80*(1), 1–9. DOI: 10.1007/s00204-005-0009-5 PMID: 16187101

Stein, A. J. (2010). Global impacts of human mineral malnutrition. *Plant and Soil*, *335*(1-2), 133–154. DOI: 10.1007/s11104-009-0228-2

Stevens, G. A., Beal, T., Mbuya, M. N., Luo, H., Neufeld, L. M., Addo, O. Y., Adu-Afarwuah, S., Alayón, S., Bhutta, Z., Brown, K. H., Jefferds, M. E., Engle-Stone, R., Fawzi, W., Hess, S. Y., Johnston, R., Katz, J., Krasevec, J., McDonald, C. M., Mei, Z., & Young, M. F. (2022). Micronutrient deficiencies among preschool-aged children and women of reproductive age worldwide: A pooled analysis of individual-level data from population-representative surveys. *The Lancet. Global Health*, *10*(11), e1590–e1599. DOI: 10.1016/S2214-109X(22)00367-9 PMID: 36240826

Stiles, L. I., Ferrao, K., & Mehta, K. J. (2024). Role of zinc in health and disease. *Clinical and Experimental Medicine*, *24*(1), 38. Advance online publication. DOI: 10.1007/s10238-024-01302-6 PMID: 38367035

Sturniolo, G. C., Leo, V. D., Barollo, M., Fries, W., Mazzon, E., & Ferronato, A. (2000). The many functions of zinc in inflammatory conditions of the gastrointestinal tract. *The Journal of Trace Elements in Experimental Medicine*, *13*(1), 33–39. DOI: 10.1002/(SICI)1520-670X(2000)13:1<33::AID-JTRA5>3.0.CO;2-K

Subhasri, D., Dutta, S., Leena, M. M., Moses, J., & Anandharamakrishnan, C. (2022). Gastronomy: An extended platform for customized nutrition. *Future Foods : a Dedicated Journal for Sustainability in Food Science*, *5*, 100147. DOI: 10.1016/j.fufo.2022.100147

Suliburska, J., Skrypnik, K., Szulinska, M., Kupsz, J., Markuszewaki, L., & Bogdanski, P. (2018). Diuretics, Ca antagonists and angiotensin converting enzyme inhibitors affect zinc status in hypertensive patients on monotherpy: A randomized trial. *Nutrients*, *10*(9), 1284. DOI: 10.3390/nu10091284 PMID: 30208601

Sun, R., Wang, J., Feng, J., & Cao, B. (2022). Zinc in cognitive impairment and aging. *Biomolecules*, *12*(7), 1000. DOI: 10.3390/biom12071000 PMID: 35883555

Swamy, B. P. M., Rahman, M. A., Inabangan-Asilo, M. A., Amparado, A., Manito, C., Chadha-Mohanty, P., Reinke, R., & Slamet-Loedin, I. H. (2016). Advances in breeding for high grain Zinc in Rice. *Rice (New York, N.Y.)*, *9*(1), 49. DOI: 10.1186/s12284-016-0122-5 PMID: 27671163

Swardfager, W., Herrmann, N., Mazereeuw, G., Goldberger, K., Harimoto, T., & Lanctôt, K. L. (2013). Zinc in depression: A meta-analysis. *Biological Psychiatry*, *74*(12), 872–878. DOI: 10.1016/j.biopsych.2013.05.008 PMID: 23806573

Swardfager, W., Herrmann, N., McIntyre, R. S., Mazereeuw, G., Goldberger, K., Cha, D. S., Schwartz, Y., & Lanctôt, K. L. (2013). Potential roles of zinc in the pathophysiology and treatment of major depressive disorder. *Neuroscience and Biobehavioral Reviews*, *37*(5), 911–929. DOI: 10.1016/j.neubiorev.2013.03.018 PMID: 23567517

Swart, R., Sanders, D., & McLachlan, M. (2008). Nutrition: A primary health care perspective: Primary health care: Programme areas. *South African Health Review*, *2008*(1), 129–147.

Szewczyk, B. (2013). Zinc homeostasis and neurodegenerative disorders. *Frontiers in Aging Neuroscience*, *5*. Advance online publication. DOI: 10.3389/fnagi.2013.00033 PMID: 23882214

Tada-Oikawa, S., Ichihara, G., Suzuki, Y., Izuoka, K., Wu, W., Yamada, Y., Mishima, T., & Ichihara, S. (2015). Zn (II) released from zinc oxide nano/micro particles suppresses vasculogenesis in human endothelial colony forming cells. *Toxicology Reports, 2*, 692–701. DOI: 10.1016/j.toxrep.2015.04.003 PMID: 28962405

Tadokoro, T., Morishita, A., Himoto, T., & Masaki, T. (2023). Nutritional support for alcoholic liver disease. *Nutrients, 15*(6), 1360. DOI: 10.3390/nu15061360 PMID: 36986091

Takagishi, T., Hara, T., & Fukada, T. (2017). Recent Advances in the Role of SLC39A/ZIP Zinc Transporters In Vivo. *International Journal of Molecular Sciences, 18*(12), 2708. DOI: 10.3390/ijms18122708 PMID: 29236063

Takeda, A. (2011). Zinc signaling in the hippocampus and its relation to pathogenesis of depression. *Molecular Neurobiology, 44*(2), 166–174. DOI: 10.1007/s12035-010-8158-9 PMID: 21161611

Takeda, T., Miyazaki, S., Kobayashi, M., Nishino, K., Goto, T., Matsunaga, M., Ooi, M., Shirakawa, H., Tani, F., Kawamura, T., Komai, M., & Kambe, T. (2018). Zinc deficiency causes delayed ATP clearance and adenosine generation in rats and cell culture models. *Communications Biology, 1*(1), 113. DOI: 10.1038/s42003-018-0118-3 PMID: 30271993

Takkar, P. N. (1996). Micronutrient research and sustainable agricultural productivity in India. *Journal of the Indian Society of Soil Science, 44*(4), 562–581.

Tan, L., Qu, M., Zhu, Y., Peng, C., Wang, J., Gao, D., & Chen, C. (2020). ZINC TRANSPORTER5 and ZINC TRANSPORTER9 function synergistically in zinc/cadmium uptake. *Plant Physiology, 183*(3), 1235–1249. DOI: 10.1104/pp.19.01569 PMID: 32341004

Tanwar, V. S., Zhang, X., Jagannathan, L., Jose, C. C., & Cuddapah, S. (2019). Cadmium exposure upregulates SNAIL through miR-30 repression in human lung epithelial cells. *Toxicology and Applied Pharmacology, 373*, 1–9. DOI: 10.1016/j.taap.2019.04.011 PMID: 30998937

Tapiero, H., & Tew, K. D. (2003). Trace elements in human physiology and pathology: Zinc and metallothioneins. *Biomedicine and Pharmacotherapy, 57*(9), 399–411. DOI: 10.1016/S0753-3322(03)00081-7 PMID: 14652165

Tarini, A., Manger, M. S., Brown, K. H., Mbuya, M. N., Rowe, L. A., Grant, F., Black, R. E., & McDonald, C. M. (2021). Enablers and barriers of zinc fortification; experience from 10 low-and middle-income countries with mandatory large-scale food fortification. *Nutrients, 13*(6), 2051. DOI: 10.3390/nu13062051 PMID: 34203987

Tessema, M., De Groote, H., & Brouwer, D., I., JM Feskens, E., Belachew, T., Zerfu, D., ... & S. Gunaratna, N. (2019). Soil zinc is associated with serum zinc but not with linear growth of children in Ethiopia. *Nutrients*, *11*(2), 221.

Thu, B. D., Schultink, W., Dillon, D., Gross, R., Leswara, N. D., & Khoi, H. H. (1999). Effect of daily and weekly micronutrient supplementation on micronutrient deficiencies and growth in young Vietnamese children. *The American Journal of Clinical Nutrition*, *69*(1), 80–86. DOI: 10.1093/ajcn/69.1.80 PMID: 9925127

Tokuyama, A., Kanda, E., Itano, S., Kondo, M., Wada, Y., Kadoya, H., Kidokoro, K., Nagasu, H., Sasaki, T., & Kashihara, N. (2021). Effect of zinc deficiency on chronic kidney disease progression and effect modification by hypoalbuminemia. *PLoS One*, *16*(5), e0251554. DOI: 10.1371/journal.pone.0251554 PMID: 33974681

Tran, C. D., Katsikeros, R., Manton, N., Krebs, N. F., Hambidge, K. M., Butler, R. N., & Davidson, G. P. (2011). Zinc homeostasis and gut function in children with celiac disease. *The American Journal of Clinical Nutrition*, *94*(4), 1026–1032. DOI: 10.3945/ajcn.111.018093 PMID: 21865333

TRIPATHI. P. (2024). Food Nutrition in Human Science. Blue Rose Publishers.

Troche, C., Aydemir, T. B., & Cousins, R. J. (2016). Zinc transporter Slc39a14 regulates inflammatory signalling associated with hypertrophic adiposity. *American Journal of Physiology. Endocrinology and Metabolism*, *310*(4), E258–E268. DOI: 10.1152/ajpendo.00421.2015 PMID: 26646099

Ugarte, M., & Osborne, N. N. (2001). Zinc in the retina. *Progress in Neurobiology*, *64*(3), 219–249. DOI: 10.1016/S0301-0082(00)00057-5 PMID: 11240307

UNICEF, M. (2019). *Comprehensive National Nutrition Survey (CNNS) 2016-2018.*

Upadhaya, S. D., & Kim, I. H. (2020). Importance of micronutrients in bone health of monogastric animals and techniques to improve the bioavailability of micronutrient supplements—A review. *Asian-Australasian Journal of Animal Sciences*, *33*(12), 1885–1895. DOI: 10.5713/ajas.19.0945 PMID: 32164057

Urbano, M. R., Vitalle, M. S., Juliano, Y., & Amancio, O. M. (2002). Iron, copper and zinc in adolescents during pubertal growth spurt. *Jornal de Pediatria*, *78*(4), 327–334. DOI: 10.2223/JPED.868 PMID: 14647765

Uriu-Adams, J. Y., & Keen, C. L. (2010). Zinc and reproduction: Effects of zinc deficiency on prenatal and early postnatal development. *Birth Defects Research. Part B, Developmental and Reproductive Toxicology*, *89*(4), 313–325. DOI: 10.1002/bdrb.20264 PMID: 20803691

USDA Food data Central. https://fdc.nal.usda.gov/fdc-app.html#/food-search?component=1095

Valberg, L. S., Flanagan, P. R., & Chamberlain, M. J. (1984). Effects of iron, tin, and copper on zinc absorption in humans. *The American Journal of Clinical Nutrition*, *40*(3), 536–541. DOI: 10.1093/ajcn/40.3.536 PMID: 6475824

Vallee, B. L., & Falchuk, K. H. (1993). The Biochemical Basis of Zinc Physiology. In *REVIEWS* (Vol. 73, Issue 1). DOI: 10.1152/physrev.1993.73.1.79

Vallee, B. L., & Auld, D. S. (1990). Zinc coordination, function, and structure of zinc enzymes and other proteins. *Biochemistry*, *29*(24), 5647–5659. DOI: 10.1021/bi00476a001 PMID: 2200508

Van Der Straeten, D., Bhullar, N. K., De Steur, H., Gruissem, W., MacKenzie, D., Pfeiffer, W., Qaim, M., Slamet-Loedin, I., Strobbe, S., Tohme, J., Trijatmiko, K. R., Vanderschuren, H., Van Montagu, M., Zhang, C., & Bouis, H. (2020). Multiplying the efficiency and impact of biofortification through metabolic engineering. *Nature Communications*, *11*(1), 1–10. DOI: 10.1038/s41467-020-19020-4 PMID: 33060603

Van Der Straeten, D., Fitzpatrick, T. B., & De Steur, H. (2017). Editorial overview: Biofortification of crops: achievements, future challenges, socio-economic, health and ethical aspects. *Current Opinion in Biotechnology*, *44*, VII–X. DOI: 10.1016/j.copbio.2017.03.007 PMID: 28342725

Van Wouwe, J. P. (1989). Clinical and laboratory diagnosis of acrodermatitis enteropathica. *European Journal of Pediatrics*, *149*(1), 2–8. DOI: 10.1007/BF02024322 PMID: 2691254

Vannucchi, H., Favaro, R. M., Cunha, D. F., & Marchini, J. S. (1995). Assessment of zinc nutritional status of pellagra patients. *Alcohol and Alcoholism (Oxford, Oxfordshire)*, *30*(3), 297–302. PMID: 7545983

Veenemans, J., Milligan, P., Prentice, A. M., Schouten, L. R. A., Inja, N., Heijden, A. C., de Boer, L. C. C., Jansen, E. J. S., Koopmans, A. E., Enthoven, W. T. M., Kraaijenhagen, R. J., Demir, A. Y., Uges, D. R. A., Mbugi, E. V., Savelkoul, H. F. J., & Verhoef, H. (2011). Effect of supplementation with zinc and other micronutrients on malaria in Tanzanian children: A randomised trial. *PLoS Medicine*, *8*(11), e1001125. DOI: 10.1371/journal.pmed.1001125 PMID: 22131908

Venugopal, V., & Gopakumar, K. (2017). Shellfish: Nutritive Value, Health Benefits, and Consumer Safety. *Comprehensive Reviews in Food Science and Food Safety*, *16*(6), 1219–1242. DOI: 10.1111/1541-4337.12312 PMID: 33371588

Ver Ploeg, M., Breneman, V., Farrigan, T., Hamrick, K., Hopkins, D., Kaufman, P., Lin, B.-H., Nord, M., Smith, T. A., & Williams, R. (2009). *Access to affordable and nutritious food: Measuring and understanding food deserts and their consequences: report to congress*. https://ageconsearch.umn.edu/record/292130/

Vicente, A. R., Manganaris, G. A., Darre, M., Ortiz, C. M., Sozzi, G. O., & Crisosto, C. H. (2022). Compositional determinants of fruit and vegetable quality and nutritional value. In *Postharvest handling* (pp. 565–619). Elsevier., https://www.sciencedirect.com/science/article/pii/B9780128228456000191 DOI: 10.1016/B978-0-12-822845-6.00019-1

Vickram, S., Rohini, K., Srinivasan, S., Nancy Veenakumari, D., Archana, K., Anbarasu, K., Jeyanthi, P., Thanigaivel, S., Gulothungan, G., Rajendiran, N., & Srikumar, P. S. (2021). Role of Zinc (Zn) in Human Reproduction: A Journey from Initial Spermatogenesis to Childbirth. *International Journal of Molecular Sciences*, *22*(4), 2188. DOI: 10.3390/ijms22042188 PMID: 33671837

Victora, C. G., Christian, P., Vidaletti, L. P., Gatica-Domínguez, G., Menon, P., & Black, R. E. (2021). Revisiting maternal and child undernutrition in low-income and middle-income countries: Variable progress towards an unfinished agenda. *Lancet*, *397*(10282), 1388–1399. DOI: 10.1016/S0140-6736(21)00394-9 PMID: 33691094

Videira, C. P. F. (2020). *Effectiveness of nutrition and WASH/malaria educational community-based interventions in reducing anemia, malnutrition and micronutrients deficiencies in preschool children from Bengo, Angola*. https://repositorio-aberto.up.pt/bitstream/10216/129251/2/419837.pdf

Vreugdenhil, M., Akkermans, M. D., Van Der Merwe, L. F., Van Elburg, R. M., Van Goudoever, J. B., & Brus, F. (2021). Prevalence of Zinc Deficiency in Healthy 1–3-Year-Old Children from Three Western European Countries. *Nutrients*, *13*(11), 3713. DOI: 10.3390/nu13113713 PMID: 34835970

Vu, T. T., Fredenburg, J. C., & Weitz, J. I. (2013). Zinc: An important cofactor in haemostasis and thrombosis. *Thrombosis and Haemostasis*, *109*(3), 421–430. DOI: 10.1160/TH12-07-0465 PMID: 23306381

Walke, G., Gaurkar, S. S., Prasad, R., Lohakare, T., & Wanjari, M. (2023). The impact of oxidative stress on male reproductive function: Exploring the role of antioxidant supplementation. *Cureus*, *15*(7). Advance online publication. https://www.cureus.com/articles/169642-the-impact-of-oxidative-stress-on-male-reproductive-function-exploring-the-role-of-antioxidant-supplementation.pdf. DOI: 10.7759/cureus.42583 PMID: 37641770

Walker, C. F., & Black, R. E. (2004). Zinc and the risk for infectious disease. *Annual Review of Nutrition*, *24*(1), 255–275. DOI: 10.1146/annurev.nutr.23.011702.073054 PMID: 15189121

Walravens, P. A., & Hambidge, K. M. (1976). Growth of infants fed a zinc supplemented formula. *The American Journal of Clinical Nutrition*, *29*(10), 1114–1121. DOI: 10.1093/ajcn/29.10.1114 PMID: 788494

Walsh, C. T., Sandstead, H. H., Prasad, A. S., Newberne, P. M., & Fraker, P. J. (1994). Zinc health effects and research priorities for the 1990's. *Environmental Health Perspectives*, *102*, 5–46. PMID: 7925188

Wang, B., Fang, T., & Chen, H. (2023). Zinc and central nervous system disorders. *Nutrients*, *15*(9), 2140. DOI: 10.3390/nu15092140 PMID: 37432243

Wang, H., Hu, Y.-F., Hao, J.-H., Chen, Y.-H., Su, P.-Y., Wang, Y., Yu, Z., Fu, L., Xu, Y.-Y., Zhang, C., Tao, F.-B., & Xu, D.-X. (2015). Maternal zinc deficiency during pregnancy elevates the risks of fetal growth restriction: A population-based birth cohort study. *Scientific Reports*, *5*(1), 11262. DOI: 10.1038/srep11262 PMID: 26053136

Wang, J., Li, Y., Yang, Y., Xiao, C., Ruan, Q., Li, P., Zhou, Q., Sheng, M., Hao, X., & Kai, G. (2023). Comprehensive analysis of OpHD-ZIP transcription factors related to the regulation of camptothecin biosynthesis in *Ophiorrhiza pumila.International Journal of Biological Macromolecules*, *242*, 124910. DOI: 10.1016/j.ijbiomac.2023.124910 PMID: 37217041

Wang, K., Zhou, B., Kuo, Y.-M., Zemansky, J., & Gitschier, J. (2002). A Novel Member of a Zinc Transporter Family Is Defective in Acrodermatitis Enteropathica. In *Am* (Vol. 71). J. Hum. Genet. DOI: 10.1086/341125

Wang, X., Valenzano, M. C., Mercado, J. M., Zurbach, E. P., & Mullin, J. M. (2013). Zinc Supplementation Modifies Tight Junctions and Alters Barrier Function of CACO-2 Human Intestinal Epithelial Layers. *Digestive Diseases and Sciences*, *58*(1), 77–87. DOI: 10.1007/s10620-012-2328-8 PMID: 22903217

Wang, X., Wu, W., Zheng, W., Fang, X., Chen, L., Rink, L., Min, J., & Wang, F. (2019). Zinc supplementation improves glycemic control for diabetes prevention and management: A systematic review and meta-analysis of randomized controlled trials. *The American Journal of Clinical Nutrition*, *110*(1), 76–90. DOI: 10.1093/ajcn/nqz041 PMID: 31161192

Wan, Y., & Zhang, B. (2022). The impact of zinc and zinc homeostasis on the intestinal mucosal barrier and intestinal diseases. *Biomolecules*, *12*(7), 900. DOI: 10.3390/biom12070900 PMID: 35883455

Wapnir, R. A. (2000). Zinc deficiency, malnutrition and the gastrointestinal tract. *The Journal of Nutrition*, *130*(5), 1388S–1392S. DOI: 10.1093/jn/130.5.1388S PMID: 10801949

Weaver, C. M., & Kannan, S. (2001). Phytate and mineral bioavailability. In *Food phytates* (pp. 227–240). CRC Press., https://www.taylorfrancis.com/chapters/edit/10.1201/9781420014419-15/phytate-mineral-bioavailability-connie-weaver-srimathi-kannan

Wegmüller, R., Tay, F., Zeder, C., Brnić, M., & Hurrell, R. F. (2014). Zinc absorption by young adults from supplemental zinc citrate is comparable with that from zinc gluconate and higher than from zinc oxide. *The Journal of Nutrition*, *144*(2), 132–136. DOI: 10.3945/jn.113.181487 PMID: 24259556

Welch, R. M., & Graham, R. D. (2004). Breeding for micronutrients in staple food crops from a human nutrition perspective. *Journal of Experimental Botany*, *55*(396), 353–364. DOI: 10.1093/jxb/erh064 PMID: 14739261

Wessells, K. R., & Brown, K. H. (2012). Estimating the global prevalence of zinc deficiency: Results based on zinc availability in national food supplies and the prevalence of stunting. *PLoS One*, *7*(11), e50568. DOI: 10.1371/journal.pone.0050568 PMID: 23209782

Wessells, K. R., Manger, M. S., Tsang, B. L., Brown, K. H., & McDonald, C. M. (2024). Mandatory large-scale food fortification programmes can reduce the estimated prevalence of inadequate zinc intake by up to 50% globally. *Nature Food*, *5*(7), 625–637. DOI: 10.1038/s43016-024-00997-w PMID: 38898330

Wessels, I., Fischer, H. J., & Rink, L. (2021). Dietary and physiological effects of zinc on the immune system. *Annual Review of Nutrition*, *41*(1), 133–175. DOI: 10.1146/annurev-nutr-122019-120635 PMID: 34255547

Wessels, I., & Rink, L. (2020). Micronutrients in autoimmune diseases: Possible therapeutic benefits of zinc and vitamin D. *The Journal of Nutritional Biochemistry*, *77*, 108240. DOI: 10.1016/j.jnutbio.2019.108240 PMID: 31841960

Weyh, C., Krüger, K., Peeling, P., & Castell, L. (2022). The role of minerals in the optimal functioning of the immune system. *Nutrients*, *14*(3), 644. DOI: 10.3390/nu14030644 PMID: 35277003

Whittaker, P. (1998). Iron and zinc interactions in humans. *The American Journal of Clinical Nutrition*, *68*(2), S442–S446. DOI: 10.1093/ajcn/68.2.442S PMID: 9701159

WHO (World Health Organization) (2006). Implementing the new recommendations on the clinical management of diarrhoea: Guidelines for policy makers and programme managers.

Wierdsma, N. J., Van Bokhorst-de van der Schueren, M., Berkenpas, M., Mulder, C., & Van Bodegraven, A. (2013). Vitamin and mineral deficiencies are highly prevalent in newly diagnosed celiac disease patients. *Nutrients*, *5*(10), 3975–3992. DOI: 10.3390/nu5103975 PMID: 24084055

Williams, P. (2007). Nutritional composition of red meat. *Nutrition & Dietetics: the Journal of the Dietitians Association of Australia*, *64*(s4), S113–S119. DOI: 10.1111/j.1747-0080.2007.00197.x

Winichagoon, P. (2008). Coexistence of micronutrient malnutrition: Implication for nutrition policy and programs in Asia. *Asia Pacific Journal of Clinical Nutrition*, •••, 17. PMID: 18296375

World Health Organization. (2006). *The international pharmacopoeia* (Vol. 1). World Health Organization.

World Health Organization. (2007). Community-based management of severe acute malnutrition: A joint statement by the World Health Organization, the World Food Programme, the United Nations System Standing Committee on Nutrition and the United Nations Children's Fund

Xie, Z., Wu, H., & Zhao, J. (2020). Multifunctional roles of zinc in Alzheimer's disease. *Neurotoxicology*, *80*, 112–123. DOI: 10.1016/j.neuro.2020.07.003 PMID: 32717200

Xu, H., Yuan, R., Liu, X., Li, X., Qiao, G., Li, C., Gedanken, A., & Lin, X. (2019). Zn-doped CuO nanocomposites inhibit tumor growth by NF-κB pathway cross-linked autophagy and apoptosis. *Nanomedicine (London)*, *14*(2), 131–149. DOI: 10.2217/nnm-2018-0366 PMID: 30394176

Xu, J., Wang, X., Zhu, H., & Yu, F. (2021). Maize genotypes with different zinc efficiency in response to low zinc stress and heterogeneous zinc supply. *Frontiers in Plant Science*, *12*, 736658. DOI: 10.3389/fpls.2021.736658 PMID: 34691112

Xu, Y., Xiao, G., Liu, L., & Lang, M. (2019). Zinc transporters in Alzheimer's disease. *Molecular Brain*, *12*(1), 106. DOI: 10.1186/s13041-019-0528-2 PMID: 31818314

Yadava, D. K., Hossain, F., & Mohapatra, T. (2018). Nutritional security through crop biofortification in India: Status & future prospects. *The Indian Journal of Medical Research, 148*(5), 621–631. DOI: 10.4103/ijmr.IJMR_1893_18 PMID: 30666987

Yagi, T., Asakawa, A., Ueda, H., Ikeda, S., Miyawaki, S., & Inui, A. (2013). The role of zinc in the treatment of taste disorders. *Recent Patents on Food, Nutrition & Agriculture, 5*(1), 44–51. DOI: 10.2174/2212798411305010007 PMID: 23305423

Yamaguchi, M. (1998). Role of zinc in bone formation and bone resorption. *The Journal of Trace Elements in Experimental Medicine, 11*(2–3), 119–135. DOI: 10.1002/(SICI)1520-670X(1998)11:2/3<119::AID-JTRA5>3.0.CO;2-3

Yamaguchi, M. (2007). Role of zinc in bone metabolism and preventive effect on bone disorder. *Biomedical Research on Trace Elements, 18*(4), 346–366.

Yamaguchi, M., & Weitzmann, M. N. (2011). Zinc stimulates osteoblastogenesis and suppresses osteoclastogenesis by antagonizing NF-κB activation. *Molecular and Cellular Biochemistry, 355*(1–2), 179–186. DOI: 10.1007/s11010-011-0852-z PMID: 21533765

Yamasaki, S., Sakata-Sogawa, K., Hasegawa, A., Suzuki, T., Kabu, K., Sato, E., Kurosaki, T., Yamashita, S., Tokunaga, M., Nishida, K., & Hirano, T. (2007). Zinc is a novel intracellular second messenger. *The Journal of Cell Biology, 177*(4), 637–645. DOI: 10.1083/jcb.200702081 PMID: 17502426

Yan, A. C., & Oboite, N. M. (2024). Nutritional disorders affecting the skin. In C. Griffiths, J. Barker, T. Bleiker, W. Hussain & R. Simpson (Eds.), ROOK'S Textbook of Dermatology (10th ed., pp. 61.25-27) John Wiley & Sons Ltd DOI: 10.1002/9781119709268.rook061

Yanar, K. (2023). Vitamin-associated elements. In *A guide to vitamins and their effects on diseases* (p. 164).

Yang, M., Li, Y., Liu, Z., Tian, J., Liang, L., Qiu, Y., Wang, G., Du, Q., Cheng, D., Cai, H., Shi, L., Xu, F., & Lian, X. (2020). A high activity zinc transporter OsZIP9 mediates zinc uptake in rice. *The Plant Journal, 103*(5), 1695–1709. DOI: 10.1111/tpj.14855 PMID: 32449251

Yan, Y. Q., & Zou, L. J. (2012). Relation between zinc, copper, and magnesium concentrations following cardiopulmonary bypass and postoperative atrial fibrillation in patients undergoing coronary artery bypass grafting. *Biological Trace Element Research, 148*(2), 148–153. DOI: 10.1007/s12011-012-9356-2 PMID: 22351155

Yao, R. Q., Ren, C., Xia, Z. F., & Yao, Y. M. (2021). Organelle-specific autophagy in inflammatory diseases: A potential therapeutic target underlying the quality control of multiple organelles. *Autophagy, 17*(2), 385–401. DOI: 10.1080/15548627.2020.1725377 PMID: 32048886

Yaqob, K. S. (2019). ZINC The Friendly and Forgotten Micronutrient. *Global Journal of Pediatrics & Neonatal Care, 1*(3). Advance online publication. DOI: 10.33552/GJPNC.2019.01.000512

Yasuda, H., & Tsutsui, T. (2016). Infants and elderlies are susceptible to zinc deficiency. *Scientific Reports, 6*(1), 21850. DOI: 10.1038/srep21850 PMID: 26912464

Younes, S. (2024). The impact of micronutrients on the sense of taste. *Human Nutrition & Metabolism, 35*, 200231. DOI: 10.1016/j.hnm.2023.200231

Yu, B.-G., Liu, Y.-M., Chen, X.-X., Cao, W.-Q., Ding, T.-B., & Zou, C.-Q. (2021). Foliar zinc application to wheat may lessen the zinc deficiency burden in rural Quzhou, China. *Frontiers in Nutrition, 8*, 697817. DOI: 10.3389/fnut.2021.697817 PMID: 34262927

Yu, S. M., & Yu, M. M. (2023). Molecular mechanisms of wound healing: The role of zinc as an essential microelement. *Research Results in Pharmacology, 9*(1), 25–40. DOI: 10.18413/rrpharmacology.9.10003

Zaman, Q. U., Aslam, Z., Yaseen, M., Ihsan, M. Z., Khaliq, A., Fahad, S., Bashir, S., Ramzani, P. M. A., & Naeem, M. (2018). Zinc biofortification in rice: Leveraging agriculture to moderate hidden hunger in developing countries. *Archives of Agronomy and Soil Science, 64*(2), 147–161. DOI: 10.1080/03650340.2017.1338343

Zand, N., Christides, T., & Loughrill, E. (2015). Dietary intake of minerals. In De La Guardia, M., & Garrigues, S. (Eds.), *Handbook of Mineral Elements in Food* (1st ed., pp. 23–39). Wiley., DOI: 10.1002/9781118654316.ch2

Zhang, X., Wang, C., Zhao, D., Chen, X., Zhang, C., Zheng, J., & Liu, X. (2020). Zinc deficiency induces abnormal development of the myocardium by promoting SENP5 overexpression. *PLoS One, 15*(11), e0242606. DOI: 10.1371/journal.pone.0242606 PMID: 33211757

Zhang, Y. Y., Stockmann, R., Ng, K., & Ajlouni, S. (2021). Opportunities for plant-derived enhancers for iron, zinc, and calcium bioavailability: A review. *Comprehensive Reviews in Food Science and Food Safety, 20*(1), 652–685. DOI: 10.1111/1541-4337.12669 PMID: 33443794

Zhang, Y. Y., Stockmann, R., Ng, K., & Ajlouni, S. (2022). Revisiting phytate-element interactions: Implications for iron, zinc and calcium bioavailability, with emphasis on legumes. *Critical Reviews in Food Science and Nutrition*, *62*(6), 1696–1712. DOI: 10.1080/10408398.2020.1846014 PMID: 33190514

Zhang, Y., Li, X., Li, J., Khan, M. Z. H., Ma, F., & Liu, X. (2021). A novel zinc complex with antibacterial and antioxidant activity. *BMC Chemistry*, *15*(1), 1–12. DOI: 10.1186/s13065-021-00745-2 PMID: 33722300

Zhang, Y., Peng, C., Zeng, Z., Zhang, X., Zhang, L., Ma, Y., & Wang, Z. (2022). Sustainable phytic acid–zinc anticorrosion interface for highly reversible zinc metal anodes. *ACS Applied Materials & Interfaces*, *14*(8), 10419–10427. DOI: 10.1021/acsami.1c24288 PMID: 35179367

Zou, P., Du, Y., Yang, C., & Cao, Y. (2023). Trace element zinc and skin disorders. *Frontiers in Medicine*, *9*, 1093868. DOI: 10.3389/fmed.2022.1093868 PMID: 36733937

Żwierełło, W., Styburski, D., Maruszewska, A., Piorun, K., Skórka-Majewicz, M., Czerwińska, M., Maciejewska, D., Baranowska-Bosiacka, I., Krajewski, A., & Gutowska, I. (2020). Bioelements in the treatment of burn injuries–The complex review of metabolism and supplementation (copper, selenium, zinc, iron, manganese, chromium and magnesium). *Journal of Trace Elements in Medicine and Biology*, *62*, 126616. DOI: 10.1016/j.jtemb.2020.126616 PMID: 32739827

About the Contributors

Ratnesh Das is a Professor in the Department of Chemistry, at Dr. Harisingh Gour Central University, Sagar, India. He has a rich experience in teaching and research for about 21 years during which he has supervised many Ph.D. students and completed many sponsored research projects. His active research areas include Heterocyclic synthesis, electrochemistry, synthesis of nano-catalysts, and green chemistry. He has authored about 80 research papers in peer-reviewed national and international journals and refereed conferences organized by professional societies worldwide.

Megha Das is working as an Assistant Professor in Department of Education, at Dr. Harisingh Gour Central University Sagar (M.P). She has completed her UGC Women's Postdoctoral Research with a fellowship from UGC, New Delhi. She has published many research papers and articles in National and International journals and published many chapters in different books related to Education and science. Lambert Academic Publishing, Germany, has published her doctoral thesis. She has participated and presented several papers at National and International Seminars/ Conferences.

***

Ankit Ab currently works at the Institute of Pharmacy, Nirma University. Ankit does research in Medicinal Chemistry, Cancer Research and Bioinformatics. Their current project is 'Small molecule Aurora Kinase Inhibitors'.

B.R. Shamanna completed his medical education at Karnatak Medical College, Hubli, and his MD in Community Medicine from the All India Institute of Medical Sciences. He also holds a double Diplomate of the National Board in Maternal & Child Health and Social & Preventive Medicine. He completed his M.Sc. from University College London with distinction in Community Eye Health. He served as a Senior Research Officer in the International Council for Control of Iodine Deficiency Disorders (ICCIDD), a WHO-PAMMUNICEF Organization, and later as a Senior Resident & Medical Officer at the Primary Health Centre in Haryana. Dr. Shamanna has been closely associated with the development and implementation of activities of two large WHO Collaborating Centres for Prevention of Blindness in India, first with the Lions Aravind Institute of Community Ophthalmology of the Aravind Eye Care System in Madurai and with the International Centre for Advancement of Rural Eye Care of the L.V. Prasad Eye Institute, Hyderabad. He is a visiting faculty member for the Masters in Public Health Eyecare at the London School of Hygiene and Tropical Medicine and an adjunct senior lecturer at the School of Visual Sciences, Faculty of Science, University of New South Wales, Sydney, Australia. He is a visiting professor at the Manipal University, India, and an adjunct faculty member with the Public Health Foundation of India.

Paran Jyoti Borpatra was born in the Lakhimpur district of Assam, India. He completed his Ph.D degree (2020) under the supervision of Prof. Pranjal Kumar Baruah at Gauhati University, Assam, working in the area of organic synthesis, especially C-H activation reactions, multicomponent reactions, etc. Dr. Borpatra completed a two-year research project as JRF under 'DBT's Twinning Program for the NE' titled "De Novo Rationally Designed Curcumin Derived Analogues for Increased Bioavailability and Its Metal Analogues for Anticancer and Protective Studies" under the guidance of Prof. Pranjal Kumar Baruah. Currently, he has been working as a D. S. Kothari Post-Doctoral Fellow (DSKPDF) under Prof. Satyendra Kumar Pandey at Banaras Hindu University, Varanasi, focusing on synthetic methodology and C-H functionalization. He has also co-authored a number of publications in journals with good impact factors.

Bhawna Chopra, Professor, Department of Pharmaceutical Chemistry, Guru Gobind Singh College of Pharmacy, Yamuna Nagar, Haryana (India), has academic and research experience of 15+ years in medicinal and pharmaceutical chemistry. She had completed PhD in Pharmaceutical Sciences from I.K. Gujral Punjab Technical University, Jalandhar, Punjab (India) in 2018. Her present areas of research include the medicinal chemistry of antimicrobial and anti-inflammatory agents and drug discovery from natural products.

Hrithik Dey is an M Pharm scholar with a specialization in pharmacology and toxicology. His expertise extends to various critical areas, including animal handling, safety pharmacology, and drug testing. With a strong foundation in these fields, Hrithik is dedicated to advancing the understanding and application of pharmacological principles to ensure the safety and efficacy of therapeutic drugs.

Ashwani K. Dhingra is presently working as a Professor and Principal at the Global Research Institute of Pharmacy, Radaur, Yamuna Nagar, Haryana, India. He is proficient in technical writing skills, analysis and interpretating of data. He has extensive knowledge of functions related to pharmacy research and development, product development, laboratory operations and documentation. His present areas of interest include the design and development of synthetic methodologies dealing with various organic transformations, multistep synthesis of medicinally active N-heterocyclic derivatives, and isolation and structural modification of bioactive natural compounds. To his credit, Dr. Dhingra has a total of 90 publications in national and international journals of repute, 10 book chapters, and 10 books. He has also published 6 design patents. He has been awarded as Bentham Science Ambassador by Bentham Science Publishers, Highly Cited Researcher from Elsevier, and Innovational Ambassador by MHRD Innovational Cell, AICTE, New Delhi. Further, he has been on review panels for various prestigious journals, including Elsevier, Springer, Bentham Science, Frontiers, Frontiers, Taylor & Francis, etc.

Suresh Gadapati completed his bachelor's degree at DR. NTR University of Health Sciences, Andhra Pradesh. And a master's degree(MPH) from the University of Hyderabad. He is pursuing his doctoral degree in Public Health at UoH. He worked for a couple of years in the healthcare sector.

Preeti Garg is a crucial figure in facilitating the transition of students from academic life to professional careers. With a blend of strategic vision, industry insight, and a student-centric approach, she plays an instrumental role in shaping the career trajectories of students. Ms. Garg is committed to ensuring that students are well-prepared, competitive, and confident as they enter the job market. Under her leadership, the institute has established strong industry connections and achieved impressive placement rates. Her efforts in organizing successful recruitment drives, providing comprehensive career counselling, and enhancing students' skills have led to positive career outcomes for many graduates.

Safdar Hussain is currently working as Head of "Molecular Genetics & Forensics" research group at Centre for Applied Molecular Biology, University of the Punjab Lahore. Dr. Hussain completed his PhD degree in 'Molecular Biology & Biochemistry' from Xi'an Jiaotong University (XJTU), China. Dr. Hussain has a vast experience of working in the field of 'Forensic DNA Typing" and has joined a formal training program at Strand Analytical Laboratories, Indianapolis, Indiana, USA. Dr. Hussain's current research work focuses on the future methodologies of Forensic DNA profiling as well as molecular characterization of congenital and hereditary diseases.

Anjali Maurya currently works as a Project Assistant under the agies of CURIE Core Grant project funded by Department of Science and Technology (DST), New Delhi, at SS Khanna Girls Degree College. She completed her PhD (Microbiology) from Sam Higginbottom University of Agriculture, Technology, and Sciences, Prayagraj, (UP). She has a deep understanding of both pharmaceutical microbiology and biotechnology techniques.

Rajesh Datt Mehta is actively involved in research in field of dermatology and in particular with nutritional disorders. Supervises the research activities by the post-graduate students of the department.

Shashwat Datt Mehta is a well-known ENT Specialist associated with Marwar Hospital, Sadul Colony. He has 12 years of experience in ENT and has worked as an expert in different cities in India. Doctor Shashwat has contributed to handling numerous complex medical cases in several hospitals. He is known for his attention to accurate diagnosis and treating patients empathetically. The speciality interests of Dr Shashwat are all types of Ear, Nose, and Throat surgeries. Dr Mehta did his graduation with MBBS and MS ENT. He has also participated in research work and various workshops under the ENT department and published many papers.

Nosheen Mushtaq has completed her PhD degree from Xian Jiaotong University, China in Microbiology and working as an Associate Professor at Department of Allied Health Sciences, Lahore University of Biological & Applied Sciences (UBAS).

Smita Narwal received the prestigious 'Nation Builder Award' from Rotary Club Radaur, Yamuna Nagar, Haryana, in recognition of her valuable contributions to nation building through teaching.

B. Shriya Saikia was born in Guwahati, Assam, India. She received her MS degree from Gauhati University. She was awarded the INSPIRE Fellowship (2019) by DST, Govt. of India, and is currently pursuing her Ph.D under Prof. Pranjal K. Baruah as an INSPIRE fellow. Her research work broadly focuses on developing novel methodologies via C–H functionalization.

Anuradha Singh is a Senior Assistant Professor in the Department of Chemistry at S.S. Khanna Girls' Degree College, University of Allahabad. She is well versed in synthetic chemistry, computer-aided drug design and other techniques used in the field of medicinal chemistry. She has been selected for the prestigious Indian National Science Academy's Visiting Scientist fellowship in 2023. She successfully led research projects funded by DST and UGC, demonstrating strong leadership and project management skills. She has been awarded with gold medal during her post graduate studies and Swarnajayanti Fellowships by National Academy of Sciences, India. Dr. Singh has published more than 30 research papers/book chapters, in addition to several articles, in journals/books of national and international repute. Dr. Singh has also demonstrated editorial expertise by editing four books. Dr. Singh's influence extends beyond research. As a CURIE Grant Nodal Officer, she secured and managed a DST grant to improve postgraduate teaching and research facilities. Her leadership at the institutional level is demonstrated by her role as the convenor of the Innovation Council, which has spurred student innovation and entrepreneurship, leading to prestigious recognition from the Ministry of Education and AICTE.

Neha Yadav is the Head of the Department at Global Research Institute of Pharmacy, Yamuna Nagar, Haryana. She completed B.Pharmacy in 2011 and M.Pharmacy (Pharmaceutical Chemistry) in 2013. She also recently completed her Doctorate in pharmaceutical sciences. She has a total of 8 years of experience in the Pharmacy field. Her goal is to create a platform where the organization can grow in sync with the recent developments of the field.

Index

A

B

D

E

F

G

H

I

N

P

S

Z

www.ingramcontent.com/pod-product-compliance
Lightning Source LLC
LaVergne TN
LVHW080859300926
849162LV00003B/482